Organizational Behavior and Management in Health and Medicine

James K. Elrod • John L. Fortenberry, Jr.

Organizational Behavior and Management in Health and Medicine

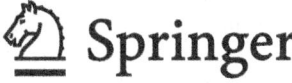 Springer

James K. Elrod
Willis Knighton Health
Shreveport, LA, USA

John L. Fortenberry, Jr.
College of Business
LSU Shreveport
Shreveport, LA, USA

Willis Knighton Health
Shreveport, LA, USA

ISBN 978-3-031-61825-3   ISBN 978-3-031-61823-9   (eBook)
https://doi.org/10.1007/978-3-031-61823-9

This Springer imprint is published by the registered company Springer Nature Switzerland AG
The registered company address is: Gewerbestrasse 11, 6330 Cham, Switzerland

If disposing of this product, please recycle the paper.

This book is dedicated to the employees of Willis Knighton Health who, through their collective contributions, positively impact the lives of patients each and every day.

Preface

When viewing the operations of healthcare institutions comprehensively, it is virtually impossible to not be awed by the complexities required for health and medical services to be delivered successfully. In well-operated healthcare establishments, when patients present for treatment, they set off a monumental array of logistics, orchestrated in careful fashion, that sees the deployment of numerous resources required for the effective provision of health and medical care. Much of this complex orchestration is highly visible to patients, with simple and complex procedures alike requiring circulation through numerous areas in and around given healthcare establishments. This exposes patients to multiple people (e.g., admissions clerks, nurses, physicians, laboratory technicians, imaging technologists, dietary aids), places (e.g., parking areas, waiting rooms, patient rooms, cafeterias, surgical suites), and things (e.g., clinical and administrative work processes, technologies, equipment, supplies), ultimately affording the care delivery experience.

But that which is seen by patients represents just the tip of the iceberg. Complementing the highly visible aspects of healthcare operations are myriad support services which are vital for making the delivery of care possible. Among a seemingly endless range of duties and responsibilities, missions and associated strategic priorities must be determined and pursued; personnel must be recruited, hired, and managed properly; equipment and supplies must be ordered, inventoried, and deployed in a timely fashion; care environments must be well designed and maintained to ensure proper form and function; policies must be monitored to ensure compliance; and services must be marketed to foster attention and awareness. Such critical and varied pursuits demand keen expertise in organizational behavior and management.

Organizational behavior and management happen to be two separate, but closely related subjects. Organizational behavior refers to the formal study of human behavior in organizations. Management refers to a range of activities (i.e., planning, organizing, staffing, directing, coordinating, reporting, and budgeting) which are carried out by formally appointed individuals (e.g., chief executive officers, vice presidents, directors, managers, supervisors) for purposes of aiding organizations in realizing their missions. Management effectively serves as the action component of organizational behavior, operationalizing associated discoveries aimed at understanding workplace aspects and interactions in a bid to generate top performance. Textbooks tend to focus on one area or the other, but due to the highly intertwined nature of the two subjects and our desire to concisely portray associated content, we decided to combine the two areas into a book that provides a general overview bridging theory and practice.

Written primarily for students of health administration, medicine, nursing, allied health, and other disciplines of the healthcare industry, *Organizational Behavior and Management in Health and Medicine* presents a series of 14 chapters featuring topics which must be mastered in order to successfully operate healthcare organizations. The content presented in this work covers a fairly broad spectrum of organizational behavior and management, including leadership, strategy, communication, motivation, organizational culture, groups and teams, and power and politics, addressing each within the context of the healthcare industry and its associated organizations. This work was written in a purposely succinct manner, permitting readers to quickly become apprised of chapter content without being drawn into extended, often exhausting portrayals common in many standard textbooks. In this regard, the book is more of a primer on organizational behavior and management, focusing on conveying core details which, if desired, can easily be explored further through readily available sources.

While the book is ideally suited for student learners following the typical cover-to-cover reading plan commonly required in college coursework, it serves a dual purpose as an excellent desk reference for anyone interested in organizational behavior and management in healthcare settings. This is facilitated by the construction of chapters, with each being designed to be read as a stand-alone document, increasing the utility of the book, especially for practicing healthcare executives desirous of occasional refreshers on various topics of organizational behavior and management. A glossary of organizational behavior and management terminology is included at the conclusion of the work, further enhancing the book's value for both prospective and current employees of the healthcare industry.

Beyond its efficient presentation of core facets of organizational behavior and management, one of the most intriguing features of the book is its inclusion of practical insights in each chapter from our experiences as leaders at Willis Knighton Health. Based in Shreveport, Louisiana, Willis Knighton Health is a nongovernmental, not-for-profit healthcare provider delivering comprehensive health and wellness services through multiple hospitals, an all-inclusive retirement community, and numerous general and specialty medical clinics. Founded in 1924, the system holds market leadership in its served region, centered in the heart of an area known as the Ark-La-Tex, where the states of Arkansas, Louisiana, and Texas converge. Through our combined service at Willis Knighton Health totaling over six decades, we have observed almost everything imaginable regarding the operation of healthcare institutions, with these insights adding particularly enlightening portrayals in the book. Termed WK Reflections, these special passages briefly step away from the primary text of each chapter and share real-world insights, often involving unique applications, innovative thinking, and other creative perspectives from practice. These viewpoints are invaluable for helping readers to ground the theoretical overviews presented in each chapter, bolstering knowledge and understanding.

It is our hope that you will find the content presented in this book useful both in your study of healthcare organizational behavior and management and in your career in the healthcare industry.

Shreveport, LA, USA   James K. Elrod
                                                                                    John L. Fortenberry, Jr.

Acknowledgments

While we would love to take full credit for the development of this learning resource, *Organizational Behavior and Management in Health and Medicine* ultimately would not have been possible without the support and encouragement of our colleagues at Willis Knighton Health and LSU Shreveport. Equal appreciation is extended to Springer for the publishing opportunity and associated expert guidance. We sincerely applaud each and every one of our supporters. Through their understanding of the value of this work, coupled with their belief in us as authors, we were able to make *Organizational Behavior and Management in Health and Medicine* a reality.

Contents

About the Authors

James K. Elrod is President Emeritus and a member of the board of directors of Shreveport, Louisiana-based Willis Knighton Health, the region's largest provider of healthcare services. A Fellow of the American College of Healthcare Executives and honoree as a Louisiana Legend by Friends of Louisiana Public Broadcasting, he holds a bachelor's degree in business administration from Baylor University, a master's degree in hospital administration from Washington University School of Medicine, and an honorary doctorate of science and humane letters from Northwestern State University of Louisiana. He served as President and Chief Executive Officer of Willis Knighton Health for 57 years, earning recognition as America's longest-tenured hospital administrator. He is the author of *Breadcrumbs to Cheesecake*, a book which chronicles the history of Willis Knighton Health.

John L. Fortenberry, Jr. is Chair of the James K. Elrod Department of Health Administration, James K. Elrod Professor of Health Administration, and Professor of Marketing in the College of Business at LSU Shreveport where he teaches a variety of courses in both health administration and marketing. He holds a BBA in marketing from the University of Mississippi; an MBA from Mississippi College; a PhD in public administration and public policy, with concentrations in health administration, human resource management, and organization theory, from Auburn University; and a PhD in business administration, with a major in marketing, from the University of Manchester in the United Kingdom. He is the author of numerous books and scholarly journal articles focusing on marketing, strategy, organizational behavior, and management. He also serves as Vice President of Marketing Strategy and Planning at Willis Knighton Health.

List of Boxes

Chapter 1
Management in Health and Medicine

Learning Objectives

After examining this chapter, readers will have the ability to:

- Define the concept of management, understand its various features and characteristics, and appreciate its essential role in the delivery of health and medicine.
- Understand the different levels of management within healthcare organizations, identify common managerial titles associated with each level, and discuss the scope of control held by managers at each level.
- Identify and discuss the source of authority from which managers derive their power within healthcare institutions, and reflect on its implications for managerial performance.
- Identify and define the 14 general principles of management as outlined by Henri Fayol, and discuss their application in health and medicine.
- Identify and define the activities of management as presented in Luther Gulick's POSDCORB model, and share insights regarding their essentiality in daily organizational life.
- Discuss the critical need for healthcare managers to acquire leadership skills, and comment on how healthcare institutions are positively impacted by managers with such proficiencies.

J. K. Elrod, J. L. Fortenberry, Jr., *Organizational Behavior and Management in Health and Medicine*, https://doi.org/10.1007/978-3-031-61823-9_1

WK Reflections: Preparing to Become a Manager

The backbone of any healthcare establishment arguably could be said to be centered on the managerial workforce responsible for overseeing institutional operations. The product of healthcare simply could not be delivered effectively without competent managers. This is not to diminish others within healthcare establishments, notably including the highly trained practitioners who deliver medicine, but it is through management that these parties are able to do their jobs proficiently. Indeed, the stage must be set and maintained to allow physicians, nurses, physical therapists, dieticians, and other personnel to properly address patients. Management, by and large, is responsible for setting and maintaining this stage [1–4].

For those who are seeking to become managers in health and medical organizations, investments must be made in acquiring and honing associated skills and abilities. Competition for the best positions in healthcare establishments typically is fierce, prompting aspiring managers to build their resumes as robustly as possible. But what exactly should individuals do to best position themselves for managerial careers in health and medical establishments? Many pathways exist, with one particularly productive array of preparatory steps, as summarized in Box 1.1, being offered by Willis Knighton Health.

Box 1.1: A Checklist for Managerial Preparation

1. Pursue formal educational initiatives (e.g., undergraduate and graduate programs in business, health administration, or related disciplines).
2. Conduct informal educational initiatives (e.g., self-study plans involving actively reading healthcare industry and management-related books and articles; staying abreast of current events by monitoring news developments applicable to the healthcare industry).
3. Acquire relevant professional certifications.
4. Join and actively participate in relevant professional societies.
5. Ensure the exemplification of professionalism in all aspects of life (e.g., actions, appearance, mannerisms, work ethic).
6. Build a successful employment track record demonstrating progressively responsible work experience; charitably contribute time and talents by volunteering in healthcare establishments to gain insights and understanding; pursue internship and residency opportunities in healthcare institutions.
7. Engage the community by being actively involved in civic associations, churches, and similar organizations.
8. Embrace personal values which align with those embraced by leading healthcare institutions.

As management is a defined discipline, possessing a significant body of ever-evolving theory and practical applications, care must be taken to acquire associated knowledge, skills, and abilities. Formal education is essential for achieving the best results, with institutions of higher learning being the primary providers of such training. One reading this particular text likely is enrolled in undergraduate or graduate training in business, health administration, or related disciplines, or increasingly, in clinical programs which are now directing attention toward management to complement training in medicine, nursing, and the like. Formal degrees, especially those at the graduate level which heavily emphasize management fundamentals (e.g., MBA, MHA), are considered to be top assets held by managerial candidates and often are required by employers. In fact, Willis Knighton Health's desire for healthcare managers to possess quality managerial training was so intense that it funded the development of the Master of Health Administration program at LSU Shreveport which is now one of the largest MHA programs in America.

Beyond formal classroom-based education, Willis Knighton Health desires seeing evidence that managerial candidates are taking steps to enhance and elevate their skills through informal means. Actively reading the latest books and journal articles on the topic of management and related areas of administration, for example, is very helpful for personal development and benefits employers, as well. This ensures that candidates possess contemporary, relevant perspectives which then can be brought into the workplace for improved performance. It is also desirable to see that managerial candidates have enacted a personal plan to remain current on political, economic, social, and technological fronts by, for example, actively reading newspapers, healthcare trade journals, industry-related websites, and the like. As healthcare institutions exist within greater environments of high complexity, possessing an awareness of what is happening in the world is essential for managerial success, especially as one advances up an organization's hierarchy.

Professional certifications in management or management-related areas also are viewed by Willis Knighton Health to be very valuable. Certification options abound, with selection and pursuit being dependent on one's desired career path. Board certification in healthcare management, for example, is offered through the American College of Healthcare Executives [5]. The Human Resource Certification Institute offers certifications for prowess in human resource management [6]. The American Marketing Association offers a range of certifications for those involved in marketing management [7]. Many more exist, spanning the gamut of management and administration. Eligibility for certifications often entails some combination of education and work experience, with this varying based on the particular certification desired. Even for those who are currently ineligible to sit for certification examinations due, for example, to a lack of work experience, steps can be initiated to prepare for acquiring given credentials, with this going a long way to demonstrate to potential employers a commitment to managerial excellence.

Related to certifications and equally beneficial is that of joining relevant professional societies. Many of these offer the certifications noted earlier, but even if those credentials are not pursued, membership in given associations offers numerous benefits. At its most basic and practical level, membership gives the holder of such the right to claim it on a resume, demonstrating to others at least some commitment to the given association and its focus. But far richer value exists by actively participating in these societies, permitting one to access learning resources, such as conferences and informational seminars, and make all-important professional contacts. As with certifications, professional societies are numerous, covering virtually any area of interest in management and administration, with selection being determined by career ambitions.

As the healthcare industry is well-known to be a professional one, its employees must carry this forward in their actions (e.g., communication, work performance), appearance (e.g., grooming, attire), and mannerisms (e.g., conduct, expressions). Something as seemingly innocent as calling a physician by his or her first name in the workplace can be catastrophic to one's career, as it is expected that employees understand and adhere to proper decorum in addressing those holding doctoral credentials. Managers especially must exemplify professionalism in all aspects of life, as they serve as prominent representatives of their given healthcare establishments, whether they are on duty or off duty. Professionalism also naturally includes maintaining a devoted work ethic, ensuring that one delivers full value for compensation earned. An employee who demonstrates professionalism is a true asset within the halls of medicine.

Prior successful, progressively responsible work experience, whether managerial or nonmanagerial, is viewed as highly desirable, especially if that experience was gained in the healthcare industry. For those without any work experience in healthcare institutions, volunteerism can be most helpful in gaining exposure to organizational operations. Health and medical establishments very often provide a wealth of opportunities for individuals interested in making a charitable contribution through their service. Even if exposure is not management-related, volunteer experiences can help one to understand health and medical institutions, those employed within them, and those served by them, with this advancing knowledge and improving employment prospects in the healthcare industry. Internships and residencies in healthcare establishments also offer opportunities for industry exposure, with these being particularly attractive to hiring parties, warranting their consideration as one prepares for a career in healthcare management.

Community engagement further benefits aspiring managers. Possessing an understanding of the wants and needs that exist in given communities is most helpful, as this influences what healthcare institutions do and do not provide, how they address patients, and so on. Without engaging communities by active involvement in civic associations, churches, and similar organizations, situational awareness will be limited, diminishing one's value to his or her employer. By having one's finger on the pulse of one's community, keen insights can be acquired and shared with colleagues, aiding healthcare institutions in capitalizing on opportunities and avoiding or eliminating threats.

Willis Knighton Health also desires seeing indications that management prospects embrace personal values which parallel institutional values. Health and medical organizations typically have very defined moral and ethical positions which are expressed notably in values statements, permitting employees and other stakeholders to understand institutional stances. Commonly expressed institutional values include integrity, professionalism, compassion, commitment, and related mindsets and attitudes. It is very beneficial for applicants to review these statements and decide if the values expressed parallel their own value sets. If they do, applicants stand an improved chance of being selected, particularly if they can provide evidence of their values being demonstrated in prior work or life experiences, for example, by referencing prior ethical dilemmas faced and actions taken in response.

The steps noted above offer those preparing to be managers excellent insights into what they should focus on as they work to position themselves for service in healthcare environments. Building resumes which feature these elements is strongly encouraged, both for advancing one's personal development and for increasing one's chances of securing desired career opportunities. On hiring, personal efforts to develop oneself must continue. At this point, however, managerial development efforts are not completely independent. Quality healthcare providers join in the development process, offering support in the form of mentorships, training seminars, continuing education opportunities, and the like to aid managers in being the best they can be.

1.1   Background

When viewing the operations of healthcare institutions comprehensively, it is virtually impossible to not be awed by the complexities required for health and medical services to be delivered successfully. In well-operated healthcare establishments, when patients present for treatment, they set off a monumental array of logistics, orchestrated in careful fashion, that sees the deployment of numerous resources required for the effective provision of health and medical care. Much of this complex orchestration is highly visible to patients, with simple and complex procedures alike requiring circulation through numerous areas in and around given healthcare establishments. This exposes patients to multiple people (e.g., admissions clerks, nurses, physicians, laboratory technicians, imaging technologists, dietary aids), places (e.g., parking areas, waiting rooms, patient rooms, cafeterias, surgical suites), and things (e.g., clinical and administrative work processes, technologies, equipment, supplies), ultimately affording the care delivery experience [1–3, 8, 9].

But that which is seen by patients represents just the tip of the iceberg. Complementing the highly visible aspects of healthcare operations are myriad support services which are vital for making the delivery of care possible. Among a seemingly endless range of duties and responsibilities, missions and associated strategic priorities must be determined and pursued; personnel must be recruited, hired, and managed properly; equipment and supplies must be ordered, inventoried, and deployed in a timely fashion; care environments must be well designed and maintained to ensure proper form and function; policies must be monitored to ensure compliance; and services must be marketed to foster attention and awareness [1–4, 10–12]. Such critical and varied pursuits represent just a few of the many practices, often unseen by outside eyes, that must be carried out in order to provide health and medical services to patients.

Quite obviously, healthcare operations are highly complex, necessitating extensive efforts to proficiently coordinate and direct vast, diverse resources in such a manner to fulfill designated missions. Robust guidance systems are required, with perhaps the most notable of these being networks of officials charged with overseeing operations. These officials are formally appointed into defined roles carrying various titles, such as chief executive officer, vice president, director, manager, coordinator, supervisor, and so on. With varying degrees of responsibility, they collectively perform what aggregately would be termed management roles. These roles are vital to healthcare institutions for many reasons, with arguably the most notable one being that managerial personnel ensure that work processes are completed in accordance with assigned directives, permitting services to be rendered effectively [1, 13, 14]. As such, anyone holding or contemplating acquiring a position of authority in health and medicine must possess a firm understanding of management, the focus of this chapter.

1.2 Defining Management

Management is defined as a range of activities (i.e., planning, organizing, staffing, directing, coordinating, reporting, and budgeting) which are carried out by formally appointed individuals (e.g., chief executive officers, vice presidents, directors, managers, supervisors) for purposes of aiding organizations in realizing their missions. It essentially serves as the action component of **organizational behavior**—the formal study of human behavior in organizations—operationalizing associated discoveries aimed at understanding workplace aspects and interactions in a bid to generate top performance. Of all administrative tools, management is the preeminent driving force of healthcare establishments, with excellence being essential for the best outcomes. Management is transactional by nature, relying on directives issued by managers to their subordinates who, in turn, are tasked with carrying out those directives to achieve desired outcomes. **Managers**—those individuals who are responsible for the management of organizations—are placed strategically throughout the hierarchies of healthcare establishments, essentially at points requiring careful oversight, permitting intensive coordination and control [15, 16]. Their quantity and scope of operation in healthcare institutions is dependent on the preferences of particular establishments, with associated decisions being heavily influenced by the depth and breadth of medical services provided and the requirements for delivering them proficiently. Some healthcare establishments might desire more robust managerial oversight, compelling them to offer more managerial positions. Others, however, might desire a leaner managerial structure, permitting employees greater autonomy, with this reducing the number of managers placed about hierarchies. The ideal array of managers within healthcare establishments typically emerges from trial and error occurring within given institutions, eventually revealing a fitting balance [17, 18].

Healthcare establishments typically have three broad levels of managers operating within them; namely, at upper, middle, and lower realms. The higher the managerial level, the more authority and responsibility the given manager possesses within the organization. While all are collectively viewed to be managers, specific titles vary based on level of authority and responsibility. **Upper-level managers**, sometimes referred to as **senior managers**, typically include the officers of given healthcare institutions. The title of president is commonly held by the top officer, with an array of vice presidents overseeing functional areas, such as operations, finance, nursing, marketing, and so on. Alternatively, and sometimes in tandem with other titling schemes, institutions might embrace C-suite designations, using titles such as chief executive officer, chief operating officer, chief financial officer, chief nursing officer, and so on. **Middle-level managers** very often consist of those carrying director or manager titles, with the former typically holding more authority and responsibility than the latter. A hospital's human resource department might, for example, be led by a director who oversees a range of managers responsible for staffing, compensation, safety, and related functional areas. Similarly, a particular nursing unit within a medical center might be led by a director of nursing with several managers operating under her supervision. **Lower-level managers** typically make up a subset of management known as **supervision** which generally focuses on a limited array of managerial activities centered primarily on personnel oversight [15, 16]. In healthcare facilities, lower-level managers typically carry titles such as supervisor or coordinator. While this particular managerial titling scheme is quite common in health and medicine, many variations exist between and among healthcare establishments.

Managers, of course, are equipped with more than mere titles as a means of accomplishing their oversight duties. Healthcare organizations also grant them authority stemming from their given positions, with this being known as position power. **Position power** specifically refers to power derived from holding a formal position of responsibility, granting an individual the legitimate authority to issue directives to others, expect compliance, and reward or penalize actions. Simply by virtue of holding a particular managerial title, an individual is able to wield power over his or her subordinates, with degree of power varying based on the managerial level of the particular individual. In many respects, managers in healthcare organizations operate in similar fashion to officers in the military where rank determines the authority of particular officers. **Subordinates**—those who directly report to managers—essentially have an obligation to comply with the reasonable requests issued by their assigned managers based solely on the fact that they occupy a superior position in the chain of command and are charged with oversight of given cadres of employees. Notably, other forms of power exist—profiled extensively in Chap. 13—and these may or may not be possessed by given managers. Position power, however, is held by all managers, courtesy of their formal roles in their respective healthcare organizations [15, 19].

1.3   Fayol's 14 General Principles of Management

Principles of management—fundamentals associated with the order and operation of the discipline of management—are ever-evolving, just as is the case in any other discipline. Executives and scholars are always at work exploring new techniques, examining existing ones, and cataloguing their findings in a bid to advance managerial knowledge. Over time, insights which have become so tried and true that they can reliably explain the discipline emerge as principles, offering guidance for organizations to follow as they seek to foster excellence in management. Despite the continual evolution of management principles and their associated refinements and advancements, a range of foundational tenets have withstood the test of time, forming an excellent basis for understanding core issues and concerns of management. These foundational principles emerged over centuries, but their systematic presentation did not occur until the publication of Henri Fayol's *General and Industrial Management* in 1916. In this work, Fayol profiled what he described as 14 general principles of management. Fayol's principles include division of work, authority and responsibility, discipline, unity of command, unity of direction, subordination of individual interest to the general interest, remuneration of personnel, centralization, scalar chain (line of authority), order, equity, stability of tenure of personnel, initiative, and esprit de corps [18, 20].

Fayol's work has been described as "the first complete theory of management" [20, p. 12]. Many of the principles he discussed indeed had been addressed by others in earlier periods of history. For example, Sun Tzu's *The Art of War*, published in 500 BC, described the necessity for hierarchical organization, interorganizational communication, and planning. Xenophon, in 370 BC, provided the earliest known account of the advantages of the division of labor. Machiavelli, in 1513, discussed the principle of unity of command in *The Discourses*. And Adam Smith, in 1776, discussed optimal organization, including the benefits of specialization, in *The Wealth of Nations*. Fayol, however, compiled selected principles into an aggregate theory of management, merging various areas of thought to form a comprehensive profile of the emerging discipline [20]. His efforts continue to influence modern-day management thought. Despite these principles being formulated over a century ago, they remain pillars of the discipline of management [18, 20]. Knowledge of such provides an excellent foundation in management.

1.3.1   Division of Work

The principle of **division of work**, or **division of labor** as it is more commonly referred to today, references the need for work to be divided in a manner to permit employees to specialize in particular areas of responsibility. Doing so allows for more and better work to be produced, courtesy of attention being devoted to specific duties rather than diluted across a range of differentiated obligations. Such concentrated focus produces keen expertise which translates into production benefits for organizations [18]. Modern organizations face unending demands to flesh out the highest performance possible, leading managers to engage in constant quests to identify productivity measures [21–25]. The principle of division of work is one such measure, as it structures work in a manner to maximize productivity, courtesy of the intensive focus created by specialization.

Division of work is common in most any complex organizational environment, but it is especially so in health and medicine where, by law, many endeavors can be performed only by those holding certain credentials (e.g., certifications, licenses). For example, a registered nurse, courtesy of his or her training and license, is legally entitled to perform particular nursing duties and responsibilities. Via his or her associated nursing credentials, however, engaging in the practice of, say, medicine or pharmacy would be prohibited. This, of course, makes perfect sense for myriad reasons, notably including that it ensures that employees concentrate their full attention on their chosen profession. Even outside of those work opportunities which mandate possession of certifications or licenses, many occupations in the healthcare industry remain structured in a manner permitting specialization. A hospital's human resource department often divides jobs by specialty, permitting employees to focus their attention on one of several defined areas, such as compensation, training, compliance, safety and health, or similar. A medical center's maintenance department might permit those broadly qualified across multiple areas to focus on a single component of work, such as painting, plumbing, electrical, and so on, to develop concentrated expertise in given specialties. Due to associated performance benefits, structuring work in such a manner is very common in health and medicine, regardless of the occupation under examination.

1.3.2   Authority and Responsibility

According to the principle of authority and responsibility, managers must be granted **authority**, that is, the right to give orders and the power to mandate compliance. But with this authority, managers also must possess **responsibility**, accepting accountability for outcomes. When either of these is not possessed by managers, the individuals holding associated roles are relegated to mere figureheads, destining them for failure and harming associated organizational productivity [18]. Failures here typically become prominent, demoralizing, and debilitating very quickly. Consider a situation where the manager of a medical clinic is charged with overseeing operations and ensuring top performance of the establishment but finds that she has no power to compel members of, say, the medical staff to work in a manner to optimize productivity. This limitation quite obviously will have a profound bearing on managerial performance and, as such, institutional performance.

Better healthcare institutions certainly will take decisive steps to properly pair authority and responsibility in their managerial positions, avoiding the risks of failure associated with doing otherwise. Creating comprehensive, accurate job descriptions serves as an excellent defense. A **job description** is a document which details the duties and responsibilities, reporting relationships, job qualifications, authority assigned, and related information for a particular job. It typically is the product of **job analysis**, an intensive investigation of the requirements of a job for the purpose of creating a comprehensive job description which aids both institutions and employees in properly understanding associated roles and responsibilities [26, 27]. The job analysis process and resulting job description can aid healthcare establishments in ensuring that they do not inadvertently neglect to incorporate both authority and responsibility into management positions. Of course, job descriptions which are properly developed must be translated accurately into practice, resulting in managers bearing both authority and responsibility. If this occurs, managerial success becomes entirely possible.

1.3.3   Discipline

The principle of **discipline** conveys the need for managers to ensure that both they and their employees conduct themselves in a manner consistent with the wishes of their organization. Pursuing directives in an obedient, energized fashion demonstrates dedication and commitment to task, permitting positive and productive business results [18]. The word **professionalism** is often used as a parallel term for the principle of discipline as described by Fayol. As indicated earlier in the chapter, professionalism is appreciated in most any industry, but it is especially cherished in health and medicine, given the sensitivity of the services rendered and its historic portrayal as a professional industry. Managerial employees, as authorities within their respective healthcare establishments, have an even greater duty than their subordinates to exemplify professionalism as they are charged with guiding and directing others. They also serve as the public face of healthcare establishments. They must lead by example, develop professionalism within their departments, and, when necessary, issue corrections to subordinates who fail to meet associated standards. Indeed, professionalism (i.e., discipline) is one of the most sought-after and expected qualities of managerial personnel serving in health and medicine [1, 28, 29].

1.3.4 Unity of Command

According to the principle of **unity of command**, employees should receive orders from only one superior. If this principle is violated, the consequences are serious. Dual command undermines authority, jeopardizes discipline, disrupts order, and threatens stability. Fayol warned that unity of command failures are very common [18]. This remains true to this day. Due to the complexity that is often found in many healthcare establishments, violations of unity of command are an ever-present threat. One of the most common situations leading to this occurs when sharing staff members between departments, something that is often by necessity due to periodic staffing gaps. While sharing helps bridge these gaps, it places an employee from one department under the supervision of a manager from another unit. This often works fine if the two managers communicate well with each other and the given employee, but occasionally, associated breakdowns can occur, resulting in the employee receiving conflicting orders and assignments. This presents very difficult dilemmas for personnel and can be detrimental to productivity [30–32]. Sometimes dual command is built into structures intentionally, as in the case of the matrix form of organization design, profiled in Chap. 9, but in such situations, safeguards are put into place to minimize potential negative effects. Great care must be taken in any case, especially when dual command emerges unintentionally, something that can happen as organizations evolve. This necessitates vigilance in efforts to ensure that proper structures and mechanisms are in place to preserve the principle of unity of command throughout institutions [18].

1.3.5 Unity of Direction

The principle of **unity of direction**, expressed by Fayol as "one head, one plan" [18, p. 56], refers to the necessity that in order to pursue an action in a concerted, focused, and coordinated fashion, employees must work under the direction of one superior following one plan. Fayol indicated that while unity of command is essential in order for unity of direction to be possible, unity of direction does not actually flow from unity of command. Instead, it results from the sound organization of the institution [18]. Errors are not uncommon. A hospital president who is constantly changing the mission of the establishment, for example, has created a moving target that plays havoc with those responsible for its achievement. Similarly, when the top executives of a retail pharmacy chain with a defined operational philosophy tolerate store managers who run their given pharmacies as they wish, mission fulfillment is hampered. In both of these cases, a clear plan does not appear to be in hand, diminishing productivity and opportunity.

Violating the principle of unity of direction is not limited to those managers serving in upper realms of healthcare organizations. It can occur at any level. A dietary manager who gives conflicting orders to dietary aides and other subordinates undermines department productivity, with this being an indication that the given individual does not possess a clear plan for accomplishing the work of the unit. A patient admissions coordinator who can never seem to schedule admission clerks properly, constantly altering their hours of work, often at the last minute, creates major hardships for employees, with this potentially revealing the person's uncertainty over the direction of the operation. Reflecting on these examples, it is easy to understand the resulting hardships and consequences associated with violating the principle of unity of direction, illustrating the importance of one head following one plan.

1.3.6   Subordination of Individual Interest to the General Interest

The principle of **subordination of individual interest to the general interest** conveys that, in organizational life, the interests of one employee or a small group of employees should not take precedent over the mission being pursued by the establishment. When the general interest is lost to individual interest, organizational performance suffers. Fostering what might aptly be described as **sacrifice** can be hastened by employing leaders who demonstrate commitment to cause and set good examples, structuring agreements as fairly as possible, and fostering productive dialogues between supervisors and subordinates [18]. The healthcare industry fortunately is teeming with examples of sacrifice where administrators, physicians, nurses, and many others go the extra mile to benefit those they serve. In such cases, these employees are placing patients—and the missions of their organizations—above themselves, a perspective which is particularly well suited and highly needed in healthcare establishments [1, 33].

When this principle goes awry, however, the consequences can be devastating. Anyone who has worked in healthcare organizations, or any other institution for that matter, likely has witnessed breakdowns where employees focus selfishly on their own wants and needs at the expense of their colleagues. A hospital administrator who constantly works his way out of weekend on-call duties, forcing his colleagues to pick up the slack, serves as an excellent example of an individual's interest trampling on the general interest. This can even occur more broadly, as in cases where entire departments battle other departments (e.g., nursing departments versus laboratory departments, maintenance departments versus housekeeping departments) instead of working collegially with each other for the benefit of themselves, their institutions, and, most importantly, the patients they serve. Given intensive needs for selfless as opposed to self-serving behaviors in health and medicine, managers throughout the hierarchies of healthcare establishments must strive to ensure that the principle of subordination of individual interest to the general interest is a constant presence within their given institutions.

1.3.7 Remuneration of Personnel

Remuneration of personnel pertains to compensation and benefits, effectively constituting employee pay. Fayol argued that pay should be fair and, as much as possible, should provide satisfaction to both the employee and the institution. He also conveyed that pay should be motivating, designing it to reward productive efforts [18]. Productive healthcare establishments are always searching for additional ways to bolster compensatory packages for their employees. Doing so is motivated by concerns for employee satisfaction and well-being and also by desires to maintain competitiveness with marketplace rivals, permitting given establishments better opportunities to recruit and retain healthcare personnel [1, 27, 34]. Healthcare managers, with the assistance of their associated human resource departments, must stay abreast of compensation trends in their given markets, ensuring that contemporary remuneration programs are in effect within their organizations. Salary surveys are helpful, but so is intelligence gained from the workforce. Given the tight-knit nature of the healthcare industry, personnel are often the first to know about increases in, say, the hourly rate of pay for nurses or other occupations at competing healthcare facilities. Knowledge of such is most helpful in fielding attractive pay schemes and performance incentives which mutually satisfy both employees and their given healthcare organizations.

1.3.8 Centralization

The concept of **centralization** refers to where decisions are formally made in institutions [17]. **Centralized organizations** concentrate power and authority at the top of their given institutional hierarchies. **Decentralized organizations** distribute power and authority, at least to some degree, throughout their institutional hierarchies. Each approach has advantages and disadvantages [17, 31]. Centralized organizations permit greater institutional control, given that autonomy is not granted to those outside of top executive ranks. This forces strict adherence to operational tenets as expressed by top officers. Such control, however, has the potential to hamper speed as managers at lower levels must first communicate with top managers and acquire permission before taking actions to address matters. Decentralized organizations grant autonomy to managers throughout the organizational hierarchy, increasing expediency in addressing organizational matters. Control, however, is diminished, with this potentially resulting in actions which deviate from that which top managers have prescribed [30].

Fayol argued that the "centralization versus decentralization" question is resolved not by simply stipulating a particular proportion but instead by determining the optimal degree required to successfully accomplish given goals and objectives. Ascertaining a proper balance is necessary for achieving the best outcomes, with this typically requiring trial and error on the part of healthcare establishments as they go about drawing and refining their organizational charts [18]. This particular principle is explored more deeply in Chap. 9.

1.3.9 Scalar Chain (Line of Authority)

The **scalar chain** or **line of authority** refers to the chain of command from the very top authority within an organization to the lowest ranks of the establishment [18, 30]. Fayol argued that formally devised lines of authority should be respected but cautioned that rigid adherence to such can be highly inefficient. Sensible decisions must be made which honor the scalar chain but also ensure permissibility of certain communications between parties not directly connected in the chain for purposes of efficiency and productivity [18]. Healthcare institutions must determine for themselves how much latitude is permitted for, say, a manager from one department to directly contact the director of another, bypassing his or her immediate supervisor, with institutional performance being the operative concern in making such determinations. Arrangements which permit managers latitude to enter dialogues with those outside of their chain of command can work effectively, but it places a premium on trust between and among parties. It also necessitates excellent communication and complete transparency as a means of ensuring that parties remain apprised of discoveries, intelligence, or any other details emanating from interactions occurring outside of lines of authority [30–32]. Given the complexity of healthcare operations, flexibility within reason is encouraged to aid health and medical organizations in maximizing productivity.

1.3.10 Order

Fayol addressed **order** on both material and human fronts. Regarding the material front, he noted the operative formula for achieving success as "A place for everything and everything in its place" [18 , p. 62]. The formula for success on the human front was described as "A place for everyone and everyone in his place" [18 , p. 62]. For success, order must be achieved on both material and human fronts, with this essentially entailing that all resources, including human resources, be suited for tasks at hand and be available and ready for deployment as needed to make respective contributions [18]. The need for order is perhaps best exemplified in surgical procedures which serve as nexus points for complex logistics involving personnel and materials, with extreme precision being necessary for success. Order, however, is required for virtually any organizational procedure within the walls of healthcare establishments, whether administrative, clinical, or technical in nature. Imagine a medical center's central supply department, for example, being led by a manager who did not value and exemplify the principle of order. Shortages of critical components for medical examinations, surgeries, and other important services likely would appear; incorrect items possibly would be distributed; and theft of valuable property would likely ensue, with these and related occurrences being disastrous for the institution and its patients. Managers indeed must maintain order regarding both its human component and its material component for there to be any hope of institutional prosperity.

1.3.11 Equity

Fayol argued that institutions should strive to ensure fairness and impartiality in the workplace at all levels of the establishment, fostering environments characterized by **equity**. Doing so requires a delicate balance which supports equity without losing sight of the mission at hand. Equity (i.e., fairness, impartiality) is generally considered to be a good thing in organizations. In work environments, legitimate disparate treatment will almost certainly result in ill will on the part of impacted employees. This diminishes the morale of personnel and their ability to positively contribute to organizational performance [18]. Even when inequitable treatment is merely an erroneous perception of those in the workforce, it can be just as powerful as reality. This amplifies the necessity for managers to communicate effectively with their subordinates in any situation where benefits granted to one might be perceived by others as favoritism of some sort. Conveyance of associated justifications can help squelch such demoralizing, counterproductive misinterpretations and resulting conflict [16, 35].

Many lapses in equity are avoided, courtesy of compliance with public policy, especially comprehensive labor law, which mandates fair treatment of employees. Certainly, healthcare organizations which abide by prevailing mandates position themselves to harbor positive environments of impartiality. But derailments are possible if health and medical providers are not careful. For example, **cliques**—small, tightly knit groups of people who possess shared interests on one or more fronts and typically are difficult for others to join—often appear in healthcare establishments. While many are harmless, some operate in sinister fashion. A hospital's pharmacy manager might perhaps have several "favorites" in the department, reserving the best schedules, highest pay raises, and other benefits for these individuals, while denying others associated advantages. In this scenario, effectively, a members-only club of sorts emerges within the pharmacy department, elevating the quality of work life of the clique, while diminishing the quality of work life of outsiders. Perhaps the pharmacy manager even encourages his or her chosen ones to gang up on those employees who are not members of the clique, further diminishing them. Such a scenario clearly violates the principle of equity and has no place in healthcare organizations. Managers must be vigilant in objectively evaluating their thoughts and actions to ensure that they do not permit their given departments to devolve, intentionally or unintentionally, into environments characterized by unfairness.

1.3.12   Stability of Tenure of Personnel

Under the principle of **stability of tenure of personnel**, in order to perform well, employees—assuming they possess requisite abilities—need time to acclimate to new work opportunities and succeed in their accomplishment. Institutions should strive to develop employees and control turnover, ensuring the capture of full value from personnel [18]. Healthcare institutions can facilitate this by taking a range of steps. Offering competitive compensation and benefits packages to employees both attracts job candidates and, once hired, aids healthcare providers in retaining them. The provision of outstanding educational opportunities, including comprehensive orientation, onboarding, and ongoing training ensures that employees have the tools they need to be successful in their careers. Proper guidance further facilitates employee success and retention, necessitating the provision of excellent managerial supervision [1]. Managers must ensure that their healthcare organizations direct these and related resources toward their personnel, permitting establishments to field stable workforces and generate satisfactory returns on associated investments.

1.3.13   Initiative

Initiative refers to the ability and drive within an individual to formulate a plan and execute it successfully. Fayol encouraged institutions to develop initiative in all employees, including managers, taking steps to instill and maintain this quality in the workforce, given the many mutual benefits afforded by such [18]. Hiring individuals who have demonstrated initiative in previous educational and employment experiences represents a good start, but once these personnel are employed, institutions must ensure that their tenacity is maintained. Properly designed jobs, excellent organizational cultures, skilled managerial guidance and direction, performance incentives, and related efforts that foster highly motivating work environments are very helpful for building and maintaining initiative. Of course, even the best of efforts on the part of healthcare organizations will do little to foster initiative unless the employees themselves possess the internal ambition necessary for them to actively engage their work. Lack of initiative is especially problematic in healthcare establishments as it reduces employee attentiveness, accuracy, and productivity, with this potentially resulting in the loss of life. As such, swift disciplinary actions must be directed toward those demonstrating uncaring dispositions. This measure of last resort unfortunately must remain a possibility to ensure that workforces are characterized by initiative. The threat of disciplinary proceedings also serves as a powerful incentive for employees to exert proper effort.

1.3.14 Esprit de Corps

Through the principle of **esprit de corps**, organizations build a sense of unity between and among the ranks, fostering teamwork that allows the workforce to direct efforts in concerted fashion toward the achievement of designated goals and objectives [18]. As the delivery of patient care results from numerous individuals with vastly different backgrounds and qualifications performing highly varied roles at the proper time and place, the principle of esprit de corps is especially important in health and medicine. This principle should be considered to be an essential ingredient of patient care, and as such, healthcare managers must build proficiencies in ensuring its proliferation. Methods for establishing esprit de corps are described in detail in the following section.

WK Reflections: Establishing Esprit de Corps

Of all of the functions of management, esprit de corps offers perhaps the widest range of latitude regarding how it is addressed. Options abound for fostering unity within healthcare organizations. Common approaches for building esprit de corps which are routinely found in health and medical establishments include instituting hiring practices which carefully vet prospective employees to identify individuals who work well with others, emphasizing in orientations and other learning experiences the importance of personnel working together to achieve goals and objectives, implementing systems which reward employees for cohesive behaviors and punish them for divisiveness, and ensuring excellent supervision aimed at unifying personnel and building camaraderie. Such standard practices indeed can build esprit de corps, but greater investments can yield even better results, warranting pursuit of advanced efforts.

For decades, Willis Knighton Health has been described by employees as having a "family feel." This perspective, where personnel feel as though they are part of a family rather than merely a component of a work group, resulted from painstaking efforts on the part of the institution to establish esprit de corps. Beyond instituting the common approaches noted earlier, Willis Knighton Health implemented a series of initiatives designed to robustly engender camaraderie between and among personnel. Several examples of this are as follows:

- Celebratory events of all kinds are held throughout Willis Knighton Health, with some being at the department level and others being systemwide. By taking opportunities to commemorate noteworthy occasions (e.g., employee birthdays, retirement celebrations, grand openings, holiday events), celebrate personal and institutional achievements (e.g., educational accomplishments, service awards, quality recognitions), and engage in similar forms of revelry and appreciation, employees are brought together, permitting socialization with peers in contexts that build pride and fuel camaraderie.

- Willis Knighton Health annually hosts WK Day, an all-day picnic and barbecue held at the Louisiana State Fair. At this event, employees and their family members are granted free admission to the fair where they enjoy free food and participate in fun games in a special tent exclusively arranged for Willis Knighton Health. They also are afforded unlimited access to rides on the midway. More than 10,000 employees and their family members routinely attend this event each year, bringing the Willis Knighton Health family together in a casual, relaxed recreational environment to foster mutual appreciation, enjoyment, and bonding.
- To assist employees facing financial hardships due to tragic events (e.g., homes destroyed by fires, tornados, or floods; domestic violence situations requiring relocation; cases of prolonged illness), Willis Knighton Health instituted the Willis Knighton Employee Benevolent Fund. The fund is administered by a committee of employees who possess the authority to approve gifts of assistance. This initiative dramatically propagates the "family feel" that characterizes Willis Knighton Health as it replicates the lifeline that families often provide their loved ones in situations of hardship. Contributions to the fund are accepted from staff members, with employee participation being exceptional, demonstrating care and concern on the part of personnel for their Willis Knighton Health family.
- Willis Knighton Health holds "dust and discover" days whenever opening a new facility or expanding service operations. During these events, employees report for duty in work clothes, wearing specially issued WK t-shirts, to help ready given facilities for service by assisting in clean-up, move-in, and associated launch processes. These work sessions have been an effective tool for developing esprit de corps, inspiring camaraderie and fueling team building.
- Comprehensive support is offered whenever a loss of life is experienced within the Willis Knighton Health family. Administrators and other employees make concerted efforts to attend all funerals and visitations, offering opportunities for Willis Knighton Health to comfort and support the families of the deceased. Flowers and memorial gifts are also regularly provided as a further demonstration of support. Contact with the deceased's family is maintained for a period of time to offer any assistance that might be required, further reinforcing Willis Knighton Health's commitment to its employees.

Through different means and contexts, these examples each bring employees together, fostering collegiality and community, unifying the workforce and advancing esprit de corps. Clearly, such programs require resources on the part of healthcare establishments, but associated expenditures should be viewed as investments as they pay significant dividends. Willis Knighton Health has observed that associated investments to build esprit de corps and foster the institution's "family feel" have increased employee morale, fostered high performance, reduced turnover rates, and advanced employee commitment, among other positive attributes [1]. Advanced initiatives which go the extra mile clearly accelerate impact potential and should be explored by progressive healthcare institutions. As esprit de corps is a defined principle of management, initiatives here should be just as robust as those associated with any other management principle.

1.4 Gulick's POSDCORB Model Profiling the Activities of Management

Whereas principles of management provide guidelines for order and operation within organizations, **activities of management** address the role of managers within organizations. Specifically, they answer the question, "What does a manager do?" As even one completely new to management could rightfully surmise, the list of activities held by managers is quite extensive. These, however, can be grouped into a memorable categorization, courtesy of the work of Luther Gulick who coined the term POSDCORB to call attention to the work of managers. **POSDCORB**, pronounced like saying the words "post" and "corb," is an acronym standing for Planning, Organizing, Staffing, Directing, Coordinating, Reporting, and Budgeting, making for a handy reference to keep the activities of management at the top of mind [36]. Importantly, the array demonstrates the comprehensive nature of management, ensuring that health and medical establishments do not inadvertently neglect key activities. It also aids managers themselves in understanding work requirements, permitting them to pursue knowledge on each front in order to perform optimally and offer their associated healthcare establishments the best oversight acumen possible. The activities of management, as identified in the POSDCORB model, are profiled as follows.

1.4.1 Planning

Planning is defined as the process of thinking through and outlining the activities necessary to accomplish a particular goal or objective [36]. Due to its frequency, it is one of the most recognized activities required of managers. Planning is routinely done on both formal and informal bases, depending on the nature of given plans and the requirements set forth by healthcare establishments. Planning appears in all managerial corners of health and medicine. Hospital administrators plan strategies for their given organizations, nurse managers plan the work schedules of staff members, dietary directors plan patient meals, marketing coordinators plan advertising campaigns, housekeeping supervisors plan the work routines of housekeeping crews, and so on.

As would be expected, the demands of planning intensify in complexity at each successive level within the hierarchy of an organization, with those at the very top of the organizational chart assuming the most challenging planning tasks, given their oversight of the establishment in its entirety. Upper-level managers primarily are concerned with **strategic planning**, planning which centers on complex, often institution-wide matters, especially those with lengthy time horizons. Managers in lower realms within healthcare organizations primarily deal with **tactical planning**, planning which aids in the accomplishment of strategic plans by focusing on one or more objectives required for their realization. Regardless of the type or level of planning at hand, managers engaged in such must have the ability to visualize a desired outcome and work backward, selecting resources, determining timelines, and coordinating logistics in order to realize the given outcome, necessitating thorough planning skills and abilities [36, 37].

1.4.2 Organizing

The management activity of **organizing** concerns matters associated with the structure and design of institutions, including their various departments and work processes [36]. Perhaps the most widely recognized facet of organizing is an establishment's **organizational chart**, a diagram which uses a series of boxes and lines to illustrate the structural arrangements of departments and people within an institution. This illustration entails numerous organizing decisions including those associated with determining lines of authority, span of control, degree of centralization, and the like [31, 38]. While overall organizational chart assembly tasks rest primarily with upper-level managers, those occupying middle and lower-level managerial realms also are engaged in organizing, albeit on more limited bases.

Arranging personnel in a manner to satisfactorily perform the work of a given unit represents an example of organizing that most any manager, regardless of level, must routinely perform [31, 39]. Consider the organizing tasks required of a housekeeping manager in a hospital. The manager must possess a firm understanding of the layout of his assigned facility, the medical services provided by the establishment, and the associated housekeeping requirements necessary for ensuring that the service environment remains clean and sanitary. With this knowledge, the housekeeping manager then must determine the arrangement of personnel required to fulfill the sanitation demands of the institution, organizing personnel into work groups with defined duties and responsibilities. This example nicely illustrates the organizing function and its important emphasis on the structure and design of work, ultimately permitting healthcare institutions to operate efficiently and effectively in the delivery of patient care.

1.4.3   Staffing

Staffing concerns all matters associated with the personnel function of organizations, with recruitment, selection, retention, training, maintaining favorable work conditions, and the like typifying the focus of this management activity [36]. While human resource departments are charged with overseeing the broad personnel management concerns of healthcare organizations, notably including policy administration and compliance, managers throughout institutional hierarchies have specific employee oversight obligations in their given work units, many of which pertain to staffing matters [3, 15]. Those responsible for managing laboratory departments in medical centers, for example, contend with a barrage of staffing issues and concerns, including hiring laboratory technologists, technicians, phlebotomists, and others; onboarding new staff members, orienting them to the workplace and its requirements; devising work schedules and assigning responsibilities; ensuring atmospheres that support individual and group performance; rewarding employees for compliant behaviors and disciplining those who commit policy violations; and handling matters associated with employee resignations and terminations. These duties all fall under what would be considered to be staffing matters. They are expected of most any healthcare manager, making staffing an essential management activity.

1.4.4   Directing

Directing centers on issuing general and specific orders to subordinates who, in turn, are charged with their fulfillment for purposes of achieving designated goals and objectives. It is an ongoing activity requiring prowess in leadership, decision-making, and communication on the part of managers [36]. Directing also requires managers to be proficient at **delegation**, turning over the authority for accomplishing particular tasks to subordinates for purposes of distributing work, developing employees showing potential, and engendering associated trust. Of all management activities, directing is perhaps the first to enter the minds of employees reflecting on the role played by managers in the workplace. This is because all employees have regular and routine exposure to the commands of their given supervisors. Further, over the course of their work lives, they almost certainly have observed the benefits of fulfilling issued directives (e.g., compliments, bonuses, promotions, and other forms of advancement), as well as the consequences associated with failing to follow orders (e.g., reprimands, demotions, terminations), leaving lasting impressions about the directing function. Orders effectively drive actions in organizations, with broad institutional dictates being broken down into more specialized issuances assigned to groups and employees across the institution, permitting the work of given establishments to be accomplished [40, 41]. Directing is an ongoing concern of managers. Without it, work would grind to a halt.

1.4.5 Coordinating

The management activity of **coordinating** refers to efforts to understand and address the interrelated components required of work, permitting it to be accomplished effectively [36]. Even simple work duties and responsibilities require extensive logistics necessary for their successful completion. Among other things, numerous resources, including people, materials, and know-how, must be called upon when and where needed in the production process, making coordination an essential skill for managers to possess. For work of great complexity, such as that required for successfully delivering healthcare services, the logistics are especially pronounced. The vast complexities of healthcare delivery necessitate extensive specialization which compartmentalizes various work components which then must be linked together to successfully provide patient care. Some of these components directly address patients (e.g., services provided by nursing, respiratory therapy, laboratory, and other clinical departments), while others do so indirectly (e.g., services provided by information technology, maintenance, security, and other nonclinical departments) [1, 3]. Given the symbiotic relationships between and among units within healthcare establishments, managers must understand the entirety of each and every one of these moving parts. This permits them to coordinate the components falling under their direct supervision and control to deliver the work for which their unit is responsible at the precise time that it is needed by other parties in the production chain, ultimately culminating in the delivery of a satisfactory patient experience.

1.4.6 Reporting

Reporting is a vital activity requiring managers to inform their supervisors of ongoing operations, activities, and developments within their assigned work units [36]. Without reporting, healthcare organizations effectively are operating blind, lacking knowledge regarding the various happenings and occurrences within given establishments. Beyond the practical value afforded by information conveyance, reporting notably aids healthcare organizations in ensuring that their managers are accountable for the productivity of their assigned work units. Proper reporting requires excellent communication abilities, with accuracy of information conveyed being absolutely essential, permitting the details transmitted to those higher up in the chain of command to be reliable and valuable. The form of reporting required of managers is up to the supervisory officials requesting the associated information but may involve both oral and written presentation methods. As with all managerial activities, reporting is essential throughout organizational hierarchies, with even chief executive officers being required to report to their supervisors in the form of the governing boards of their given institutions.

1.4.7   Budgeting

Budgeting concerns all matters of fiscal planning, accounting, and financial control within an organization [36]. It is an area deserving of extreme attention as the financial viability of healthcare establishments must be assured in order for health and medical services to be offered. Maintaining financial viability is the responsibility of managers throughout the hierarchies of healthcare establishments, as they all must operate the units under their direction in a responsible manner that adheres to designated budgets. Common tasks include preparing budgets for forthcoming periods, monitoring operations to ensure compliance and avoid cost overruns, and proactively surveilling work environments to identify and remedy any discovered wasteful practices. Budgeting responsibilities are important in any organization, but they are particularly so in the healthcare industry, where uncertainty is high and competition is fierce [1, 3, 42]. In such environments, financial missteps are especially caustic, placing institutions in extreme jeopardy, even if all other operations outside of budgetary matters are prudent and sound. As such, great care must be taken by managers to competently address budgeting activities.

WK Reflections: Managerial Immersion Within Work Environments

Gulick's POSDCORB model aptly itemizes the things that managers are responsible for doing. While many variables impact the ability of managers to successfully accomplish these activities, Willis Knighton Health has discovered an important ingredient for success: Managers must be immersed within their given work environments, permitting them to observe operations firsthand. Managerial immersion within work environments is essential as it aids managers in understanding operations from the perspective of those responsible for producing the required work. Such close proximity also affords opportunities to properly guide and direct subordinates, troubleshoot issues, and monitor resource usage, things which are more difficult to accomplish at a distance. Further, it assists managers in understanding the deliverables produced by their given units, aiding them in ensuring that associated efforts meet the expectations of their healthcare establishments. Ultimately, being near those one manages improves one's ability to engage in each of the activities of management.

The notion that workplace immersion is beneficial for managers might seem patently obvious, and, in fact, it is. However, the healthcare industry is burgeoning with examples where managers are detached from those they are responsible for managing. Sometimes this occurs inadvertently, as in cases where space restrictions, perhaps due to quick growth, might force a manager to be officed out of direct proximity to the specific work environment he or she supervises. But it also can occur by design, as in cases where a medical office building is constructed to house executives in relative isolation from the work environments over which they have responsibility. These arrangements indeed can be productive, but from Willis Knighton Health's experiences, they are not optimal, as they limit engagement opportunities.

Willis Knighton Health's commitment to ensuring managerial immersion is perhaps best exemplified by the location of the office of its president and chief executive officer, which is literally a few steps away from Willis Knighton North's Emergency Department. This arrangement essentially places the top officer of Willis Knighton Health and all of his assistants immediately adjacent to the busiest unit within the institution, making it very easy to maintain an awareness of hospital operations. Administrators for each of Willis Knighton Health's campuses also are located in their respective hospitals rather than in buildings offsite, affording these managers with complete immersion and associated direct oversight opportunities. The same goes for lower managerial ranks.

Close proximity, of course, is of limited value if managers hide in their offices and avoid circulating within their assigned work environments, missing out on opportunities to interact with the people they are responsible for managing. Managerial immersion within work environments does, however, make it easier for dedicated managers to ensure their productive exposure to operations, assisting them in addressing the activities of management. As such, healthcare providers should give careful consideration to the managerial proximity issue when they build or renovate their institutions, selecting pathways that permit managers to perform optimally, fulfilling their greatest potential.

1.5   Management and the Leadership Imperative

After reviewing the activities of management, one cannot help but to realize that conducting the activities properly requires numerous personal skills and abilities. Dedicated managers work throughout their careers to shape and hone their skill sets in an effort to deliver their maximum potential. The list of proficiencies beneficial to managers is quite extensive, essentially entailing anything and everything that can help them more adequately conduct the activities of management. Conceptual skills, for example, are vital, essentially enabling managers to identify, analyze, and resolve complex problems successfully. The same is true of interpersonal skills which permit managers to interact with, understand, and relate to others effectively. Communication and decision-making are also essential skills that managers must possess. But of all skills of importance to managers, none arguably is more essential than that of leadership [1].

Leadership is defined as a skill, composed of a series of appealing qualities, which permits a person to establish productive relationships with others, affording opportunities to influence them in a manner to achieve goals and objectives. The qualities of leaders (e.g., vision, charisma, honesty, intelligence, ambition, etc.) are attractive to others, compelling followership. This affords leaders with the ability to influence their followers, compelling them to embrace particular directives as their own, resulting in a collaborative, inspired, and voluntary pursuit of the mission at hand. Such a skill has obvious benefits for those holding managerial roles, but why is leadership viewed to be imperative for managers? Because leadership has a way of magnifying all other skills. A manager who can conceptualize with precision, engage others meaningfully, communicate well, and make decisions quickly and effectively will not be able to derive maximum benefit from those particular attributes without also possessing the ability to lead others, that is, to compel them to action, courtesy of their personal qualities which prompt followership. Managers who possess leadership skills almost certainly will see improvements across the entire range of managerial activities, making acquisition of associated skills essential [1, 30, 39, 41, 43, 44].

Often confused as being one and the same as management, leadership is a very different concept, as can be ascertained by comparing the two definitions. The two are even distinguished on the basis of the type of authority from which their associated power is derived. Unlike management, which derives its authority from position power, leadership derives its authority from **personal power**, that is, power derived from possessing appealing characteristics or attributes, compelling the admiration, respect, and followership of others [45, 46]. Chapter 2 explores the concept of leadership and its importance to healthcare managers and their organizations more deeply. For now, however, readers should understand the leadership imperative for those serving in positions of management within healthcare institutions and recognize the need for devoting extensive time and energy toward developing leadership skills to bolster managerial performance.

1.6 Summary and Conclusions

The complexities of healthcare institutions demand intense oversight in order to ensure that operations are conducted successfully, with management being a vital mechanism for doing so. Management effectively serves as a guidance system for healthcare establishments where managerial staff members endeavor daily to direct people, places, and things within health and medicine toward the ultimate goal of delivering high-quality patient care. This noble cause requires coordinated efforts from multiple parties engaged in environments of extreme diversity, complexity, perpetual change, and constant uncertainty, representing one of the most challenging work settings of any industry. Exceptional management brings order to what might be viewed by many as being an impossible pursuit. Courtesy of the extensive history of management, leaping forward with Henri Fayol's presentation of its 14 general principles, advancing further with Luther Gulick's identification of its key activities, and continuing its development through modern-day research efforts, healthcare establishments are afforded prudent pathways for overseeing operations and achieving success. Concerted attention directed toward ensuring managerial prowess should be a top priority for healthcare organizations far and wide.

Key Terms

- Activities of Management
- Authority
- Budgeting
- Centralization
- Centralized Organization
- Clique
- Coordinating
- Decentralized Organization
- Delegation
- Directing
- Discipline
- Division of Labor
- Division of Work
- Equity
- Esprit de Corps
- Fayol's 14 General Principles of Management
- Gulick's POSDCORB Model Profiling the Activities of Management
- Initiative
- Job Analysis
- Job Description
- Leadership
- Line of Authority
- Lower-Level Manager
- Management
- Manager
- Middle-Level Manager
- Order
- Organizational Behavior
- Organizational Chart
- Organizing
- Personal Power
- Planning
- POSDCORB
- Position Power
- Principles of Management

- Professionalism
- Remuneration of Personnel
- Reporting
- Responsibility
- Sacrifice
- Scalar Chain
- Senior Manager
- Stability of Tenure of Personnel
- Staffing
- Strategic Planning
- Subordinate
- Subordination of Individual Interest to the General Interest
- Supervision
- Tactical Planning
- Unity of Command
- Unity of Direction
- Upper-Level Manager

Exercises

1. In your own words, define the concept of management, discuss its various features and characteristics, and reflect on its essential role in the delivery of health and medicine.
2. Identify the different levels of management in healthcare organizations, note common managerial titles tied to each level, and discuss the scope of control held by managers at each level. Then, reflect on a recent work experience and examine the titling scheme used for managers across the organizational hierarchy. Compare this titling scheme to the examples provided in the chapter, and indicate any observed likenesses and differences. Do you have any suggestions for improving the titling scheme in your workplace? If so, indicate what they are and why they are suggested. If not, explain why you do not believe improvements are needed.
3. Box 1.1 presented a checklist for managerial preparation as derived from the insights and experiences of Willis Knighton Health. While the associated discussion focused on aspiring managers, the items in the checklist are equally applicable for aiding the advancement of healthcare managers regardless of their level of experience. Taking the eight items presented in the checklist, perform a self-assessment, preparing a brief narrative which describes your efforts on each of these fronts. Do you notice any opportunities for improvement? If so, identify them and indicate how you plan to proceed.
4. Identify and define the 14 general principles of management as outlined by Henri Fayol, and discuss their application in health and medicine. Which of the 14 principles do you view to be most critical, which do you view to be least critical, and why?

5. Assume that you have been appointed as the president of a newly established hospital. Knowing the importance of the principle of esprit de corps, discuss specific tools and techniques that you would implement to foster its proliferation throughout the institution.
6. Identify and define the seven activities of management as presented in Luther Gulick's POSDCORB model. Reflect on a recent work experience and describe your level of exposure to each of the seven activities. Which activities do you consider to be your strengths, and which do you consider to be your weaknesses? What steps do you plan to take to maintain your strengths and eliminate your weaknesses?
7. Reporting—the R in the POSDCORB model—constitutes one of the seven activities of management. Think about your current work role and describe the reporting required of you by your supervisor and the reporting that you require of your subordinates. Communicate, for example, what types of reports are required and how and when they are to be delivered. What do you view to be the strengths and weaknesses of your organization's reporting system?
8. Managers in health and medicine must develop leadership skills in order to perform optimally in their assigned roles. How do you plan to ensure that you never lose sight of the leadership imperative in your managerial career? Provide a brief narrative sharing your associated thoughts.

References

1. Elrod, J. K. (2013). *Breadcrumbs to cheesecake*. R&R Publishers.
2. Shi, L., & Singh, D. A. (2023). *Essentials of the US health care system* (6th ed.). Jones and Bartlett.
3. McConnell, C. R. (2020). *Hospitals and health systems: What they are and how they work*. Jones and Bartlett.
4. Ginter, P. M., Duncan, W. J., & Swayne, L. E. (2013). *Strategic management of health care organizations* (7th ed.). Jossey-Bass.
5. American College of Healthcare Executives. (2023). *FACHE: Become a recognized leader among executives in healthcare management by becoming a Fellow of the American College of Healthcare Executives*. Retrieved March 2, 2023, from https://www.ache.org/fache
6. HR Certification Institute. (2023). *Individual certifications*. Retrieved March 2, 2023, from https://www.hrci.org/certifications/individual-certifications
7. American Marketing Association. (2023). *Professional certifications*. Retrieved March 2, 2023, from https://www.ama.org/certifications
8. Ziebland, S., Coulter, A., Calabrese, J. D., & Locock, L. (Eds.). (2013). *Understanding and using health experiences: Improving patient care*. Oxford University Press.
9. Perez, O. J. (2009). *The patient experience: A guide to creating a meaningful patient experience in every healing encounter*. Florida Hospital Publishing.
10. Flynn, W. J., Valentine, S. R., & Meglich, P. A. (2022). *Healthcare human resource management* (4th ed.). Cengage.
11. Wilensky, S. E., & Teitelbaum, J. B. (2023). *Essentials of health policy and law* (5th ed.). Jones and Bartlett.

12. Kotler, P., Stevens, R. J., & Shalowitz, J. (2021). *Strategic marketing for health care organizations: Building a customer-driven health system* (2nd ed.). Wiley.
13. Dunn, R. T. (2021). *Dunn and Haimann's healthcare management* (11th ed.). Health Administration Press.
14. Buchbinder, S. B., Shanks, N. H., & Kite, B. J. (2021). *Introduction to health care management* (4th ed.). Jones and Bartlett.
15. Griffin, R. W. (2022). *Management* (13th ed.). Cengage.
16. Kinicki, A., & Soignet, D. B. (2022). *Management: A practical introduction* (10th ed.). McGraw-Hill.
17. Colquitt, J. A., Lepine, J. A., & Wesson, M. J. (2019). *Organizational behavior: Improving performance and commitment in the workplace* (6th ed.). McGraw-Hill.
18. Fayol, H. (2016). General principles of management. In J. M. Shafritz, J. S. Ott, & Y. S. Jang (Eds.), *Classics of organization theory* (8th ed., pp. 53–65). Cengage.
19. Schermerhorn, J. R., Jr., & Bachrach, D. G. (2019). *Management* (14th ed.). Wiley.
20. Shafritz, J. M., Ott, J. S., & Jang, Y. S. (Eds.). (2016). *Classics of organization theory* (8th ed.). Cengage.
21. Peters, T. J., & Waterman, R. H., Jr. (2004). *In search of excellence: Lessons from America's best-run companies*. HarperBusiness.
22. Blanchard, K. (2019). *Leading at a higher level: Blanchard on leadership and creating high performing organizations* (3rd ed.). FT Press.
23. Gorder, C. V. (2015). *The front-line leader: Building a high-performance organization from the ground up*. Jossey-Bass.
24. Luke, R. D., Walston, S. L., & Plummer, P. M. (2004). *Healthcare strategy: In pursuit of competitive advantage*. Health Administration Press.
25. Berry, L. L. (1999). *Discovering the soul of service: The nine drivers of sustainable business success*. The Free Press.
26. Snell, S., & Morris, S. (2023). *Managing human resources* (19th ed.). Cengage.
27. Niles, N. J. (2020). *Basic concepts of health care human resource management* (2nd ed.). Jones and Bartlett.
28. Makely, S., Austin, V. J., & Kester, Q. (2017). *Professionalism in health care: A primer for career success* (5th ed.). Pearson.
29. Cornock, M. (2023). *Accountability and professionalism in nursing and healthcare*. Sage.
30. Robbins, S. P., & Judge, T. A. (2019). *Organizational behavior* (18th ed.). Pearson.
31. Anderson, D. L. (2019). *Organization design: Creating strategic and agile organizations*. Sage.
32. Newman, A. (2017). *Business communication: In person, in print, online* (10th ed.). Cengage.
33. Elrod, J. K., & Fortenberry, J. L., Jr. (2018). Am I seeing things through the eyes of patients? An exercise in bolstering patient attentiveness and empathy. *BMC Health Services Research, 18*(Suppl 3), 41–44.
34. McConnell, C. R. (2021). *Human resource management in health care: Principles and practice* (3rd ed.). Jones and Bartlett.
35. Liddle, D. (2017). *Managing conflict: A practical guide to resolution in the workplace*. Kogan Page.
36. Gulick, L. (2016). Notes on the theory of organization. In J. M. Shafritz, J. S. Ott, & Y. S. Jang (Eds.), *Classics of organization theory* (8th ed., pp. 84–92). Cengage.
37. David, F. R., David, F. R., & David, M. E. (2020). *Strategic management: A competitive advantage approach* (17th ed.). Pearson.
38. Galbraith, J. R. (2014). *Designing organizations: Strategy, structure, and process at the business unit and enterprise levels* (3rd ed.). Jossey-Bass.
39. Konopaske, R., Ivancevich, J. M., & Matteson, M. T. (2018). *Organizational behavior and management* (11th ed.). McGraw-Hill.
40. Morgeson, F. P., Brannick, M. T., & Levine, E. L. (2020). *Job and work analysis: Methods, research, and applications for human resource management* (3rd ed.). Sage.

41. Griffin, R. W., Phillips, J. M., & Gully, S. M. (2020). *Organizational behavior: Managing people and organizations* (13th ed.). Cengage.
42. Fortenberry, J. L., Jr. (2010). *Health care marketing: Tools and techniques* (3rd ed.). Jones and Bartlett.
43. McShane, S. L., & Von Glinow, M. A. (2019). *Organizational behavior* (4th ed.). McGraw-Hill.
44. Hitt, M. A., Miller, C. C., Colella, A., & Triana, M. D. C. (2018). *Organizational behavior* (5th ed.). Wiley.
45. Northouse, P. G. (2022). *Leadership: Theory and practice* (9th ed.). Sage.
46. Kotter, J. P. (1990). *A force for change: How leadership differs from management*. The Free Press.

Chapter 2
Leadership in Health and Medicine

Learning Objectives

After examining this chapter, readers will have the ability to:

- Define the concept of leadership and recognize its vital role in achieving operational excellence in health and medicine.
- Distinguish leadership from management by being able to properly define and discuss both terms.
- Define trait, behavioral, and contingency theories of leadership and discuss their contributions to the knowledge base of leadership.
- Recognize and appreciate contemporary approaches to leadership, including charismatic and servant leadership perspectives.
- Understand the need for and be capable of organizing leadership development programs in healthcare establishments.

2.1 Background

As highly complex establishments teeming with employees from all walks of life pursuing vastly different occupations, healthcare organizations rely heavily on individuals who possess the ability to engage others and compel them to action [1–4]. Without this, health and medical establishments could never hope to deliver patient care effectively. To engage and compel, some managers choose to rely solely on the authority granted to them by their formal titles, issuing orders and expecting compliance, accordingly. Relying solely on this, however, is not the most effective pathway for achieving a highly motivated, productive workforce and could even prove to be demoralizing and discouraging. A notable improvement can be achieved by pairing excellent managerial skills and abilities with excellent leadership skills and abilities. This grouping of expertise yields tremendous synergies, elevating

J. K. Elrod, J. L. Fortenberry, Jr., *Organizational Behavior and Management in Health and Medicine*, https://doi.org/10.1007/978-3-031-61823-9_2

managerial performance and improving organizational outcomes. The infusion of leadership amplifies managerial results [1, 5–9]. As such, individuals who follow this pathway become assets of their respective healthcare organizations, representing a worthy pursuit for managers and their respective employers.

To some, the information presented in the preceding paragraph might come as somewhat of a surprise. Leadership, after all, is just a fancy word for management, right? Wrong! The two concepts are very different, with leadership referencing the particular qualities of an individual and management concerning the formal position held by a person [10–12]. Incorrectly equating the two terms is fairly common, though, as leadership and management are often used interchangeably in society and sometimes even in the workplace. Precision, however, is essential in overseeing healthcare operations, and this extends to accuracy in the use of terminology. If one uses these two distinctive terms interchangeably, he or she might not realize their unique attributes and, as such, would miss out on developmental opportunities and potential competitive advantages that otherwise could be captured. This particular chapter will clarify what leadership is, what it is not, and what individuals can do to develop their potential in this vital area of healthcare organizational behavior and management.

2.2 Defining Leadership

Leadership is defined as a skill, composed of a series of appealing qualities, which permits a person to establish productive relationships with others, affording opportunities to influence them in a manner to achieve goals and objectives. This definition draws attention to a number of important aspects which distinguish the concept. As notably conveyed, leadership is a **skill**—a defined talent or ability—possessed by an individual, making the person a **leader**. It is multifaceted, involving a range of qualities, sometimes referred to as attributes, characteristics, or something similar. Importantly, these qualities are attractive to others, compelling them to establish relationships with the leader and become **followers**. Often cited qualities associated with leadership include vision, charisma, honesty, intelligence, and ambition, but many more possibilities exist [1, 5, 6, 13–15]. The particular combination of attributes possessed by leaders varies widely between and among individuals due to differences in backgrounds, education, experience, and related characteristics. While there are many desirable leadership qualities, a universally accepted array does not exist. Different contexts very often call for different qualities.

Leaders are able to influence their followers to embrace particular directives as their own, resulting in a collaborative, inspired, and voluntary pursuit of the mission at hand. This naturally fosters **commitment**, a highly desired state in organizational life realized when individuals dedicate themselves to mission fulfillment, essentially becoming champions of their given organizations. Followers are compelled to pursue the directives issued by leaders not because they have to but because they want to. A unique bond is forged between leader and follower. Effectively, the leader's desires become the follower's desires, uniting both in associated quests. And enhanced commitment is not the only benefit possible. Research also indicates that excellent leadership can enhance employee morale, improve workforce productivity and development, facilitate change, encourage employee creativity, and bolster innovation [1, 5, 6, 13–15].

Leadership, as a practice, is age-old. From time immemorial, it has been a distinguishing feature of successful pursuits across multiple fronts. Excellence in leadership has been cited as the key to military victories, the development of nations, the success of political campaigns, the prosperity of communities, and the fortunes of business and industry, including those engaged in health and medicine [1, 3, 8, 16]. At face value, leadership might appear to be simple, but in actuality, it is a highly complex subject. To foster associated understanding, literally thousands of empirical studies on leadership have been conducted, with scores of books also being written [7, 8, 12]. Efforts span the gamut, from formulating underlying theories to identifying best practices. Despite this attention, many questions remain unanswered, prompting scholar James MacGregor Burns to famously declare that "Leadership is one of the most observed and least understood phenomena on earth" [16, p. 2]. This assertion rings true to this day, with executives and scholars alike endeavoring to better grasp the concept in an effort to capitalize on its many benefits.

2.3 Leadership Versus Management

A common misconception regarding leadership is that it is one and the same as management. In truth, the two concepts are quite distinct. **Management** is formally defined as a range of activities (i.e., planning, organizing, staffing, directing, coordinating, reporting, and budgeting) which are carried out by formally appointed individuals (e.g., chief executive officers, vice presidents, directors, managers, supervisors) for purposes of aiding organizations in realizing their missions. Management is transactional by nature, relying on directives issued by managerial personnel to their subordinates who, in turn, are tasked with carrying out those directives to achieve desired outcomes. Notably, the authority of managers is derived from **position power** (i.e., power derived from holding a formal position of responsibility, granting an individual the legitimate authority to issue directives to others, expect compliance, and reward or penalize actions); the authority of leaders is derived from **personal power** (i.e., power derived from possessing appealing characteristics or attributes, compelling the admiration, respect, and followership of others) [5–12, 17]. The transactional, exchange-oriented, position-bound characteristic of management extends to all managerial roles within institutions regardless of their level in organizational hierarchies [18–21].

Leadership is a quality that is independent of management, meaning that it can exist without the requirement of holding a managerial role. When leadership happens to be possessed by those in management roles, however, it serves to enhance associated productivity and success, as one's management duties and responsibilities are infused with the relational augmentations afforded by leadership. Effectively, leadership turns the transactional nature of management into a transformational experience by introducing powerful, supplementary attributes into managerial activities and processes [1, 5–9, 22].

To aid in ensuring that leadership and management are viewed distinctively, remembering the following adage can be helpful: *Managers may or may not be leaders and leaders may or may not be managers.* But given the appealing nature of leadership and the benefits afforded, health and medical providers must endeavor to ensure that those holding formal management roles acquire and display leadership skills and abilities. Developmental opportunities also should be provided for those who display leadership potential but are not currently serving in management roles as part of succession planning efforts. Ultimately, healthcare providers should take every opportunity to ensure the proliferation of leadership within their given institutions [1].

2.4 Traditional Perspectives of Leadership

In the formative years of leadership research, a number of perspectives were put forth and studied in a quest to better understand this important area of organizational behavior and management. These early perspectives are now considered to be classics which helped to advance knowledge associated with leadership, and they remain relevant to this day. Trait theories, behavioral theories, and contingency theories offer essential foundational information concerning leadership.

2.4.1 Trait Theories of Leadership

When most anyone reflects on an individual who they consider to be a leader, they invariably will offer descriptions of the things that characterize this person. A nursing home administrator praises his system president's charisma, passion, and strategy skills. A nurse supervisor admires her director of nursing's professional appearance, self-confidence, sincerity, and work ethic. A dietary aide appreciates her department manager's motivational capabilities, speaking skills, team-building abilities, and workplace knowledge. These and similar characteristics reference traits held by the given leaders, so it makes sense that significant efforts have been and continue to be directed toward understanding leadership through the lens of one's personal characteristics, with this particular focus generating what are known as trait theories of leadership.

Trait theories of leadership postulate that one's leadership ability is predicated on that particular individual's personal characteristics or traits. They emerged during the first part of the twentieth century, endeavoring to formally explain leadership. Trait theorists specifically view that certain innate qualities, such as physical characteristics, health status, confidence, communicative abilities, and intelligence, foster leadership ability and that people possessing such qualities will be effective leaders. This view considers leaders to be born, rather than made. Trait theories have their origins in **great man theory** which surfaced from investigations of great leaders of the past. Researchers sought to determine what made these leaders great, with particular traits emerging as potential universal indicators of leadership ability. Trait theorists initially were highly motivated by the prospect of successfully identifying traits that yield leadership excellence, permitting the selection of leaders to be hastened. The thought was that if one could identify individuals possessing those traits, excellent leadership would, at least in theory, be assured [23–25].

This pursuit, however, proved to be overly ambitious, with research over time rendering these early views to be oversimplifications of the concept of leadership. Perhaps the most notable flaw of such concerned failures to take into account environmental factors and their associated influences on leader effectiveness [23, 24]. Even at face value, the notion that individuals possessing certain attributes are natural leaders was obviously problematic. Most anyone with even minimal work experience likely has encountered employees who indeed possessed leadership traits but exhibited no leadership desire or ability. And what about those situations where an employee does not possess any discernable leadership traits, yet in practice, capably leads?

Despite such setbacks, trait theory made a positive contribution to the knowledge base of leadership, and it continues to influence perspectives to this day. While the universality of trait theory did not hold up to scrutiny, it is well-known that particular traits or qualities certainly can facilitate one's ability to be an excellent leader [1, 5–9, 23]. Consider excellent communication abilities. While possessing these does not automatically endow one with leadership prowess, it clearly is a helpful skill for leaders to possess, which, in turn, can improve their leadership abilities. That said, value exists in investigating and identifying traits conducive to excellent leadership, especially when considered in tandem with prudent behaviors and contextual factors. Ultimately, personal traits and characteristics do not guarantee leadership effectiveness, but they can be an indicator of associated potential.

2.4.2 Behavioral Theories of Leadership

So if leaders are not necessarily born, can they instead be developed? That particular question motivated what became known as behavioral theories of leadership. Specifically, **behavioral theories of leadership** view the behaviors or actions of individuals to be the prevailing determinant of their leadership potential. Emerging in the 1940s, behavioral theories postulated that leaders are made; that leadership is a learned quality, not one that is merely bestowed at birth. Behavioral theorists viewed leadership to be capable of being possessed by anyone willing to learn leadership skills and abilities and deploy them, accordingly [23, 24].

Early foundational studies conducted by the University of Michigan and the Ohio State University provided indications of the influence of behaviors on leadership [23, 24], with scores of behavioral studies following these classic efforts. Notably among these quests, researchers endeavored to identify a certain array of behaviors that would evoke effective leadership universally. Such a result, however, proved to be elusive. As with early trait theory renditions, early behavioral perspectives viewed the concept of leadership too restrictively, likewise failing to factor in matters of context on, in this case, the behaviors expressed by leaders. Still, much was learned, leading to tempered perspectives which acknowledge the critical role of behaviors on leadership while not overextending their associated influence. Healthcare institutions broadly have taken note of the impact of behaviors on leadership, evidenced by scores of leadership development programs which endeavor to advance the leadership capabilities of staff members. It now is well understood that both traits and behaviors play vital roles in leadership effectiveness, but in isolation, they are not powerful enough to guarantee optimal leader performance universally [23, 24].

2.4.3 Contingency Theories of Leadership

With both trait and behavioral theories of leadership being criticized for failing to take into consideration contextual factors and their influences on leadership effectiveness, it was only natural that efforts were directed to address this weakness. Emerging in the 1960s, **contingency theories of leadership**, which are also known as **situational theories of leadership**, postulated that factors unique to each situation encountered dictate which leader traits and behaviors are necessary to realize success. Specifically, contingency theorists believed that the attributes and actions required for leadership effectiveness were contingent on the matter at hand; the particular formula for success depends on the situation. The goal is to try to determine which leadership style is optimal to use in the context of the circumstances faced. This suggests that a one-size-fits-all leadership style does not exist. Instead, one must adapt to the circumstances [23–25].

Many contingency theories have been developed. Fred Fiedler's contingency theory, a foundational effort credited with ushering in the contingency management era, viewed leadership effectiveness to be predicated on achieving a match between a leader's style and the demands of the situation at hand. Fiedler arrived at his theory by conducting studies investigating leader style and situational demands, with findings indicating that some leadership styles were better at addressing particular situations than others, essentially validating core tenets of contingency theory as it is known today [26]. In the 1970s, Robert House advanced contingency perspectives by formulating path-goal theory which emphasized adaptability as a key ingredient of leadership success. His research specifically indicated that it was imperative for a leader to adapt his or her particular style to meet the demands of the situation at hand, supplying another perspective shoring up contingency theories [27]. Similarly,

Paul Hersey and Kenneth Blanchard's situational leadership theory emphasized the need for leadership styles to be adapted to particular contexts faced, with this effort focusing special attention on the need for supervisors to understand their subordinates and select a compatible leadership style in order to optimize performance [28].

Contingency theories greatly advanced the state of leadership knowledge, complementing earlier trait and behavioral contributions by adding the all-important element of context into the leadership equation. By focusing attention on situational influences and their impact on leadership style and ultimate outcomes, contingency perspectives addressed the chief criticisms associated with trait and behavioral views [23–25]. Contingency theories, in many respects, illustrate the complexities of leadership, reminding health and medical providers that they must consider traits, behaviors, and contextual situations when addressing institutional leadership requirements. The contributions of contingency theory and its predecessors clearly advanced the knowledge base of leadership, also setting the stage for the exploration of contemporary perspectives of leadership that continue to bolster attention and understanding.

2.5 Contemporary Perspectives of Leadership

As a thriving component of organizational behavior and management, leadership continues to generate significant attention from both scholars and executives, with these efforts producing a wealth of modern perspectives. Two particularly robust efforts center on charismatic leadership and servant leadership.

2.5.1 Charismatic Leadership

Exceptional leaders frequently are described as being charismatic. Charisma—a word derived from the Greek term for "gift"—is such a notable component of leadership that a contemporary perspective centers on the topic. **Charismatic leadership** is defined as an approach to leadership expressed by a leader with highly alluring qualities, notably including great confidence and optimism, extreme devotion to the pursuit and realization of a compelling vision, enthusiastic and inspiring communication abilities, and unyielding commitment to followers. Courtesy of these "gifts," charismatic leaders are viewed to be extraordinary, walking in a different realm than their peers, garnering widespread, intensely loyal followership. Their notable qualities permit charismatic leaders to be extremely effective influencers. In fact, they can be so inspiring that they invoke blind faith in their followers. This can prove to be good or bad, depending on the character of the leader in question, but assuming proper mindsets, such devotion certainly can prove beneficial for accomplishing missions [5, 6, 14, 29–33].

While charisma is often viewed as a trait bestowed upon one at birth, opportunities to develop charismatic leadership skills are possible even for those who are not naturally charismatic [5]. At least some of the common traits ascribed to charismatic leaders lend themselves well to being taught. Excellent communication abilities, a hallmark of the charismatic, certainly can be developed in most anyone via managerial communication training programs. Individuals also can be encouraged to actively show their passion for the mission, vision, and values of their given organizations, demonstrating enthusiasm which can generate excitement throughout the ranks. Development opportunities indeed are possible.

Charismatic leadership has received significant attention in the literature, evidenced by the availability of scores of books and articles focused on the topic. Many of these works are descriptive, supplying detailed accounts of individuals viewed to be charismatic leaders. Studies exploring the meaning and impact of charismatic leadership, however, are relatively rare, limiting the availability of findings revealing the capabilities and contributions of this leadership style [6]. Anecdotal evidence, however, supports the notion that charismatic leadership positively impacts organizations [6, 14]. Given the apparent benefits of charismatic leadership, health and medical organizations certainly should consider seeking charismatic leaders in their recruitment efforts and developing associated qualities within managerial ranks.

2.5.2 Servant Leadership

A contemporary leadership perspective known as **servant leadership** should be particularly appealing to those serving in health and medicine, given its unique view and treatment of the role of leadership. Specifically, those who embrace this philosophy express a kind of servitude toward others, routinely sacrificing their own privileges and conveniences for the benefit of those they willfully have decided to place before themselves, with the most notable party being their subordinates. Essentially, servant leadership emphasizes that leaders are to serve their followers, with this contrasting sharply with traditional views which stress the reverse. Those who practice servant leadership are well-known to their subordinates and easily identifiable by virtually anyone, courtesy of their overtly compassionate expressions and actions [14, 31, 34–36].

Consider the following examples of servant leadership: a patient accounts manager offers to work the weekend shift for an admissions clerk to permit her to spend time with a sick child, a nurse supervisor asks for feedback from his staff nurses before making a decision about a new scheduling method, a medical clinic administrator takes the time to get to know her subordinates' career aspirations so she can help develop them as employees, a housekeeping supervisor brings donuts to work each week as an expression of gratitude for the work his housekeepers have done over prior days, and a dietary manager works right alongside her cooks in the kitchen as they collectively prepare meals for patients and hospital staff members. In each of these cases, the noted leaders are engaging in activities that technically fall outside of their formally assigned duties and responsibilities. Operations would continue even without extending such gestures, yet they decided to make enhanced investments in their subordinates out of care and concern for these employees. Such expressions of service to others are quite fitting in healthcare establishments, with servant leadership philosophically paralleling the missions of many health and medical organizations. It arguably is the most compassionate approach to leadership possible.

2.6 Establishing Leadership Development Programs

As leadership excellence requires a commitment to lifelong learning, organizations must provide opportunities for workforce development [1, 7, 8, 37–39]. Many choose to establish formal **leadership development programs**, educational offerings designed to advance the leadership skills and abilities of individuals, informing and enlightening them on myriad facets of leadership which they then apply in their work lives. These programs often are managed by human resource departments as part of their greater workforce development initiatives, although placement can be elsewhere, such as in an office dedicated to leadership development. Assembly of these programs is not terribly complex, but it does require significant thought and reflection. The following six-step process provides a helpful framework for realizing a leadership development program in health and medical environments.

2.6.1 Step 1: Secure Foundational Assets Necessary for the Successful Operation of the Leadership Development Program

A leadership development program requires foundational assets similar to those required by most any significant organizational undertaking. These resources include (1) top leadership support and commitment, (2) financial resources sufficient for funding the initiative, and (3) competent employees charged with managing the operation. As the viability of leadership development endeavors largely depends on the availability and adequacy of foundational assets, healthcare organizations must take steps to secure these resources prior to initiating program development.

2.6.2   Step 2: Determine the Subject Matter to be Featured in the Leadership Development Program

With sufficient foundational assets in hand, healthcare providers next determine the subject matter to be featured. Specifically, healthcare organizations must identify the precise leadership qualities which are expected of managers. This knowledge can then be used to develop applicable learning opportunities. Arriving at such information requires a thorough needs assessment. Interviews with senior executives, for example, can be most helpful in determining learning priorities as these individuals are best positioned to understand institutional leadership requirements. Surveys which ask managers to provide self-assessments of their leadership skills and inquire about leadership topics of interest also offer opportunities for determining subject matter. Additionally, trending leadership topics can be explored in trade and scholarly journals, books, and other publications, revealing critical areas of focus for inclusion in the program. The curricula of leadership degrees offered by colleges and universities, too, can be explored for insights on key topics to be featured. And certainly, when and where possible, one should examine leadership development programs offered by other institutions, both within and outside of the healthcare industry, for associated insights. By the conclusion of this step, healthcare providers should possess a firm understanding of the subject matter to be featured in associated leadership development programs.

2.6.3   Step 3: Determine the Methods which Will be Used to Deliver Leadership Development Training

With an understanding of the subject matter to be featured, healthcare organizations next concentrate attention on determining the particular delivery methods which will be used to convey leadership knowledge. Common delivery methods include special discussions about leadership during employee orientation and onboarding sessions, workshops dedicated to one or more aspects of leadership, mentorships between senior and junior managers which permit an ongoing leadership development dialogue, formal retreats designed to build leadership skills, certificate programs offered by leadership institutes, and formal courses and degree programs in leadership and related areas offered by colleges and universities. Options abound, and it is up to given healthcare organizations to make selections prudent for institutional and individual advancement.

2.6.4   Step 4: Determine Program Placement, Responsible Parties, and Related Matters of Organization Design

With subject matter and methods of delivery determined, healthcare institutions next must focus on matters of organization design, notably including the manner in which the leadership development program is structured (i.e., its placement within the organization) and the departments and personnel responsible for program oversight and management. Will the program be managed by a single department or will components be distributed across two or more units? If more than one department will manage the program, how will the units interact with one another to ensure successful program delivery? Which individuals within designated units will be responsible for program operations? Such determinations are situation-dependent, based on the capabilities and preferences of given healthcare organizations.

2.6.5   Step 5: Organize Leadership Development Opportunities and Prepare an Academic Calendar

In similar fashion to that of a college or university organizing and scheduling activities and events for the coming term, healthcare organizations must organize and schedule their leadership development initiatives, placing them on an academic calendar, accordingly. This is an essential activity as many leadership development programs draw together wide varieties of learning opportunities, both internal and external, necessitating careful coordination. An academic calendar permits those responsible for educational planning to easily view the placement of various learning opportunities. This is most helpful for ensuring a conflict-free schedule and also aids in distributing opportunities evenly over time. The period of time covered by academic calendars is dependent on the preferences of given healthcare organizations. Once finalized, academic calendars can be used to convey learning opportunities to personnel.

2.6.6   Step 6: Operationalize the Leadership Development Program

Having completed the prior developmental steps, healthcare institutions have in their possession a leadership development program framework ready for implementation. At this point, operationalization simply involves launching the framework, bringing the leadership development program to life. Once launched, as with any operational endeavor, leadership development programs should periodically be reviewed to determine if they are meeting their intended goals and objectives, with revisions being initiated when and where needed. Attentiveness to this quality control measure sets the stage for leadership development programs to continually engage and inspire, guiding managers down pathways that will see them emerge and advance as leaders.

WK Reflections: The Role Model as a Leadership Development Tool

One often overlooked leadership development tool is passive in that it is not a purposely designed educational method but possesses all of the potential of the best active solutions traditionally housed within leadership development programs. That particular tool centers on the workplace presence of leadership role models, those managers who are maximizing their potential by exemplifying leadership excellence. These individuals serve as perfect candidates for emulation, exposing subordinates and others in given healthcare institutions to talented leaders, hastening leadership skills development and enhancing succession planning efforts. Willis Knighton Health has observed that the mere presence and operation of leadership role models in work environments plays a significant role in conveying to subordinates desired skills and abilities that are necessary to assume greater responsibility within the health system. Unlike overt leadership development methods, such as coaching, mentorships, seminars, and the like, this is a passive mechanism, requiring little to no effort on the part of healthcare organizations, with the exception of ensuring that managerial roles indeed are filled by competent leaders. Candidates for managerial roles must be scrutinized heavily to ensure that they possess the requisite leadership qualities. Proper vetting will produce a steady stream of leadership-oriented managers, capable of influencing others within their given healthcare organizations, prompting many to mirror their words and actions, with this impacting and enhancing leadership development efforts.

2.7 Summary and Conclusions

Leadership is a multifaceted, often misunderstood, vital concept, with its mastery being essential in order to achieve the best administrative and clinical outcomes in health and medicine. Due to its overarching influence on virtually every aspect of operation, healthcare providers must dedicate significant efforts toward acquiring, developing, and advancing leadership prowess within their respective institutions. Indeed, in the highly competitive, ever-changing healthcare industry, management prowess alone is insufficient; it must be complemented by leadership skills and abilities which amplify efforts and outcomes. By directing devoted attention toward leadership, health and medical providers set the stage for operational excellence, ultimately hastening mission fulfillment.

Key Terms

- Behavioral Theories of Leadership
- Charismatic Leadership
- Colleague
- Collegiality
- Commitment
- Communication
- Competence
- Contingency Theories of Leadership
- Empathy
- Follower
- Generosity
- Great Man Theory
- Honesty
- Humility
- Leader
- Leadership
- Leadership Development Program
- Management
- Mentee
- Mentor
- Mentoring
- Passion
- Personal Power
- Position Power
- Servant Leadership
- Situational Theories of Leadership
- Skill
- Trait Theories of Leadership
- Vision

Exercises

1. In your own words, define the concept of leadership and discuss its critical role in achieving operational excellence in health and medicine.
2. Prepare a brief narrative distinguishing leadership from management. Why do you believe the two terms often and incorrectly are used interchangeably?
3. Select an individual you personally know who you view to exemplify leadership excellence. Prepare a brief narrative describing this person, noting his or her leadership qualities and associated leadership style. How has this individual impacted your own leadership style?

4. Demonstrate your understanding of trait theories of leadership by performing a self-assessment, identifying leadership traits which you believe you possess. What evidence do you have to support your claims?
5. Based on your understanding of charismatic leadership, identify and describe an individual you personally know who you believe exhibits charisma. How would you rank this person's leadership performance? Why?
6. In your own words, define servant leadership, and discuss why this perspective is very fitting in health and medical organizations.
7. Think deeply about the various methods which healthcare organizations can use to deliver leadership development training. Identify at least five methods which you believe to be best suited for inclusion in a healthcare establishment's leadership development program. Be sure to justify your selections.
8. Investigate the leadership development opportunities provided by your current employer. Prepare a brief narrative detailing your findings and associated perspectives.

References

1. Elrod, J. K. (2013). *Breadcrumbs to cheesecake*. R&R Publishers.
2. Shi, L., & Singh, D. A. (2023). *Essentials of the US health care system* (6th ed.). Jones and Bartlett.
3. McConnell, C. R. (2020). *Hospitals and health systems: What they are and how they work*. Jones and Bartlett.
4. Flynn, W. J., Valentine, S. R., & Meglich, P. A. (2022). *Healthcare human resource management* (4th ed.). Cengage.
5. Robbins, S. P., & Judge, T. A. (2019). *Organizational behavior* (18th ed.). Pearson.
6. Griffin, R. W., Phillips, J. M., & Gully, S. M. (2020). *Organizational behavior: Managing people and organizations* (13th ed.). Cengage.
7. Northouse, P. G. (2022). *Leadership: Theory and practice* (9th ed.). Sage.
8. Bass, B. M. (2008). *The Bass handbook of leadership: Theory, research, and managerial applications* (4th ed.). The Free Press.
9. Kotter, J. P. (1990). *A force for change: How leadership differs from management*. The Free Press.
10. Kotter, J. P. (2001). What leaders really do. *Harvard Business Review, 79*(11), 85–97.
11. Heifetz, R. A., & Laurie, D. L. (2001). The work of leadership. *Harvard Business Review, 79*(11), 131–141.
12. Bennis, W., & Nanus, B. (2007). *Leaders: Strategies for taking charge* (2nd ed.). HarperBusiness.
13. McShane, S. L., & Von Glinow, M. A. (2019). *Organizational behavior* (4th ed.). McGraw-Hill.
14. Hitt, M. A., Miller, C. C., Colella, A., & Triana, M. D. C. (2018). *Organizational behavior* (5th ed.). Wiley.
15. Konopaske, R., Ivancevich, J. M., & Matteson, M. T. (2018). *Organizational behavior and management* (11th ed.). McGraw-Hill.
16. Burns, J. M. (1978). *Leadership*. Harper and Row.
17. Gulick, L. (2016). Notes on the theory of organization. In J. M. Shafritz, J. S. Ott, & Y. S. Jang (Eds.), *Classics of organization theory* (8th ed., pp. 84–92). Cengage.
18. Leonard, E. C., Jr., & Trusty, K. A. (2016). *Supervision: Concepts and practices of management* (13th ed.). Cengage.

19. Certo, S. C. (2019). *Supervision: Concepts and skill-building* (10th ed.). McGraw-Hill.
20. Griffin, R. W. (2022). *Management* (13th ed.). Cengage.
21. Kinicki, A., & Soignet, D. B. (2022). *Management: A practical introduction* (10th ed.). McGraw-Hill.
22. Goleman, D. (2001). *Harvard Business Review on what makes a leader.* Harvard Business School Publishing.
23. Schermerhorn, J. R., Jr., Hunt, J. G., & Osborn, R. N. (1998). *Basic organizational behavior* (2nd ed.). Wiley.
24. Barnett, T. (2000). Leadership. In M. M. Helms (Ed.), *Encyclopedia of management* (4th ed., pp. 490–495). Gale Group.
25. Handy, C. (1999). *Understanding organizations.* Penguin.
26. Fiedler, F. E. (1967). *A theory of leadership effectiveness.* McGraw-Hill.
27. House, R. J. (1971). A path goal theory of leader effectiveness. *Administrative Science, 16*(3), 321–339.
28. Hersey, P., & Blanchard, K. H. (1988). *Management of organizational behavior.* Prentice Hall.
29. Murray, K. (2020). *Charismatic leadership: The skills you can learn to motivate high performance in others.* Kogan Page.
30. Conger, J. A. (1991). *The charismatic leader: Behind the mystique of exceptional leadership.* Jossey-Bass.
31. Lussier, R. N., & Achua, C. F. (2022). *Leadership: Theory, application, and skill development* (7th ed.). Sage.
32. Hansen, S. D., Miller, D. R., & Noack, D. (2020). The impact of charismatic leadership on recruitment, development and firm performance. *Journal of Managerial Issues, 32*(2), 215–229.
33. Conger, J. A., & Kanungo, R. N. (1987). Toward a behavioral theory of charismatic leadership in organizational settings. *Academy of Management Review, 12*, 637–647.
34. Greenleaf, R. K. (1977). *Servant leadership: A journey into the nature of legitimate power and greatness.* Paulist Press.
35. Eva, N., Robin, M., Sendjaya, S., Van Dierendonck, D., & Liden, R. C. (2019). Servant leadership: A systematic review and call for future research. *The Leadership Quarterly, 30*(1), 111–132.
36. Chiniara, M., & Bentein, K. (2018). The servant leadership advantage: When perceiving low differentiation in leader-member relationship quality influences team cohesion, team task performance and service OCB. *The Leadership Quarterly, 29*(2), 333–345.
37. Peters, T. J., & Waterman, R. H., Jr. (2006). *In search of excellence: Lessons from America's best-run companies.* HarperBusiness.
38. Collins, J. (2001). *Good to great: Why some companies make the leap and others don't.* HarperCollins.
39. Tichy, N. M. (2007). *The leadership engine: How winning companies build leaders at every level.* HarperCollins.

Chapter 3
Motivation in Health and Medicine

Learning Objectives

After examining this chapter, readers will have the ability to:

- Understand the concept of motivation and its essential role in encouraging health and medical personnel to deliver their very best.
- Distinguish intrinsic motivation from extrinsic motivation.
- Understand the impact of workplace stress and employee burnout on motivation.
- Identify common methods used by health and medical establishments to motivate their employees.
- Define and discuss content and process theories of motivation, identify examples of each, and explain their impact on the knowledge base of motivation.
- Appreciate the value of motivation frameworks and understand techniques for their assembly and implementation in health and medicine.
- Recognize the utility of motivation audits and understand methods for conducting them in healthcare organizations.

WK Reflections: Motivators as Tools for Capturing Competitive Advantages

Of the many topics of motivation discussed over the pages of this chapter, one which undoubtedly will draw significant interest and attention concerns the selection of **motivators**, those tools, techniques, and incentives which are deployed by organizations to compel employees to action. These are important over the entire lifecycle of employment, including also recruitment. Things such as salary, benefits, working conditions, leadership quality, and more dictate whether one will be prompted to pursue given courses of action set forth by an organization (e.g., accept a job offer, agree to work a weekend

J. K. Elrod, J. L. Fortenberry, Jr., *Organizational Behavior and Management in Health and Medicine*, https://doi.org/10.1007/978-3-031-61823-9_3

shift, volunteer for a challenging project, give their very best in their work). Selection of these mechanisms, a process described in detail later in the chapter, is vital as a motivated healthcare workforce is mandatory for delivering excellent patient care and achieving institutional prosperity. In this pursuit, creative thinking, in particular, is encouraged, as motivators, if well devised, can lead to competitive advantages. Indeed, if unique motivators can be identified which distinguish a healthcare institution from its competitors, the stage is set for capturing advantages across the spectrum of operations.

Consider the following example from Willis Knighton Health. As the leading healthcare enterprise in its region of operation, Willis Knighton Health prides itself in offering an exceptional series of motivators which have proved over time to be very effective. Some motivators are highly unique, with perhaps the best example of this being its defined-benefit pension plan. Once a common benefit in large, nongovernmental establishments, traditional pensions have largely given way to defined-contribution plans (e.g., 401K programs, 403B programs) which are less costly for organizations to operate. Such programs, however, do not deliver the reliability of income afforded by traditional pensions, with this compelling Willis Knighton Health to retain its defined-benefit pension plan even as its nongovernmental peers dropped them. In the case of this motivator, its uniqueness emerged as traditional pensions fell out of favor due to corporate desires to cut costs. While such pensions continue to be available in government organizations, they are now a rarity in nongovernmental ones, providing Willis Knighton Health with a unique and powerful motivator that helps to drive everything from recruitment to retention.

This example illustrates the benefits that can be afforded by journeying off the beaten path, fielding unique motivators capable of encouraging individuals, bolstering their resolve to join and remain productive members of given organizations. Like no other component, motivators bring the concept of motivation to life. Readers are encouraged to reflect on motivators as they examine the chapter's content, being sure to also consider "outside of the box" ideas that can generate significant interest and attention on the part of prospective and current employees, motivating them, accordingly. Intensive efforts directed toward building a viable pool of motivators, including at least some that are unique, almost certainly will afford competitive advantages and pay significant dividends. Associated tools and techniques and much more await over the pages that follow.

3.1 Background

The range of occupations required by health and medical institutions to deliver patient care is epic. In simple and complex healthcare establishments alike, the immense variety of disciplines represented within sole institutions is readily apparent, even on cursory examination. The most obvious and well-known pursuits are those tied directly to the delivery of care, but scores of not-so-obvious, less publicized pursuits complement the more visible roles of health and medicine, serving as vital contributors to the end product of patient care. Linkages between and among departments and the personnel within them must be seamless in order to deliver the best patient experiences possible. As the delivery of care occurs via a complex chain of diverse activities and actions, breakdowns in even a single area can be detrimental and possibly even life-threatening [1–5]. This obviously requires each and every individual to be qualified for assigned roles and ready to serve, but it also requires significant work on the part of institutions to ensure that staff members are inspired to perform optimally at all times [1, 3, 6]. In essence, health and medical providers must make certain that their employees are motivated.

It must be remembered that in addition to the complex logistics of the industry, in modern healthcare establishments, demands are rigorous and challenging, obligations are significant and ever-increasing, staffing shortages are very common, and shifts can be lengthy and tiring, diminishing the mettle and morale of even the most dedicated staff members. This can especially reflect negatively on patients and their perceptions of quality care, given their extensive exposure to healthcare personnel. Unmotivated, uninspired healthcare workers erode patient confidence in services rendered, potentially detrimentally impacting operations and even institutional viability [1, 7–10]. As such, healthcare providers must devote significant time and attention toward the concept of motivation, understanding its foundations and applications in order to generate sustained levels of inspiration across the entire workforce. This particular chapter sheds light on this important topic.

3.2 Defining Motivation

Formally defined, **motivation** refers to a state whereby an individual is compelled to pursue a goal or objective to satisfy a particular **want** (i.e., something desired) or **need** (i.e., something required; a necessity) [10]. The term is derived from the Latin word *movere* which means "to move" [11]. An individual described as being motivated essentially has identified something that he or she wishes to gain or possess and has decided to move toward its acquisition. A motivated individual would be said to be in an active, as opposed to a passive or dormant state, directing energies aimed at fulfillment [12]. A nurse desirous of a promotion might decide to work extra shifts, earn a specialized certification, or take similar actions in an effort to increase her chances of being promoted. A physician who wishes to better understand management practices within his healthcare establishment might decide to pursue an MBA or MHA degree in order to build associated knowledge. A compensation manager who desires additional opportunities to interact with others might decide to volunteer to serve on particular committees or task forces. A housekeeper who desires extra pay might decide to work premium-paying, weekend or evening shifts in order to increase his compensation. Objects of desire are vast, and their attractiveness is dependent on the individual and his or her particular circumstances. What motivates one may or may not motivate another [13].

Motivation, in and of itself, is not a directly observable characteristic. It, instead, is inferred from one's actions, that is, the stream of behaviors taken by an individual as he or she pursues an identified goal or objective in hopes of satisfying a given want or need. The primary effect of motivation is on behavior. Far from being a fixed attribute within an individual, motivation is a dynamic, variable state that is impacted by the interplay between the individual and various environmental factors [14]. Something that motivates an individual today might not do so tomorrow. For example, a nurse whose car breaks down and is in need of money for the repair might be motivated to work extra shifts until the repair costs are covered, but not have any desire to do so afterward.

Motivation is an essential attribute for individuals to possess across all areas of life. Without ambition, drive, willingness, and action, even the most routine of personal duties and responsibilities could never be accomplished, let alone complex work assignments. In the workplace, employers expect their staff members to be motivated. They have been hired to deliver value and must do so in order to maintain their employment and advance within the ranks. By accepting compensation, they have obligated themselves to deliver results. As such, employees bear responsibility for their own motivation to accomplish designated goals and objectives put forth by their employers. But employees are not alone in this. Organizations, too, bear responsibility for motivating those in their employ. The very best institutions, in fact, dedicate significant efforts toward ensuring a motivated workforce.

While proper compensation is perhaps the first thing that comes to mind in shoring up motivation, options far beyond wages and salaries abound. Other forms of motivation frequently used by healthcare organizations to inspire workers include health insurance plans, retirement plans, employee appreciation programs, comfortable working environments, engaging work assignments, access to the latest technologies, excellent and inspirational leadership, collegial atmospheres, educational advancement opportunities, and much more. While assembling motivational opportunities (i.e., motivators) can be costly, if selections are well devised and implemented, associated expenditures can be considered investments. An inspired, enthusiastic labor force is one of the greatest assets that can be held by a healthcare organization [1, 11–13].

Research suggests that a motivated workforce delivers high levels of productivity, exhibits a strong commitment to employers, provides excellent customer service, fosters teamwork between and among staff members, and realizes high levels of employee satisfaction, with these characteristics being essential in order for establishments to excel [13–18]. Given this, healthcare providers must bolster their understanding of motivation and ensure that motivational tools, techniques, and incentives are deployed robustly and properly, permitting given institutions to realize an inspired, enthusiastic workforce and its many benefits.

3.3 Intrinsic Versus Extrinsic Motivation

Motivation is sometimes described as being intrinsic or extrinsic. **Intrinsic motivation** emerges from internal, personal influences. An LPN who personally desires to become an RN and takes steps to enter an LPN-to-RN training program to realize this goal would be considered to be intrinsically motivated. So too would an individual working outside of the healthcare industry who desires contributing to the noble cause of delivering patient care and decides to seek employment at a local hospital. Intrinsic motivation essentially is fueled by inspiration from within, as opposed to being prompted by outside forces [11, 12]. **Extrinsic motivation** emerges from external influences, such as a productivity bonus put forth by an employer which compels an employee to take a particular action in order to achieve the given incentive. Similarly, a compelling leader or even a personal friend who encourages an individual to seek a promotion would constitute a form of extrinsic motivation. In these and similar cases, the inspiration emerges from outside forces which, in turn, motivate others to take action [11, 12].

It is important for healthcare organizations to acknowledge and understand these two sources of motivation. Regardless of the origin of motivation, managers have the potential to offer associated support. This is very obvious in the case of extrinsic motivation as healthcare organizations routinely devise mechanisms to motivate staff members, with these being used by managers to encourage action. As for intrinsic motivation, opportunities for managerial influence are more limited, but remain, resting with the provision of support to help dedicated employees achieve their aspirations. Assume, for example, that a housekeeping director learns that a particular employee desires moving into a supervisory role. To reinforce the intrinsic motivation compelling the housekeeper, the director could choose to add sources of extrinsic motivation. He could recommend the housekeeper for a managerial training program, encourage his enrollment in college coursework on the topic of supervision, forward challenging assignments to build his skills, and so on, creating intrinsic and extrinsic motivation synergies. Doing so quite obviously requires managers to work diligently to acquire an understanding of their subordinates. With such knowledge, skilled managers can work to identify and devise plans that benefit staff members and organizations alike.

3.4   Content Theories of Motivation

Given the importance of motivation, researchers have long sought to understand its impact and influence on institutional performance. Starting in the 1940s, especially intensive attention began being directed toward understating the concept, with this period seeing the introduction of what are known as content theories of motivation. Focusing attention on human needs, **content theories of motivation** specifically investigate and seek to explain internal desires within individuals and the impact of those particular desires on behavior. Also known as **needs-based theories** [19] or simply **needs theories** [20], content theories shed light on motivation from the perspective of the person. Four of the most popular content theories are Maslow's hierarchy of needs theory, Alderfer's ERG theory, Herzberg's two-factor theory, and McClelland's acquired needs theory. Brief overviews of these content theories are provided as follows.

3.4.1   Maslow's Hierarchy of Needs Theory

In the 1940s, Abraham Maslow made an important contribution to the study of motivation by introducing **hierarchy of needs theory**. This theory postulates that all human needs can be grouped into one of five hierarchical categories: physiological, safety, social, esteem, and self-actualization. Physiological needs are situated at the base of the hierarchy and entail the most basic of human needs required for survival, including air, food, and water. Safety needs occupy the next hierarchical level, with this particular category centering on human needs for security and protection. Social needs follow, with this level involving human needs for love, friendship, affiliation, and acceptance. Esteem needs are next, entailing human needs for pride, prestige, attention, and recognition. Self-actualization needs are situated at the top of the hierarchy and represent the most advanced category, centering on human needs for personal growth and fulfillment [21].

Maslow theorized that needs at one level will not motivate an individual until needs at the preceding level are satisfied. In essence, physiological needs must be satisfied before safety needs will become motivators, safety needs must be satisfied before social needs will become motivators, and so on up through the hierarchy. This pattern was viewed to generally hold, although Maslow acknowledged that variations are possible. Maslow's research suggests that institutions must ensure that they adequately address lower-level needs in order for higher-level needs to motivate employees. Employees must, for example, be compensated adequately, be provided safe environments in which to work, and possess job security before they will be motivated by challenging work assignments, increased duties and responsibilities, enhanced prestige, and the like [19–21]. This theory supplied important details for consideration when structuring motivational opportunities in organizations. Now decades old, Maslow's hierarchy of needs theory continues to influence motivational arrays to this day.

3.4.2 Alderfer's ERG Theory

In the late 1960s and early 1970s, Clayton Alderfer introduced **ERG theory**, a theory of motivation which contained three levels: existence (i.e., human needs for physiological and material well-being), relatedness (i.e., human needs for satisfying interpersonal relationships), and growth (i.e., human needs for personal development). This framework essentially condenses Maslow's five components into three, with Alderfer's existence needs paralleling Maslow's physiological and safety needs, relatedness needs paralleling Maslow's social and esteem needs, and growth needs paralleling Maslow's self-actualization needs. ERG theory, however, operates quite differently than hierarchy of needs theory in that it does not presume that lower-level needs must be fully satisfied before higher-level needs become motivating. Needs from any of the three categories can prove motivating at any time. In employment contexts, per ERG theory, institutions should focus on providing employees with opportunities across all three needs categories, allowing them to gravitate toward those avenues which they personally view to be motivating at the given time [20, 22, 23].

3.4.3 Herzberg's Two-Factor Theory

Frederick Herzberg's introduction of **two-factor theory** in the late 1950s and early 1960s further bolstered foundations of motivation, ushering in a somewhat different perspective. According to two-factor theory, a particular pair of variables—motivators and hygiene factors—have performance implications for workers and ultimately determine one's level of motivation. As such, two-factor theory is also referred to as **motivator-hygiene theory**. Motivators include status, recognition, challenging work assignments, involvement in workplace decisions, autonomy, and similar things that lead to job enrichment. These closely parallel higher-level needs in the motivation theories offered by Maslow and Alderfer. *(Note that Herzberg's definition of motivators differs from the more general one provided earlier in the chapter which better reflects common usage of the term.)* Hygiene factors include things such as fair compensation and benefits, job security, safe working conditions, and the like. They were termed hygiene factors because Herzberg viewed such factors to address the maintenance needs of employees. They are very similar to lower-level needs in the typologies offered by Maslow and Alderfer [19, 20, 24, 25].

According to two-factor theory, hygiene factors must be present, as without them, worker dissatisfaction will result. They are not, in and of themselves, motivating. Essentially, through their provision, a neutral state—not dissatisfied and not satisfied—is obtained. In order to reach a satisfied state, a different set of factors—motivators—must also be provided. If offered, employees then can achieve states of satisfaction, permitting them to serve in an inspired manner. In essence, institutions must ensure the presence of hygiene factors so that employees are not dissatisfied, supplementing these with motivators to bring employees to states of satisfaction so that they perform to the best of their abilities [19, 20, 24, 25].

3.4.4 McClelland's Acquired Needs Theory

In the early 1960s, David McClelland introduced **acquired needs theory**. This particular perspective emerged from motivation research which identified three important human needs: the need for achievement (nAch), the need for affiliation (nAff), and the need for power (nPower). McClelland viewed these needs not to be inherent but instead learned over time, based on one's life experiences. The need for achievement involves desires to perform well and resolve any problems encountered, the need for affiliation involves desires for forming personal relationships, and the need for power involves desires to oversee and influence others [19, 20, 26, 27].

McClelland urged managers to learn about the particular needs of their given subordinates and strive to structure work in a manner that leads to the fulfillment of those needs, as doing so will prove to be motivating. For example, an employee with a high need for achievement might desire work involving individual goals and significant performance feedback, an employee with a high need for affiliation might desire team assignments featuring robust interactions with others, and an employee with a high need for power might desire assignments permitting opportunities to supervise others and gain recognition [19, 20, 26, 27]. This perspective notably directed attention toward the motivational possibilities of adopting a tailored approach in pairing individuals with their work, supplying yet another important content theory.

3.5 Process Theories of Motivation

Focusing on human reasoning, **process theories** consider motivation to be the result of conscious decision processes. They also are termed **cognitive theories** of motivation, as they explore the thought processes of individuals as they relate to desire and other aspects of motivation [19]. Whereas content theories ask the "what" questions of motivation, process theories ask the "why" and "how" questions [20]. Three prominent process theories are Vroom's expectancy theory, Adams' equity theory, and Locke's goal-setting theory. Concise profiles of each of these theories are provided below.

3.5.1 Vroom's Expectancy Theory

Introduced by Victor Vroom in the 1960s, **expectancy theory** postulates that one's motivation to engage in a particular pursuit is based on an assessment of three factors—expectancy, instrumentality, and valence—with motivation being the product of this trio. Expectancy concerns the potential for success. It is assessed by asking, "If I exert the effort to achieve a particular goal, is success expected?" Instrumentality concerns the prospects of being rewarded. It is evaluated by asking, "If I achieve the goal, will I receive a reward?" Valence concerns the desirability of the reward. It is assessed by asking, "Is there value to me personally in the anticipated reward?" A "no" answer effectively results in the given factor receiving a score of zero. Mathematically, as motivation is the product of the three noted factors, if any single factor scores a zero, motivation also will be zero (i.e., the person will not be motivated) [13, 14, 20, 28].

Expectancy theory shed significant light on the multidimensionality of motivation, courtesy of its multifactor framework. This portrayal readily conveys that motivation requires more than simply presenting an enticement before those one seeks to motivate and expecting immediate and automatic inspiration. Instead, institutions must reflect on the thought processes underlying motivation as they craft associated opportunities, envisioning how employees might answer the three operative questions of expectancy, instrumentality, and valence as they assess given goals. Such role-playing efforts can help to increase answers of "yes" across the three factors of expectancy theory and greatly improve the impact of resulting motivational avenues [13, 14, 20, 28].

3.5.2 Adams' Equity Theory

Offered by J. Stacy Adams in the 1960s, **equity theory** focuses on the concept of fairness and comparisons of equity in work environments. According to this theory, fairness is desired by employees and, when realized, it brings out their very best. Employees essentially want to see a balance between their given inputs (e.g., skills and abilities, dedication, productivity) and outputs (e.g., salary, benefits, recognition). This particular outcome is viewed as being a fair and equitable result for work performed. But comparisons do not end there. Employees also want to see their work rewarded equivalently to that of their peers. If one believes that a peer is receiving greater rewards for delivering comparable work, a state of inequity will emerge. This, in turn, compels efforts to resolve the unfair treatment. Possible actions might include reducing work output to match diminished rewards, requesting that the inequity be eliminated by demanding a pay increase or similar remedy, or bringing employment to a conclusion through resignation. Quite obviously, feelings of unfair treatment can redirect employee energies from the work at hand to their own frustrations, impacting performance [19, 29, 30].

Through Adams' contribution, employers are reminded that states of inequity have consequences which influence motivation. In particular, equity theory encourages employers to think about the rewards issued to employees, ensuring that they match associated contributions, maintaining proper balance. It also directs attention toward ensuring equitable treatment between and among employees. If this is done, the stage is set for staff members to view treatment on both individual and group levels to be equitable. It must be remembered, though, that states of inequity often are based on employee perceptions which may or may not equate with reality. To avoid unjustified claims of inequity, institutions might consider disclosures, when and where possible, which reveal and justify decisions to ensure that they are correctly perceived. For example, if several employees work in equivalent capacities and do comparable work but one edges out the others in terms of productivity and is granted a promotion, the institution could announce the person's achievement to the work group, along with associated justifications, diminishing circulation of false narratives. Such proactivity aids in transparency and fosters notions of fairness in the workplace, helping to ensure that employees maintain productive mindsets and behaviors [19, 29, 30].

3.5.3   Locke's Goal-Setting Theory

In the late 1960s, Edwin Locke added to process theories of motivation by offering **goal-setting theory**. Through his research, Locke discovered that challenging goals proved to be more motivating than easy goals. The associated challenges had to be demanding, but not too demanding. Goals essentially had to be attainable yet require concerted effort in order for success to be realized. He viewed the motivating effects of such to stem from the fact that the accomplishment of challenging goals necessitated genuine, personal determination and exertion, carrying a greater sense of fulfillment than that possible by accomplishing an easy goal which could have been achieved without hardship by virtually anyone [19, 31–33].

Locke's work greatly informed methods for structuring goals in the workplace, aiding institutions in ensuring that opportunities prove to be motivating. He further bolstered associated knowledge by identifying five goal-setting principles which foster achievement, namely, clarity (i.e., ensuring that the goal is properly described with desired outcomes being clearly understood), challenge (i.e., ensuring that the goal requires exertion to achieve, yet remains in the realm of attainability), commitment (i.e., ensuring that the individual tasked with accomplishing the goal is dedicated to its achievement), feedback (i.e., ensuring that a supportive dialogue is provided as goals are being pursued), and task complexity (i.e., ensuring that the tasks required for completion are reasonable and not overly burdensome) [19, 31–33]. These insights bolstered the body of knowledge of motivation.

3.6   Developing a Motivation Framework

When viewing motivation theories collectively, a pattern emerges dictating steps that healthcare organizations can take to foster a motivated workforce. Specifically, these efforts reveal that in order to motivate employees, one first must understand those employees. And when one comes to understand those employees, it is quickly realized that what motivates one will not necessarily motivate another. Given this workforce characteristic, healthcare establishments must make available to managers a range of motivational tools, techniques, and incentives (i.e., motivators as defined in the general sense) permitting them sufficient options to inspire employees both individually and collectively.

The motivational tools, techniques, and incentives provided by healthcare organizations typically emerge in somewhat of a haphazard fashion, originating from different sources institutionally. Human resource departments supply some things, administrative and clinical departments others, corporate offices still others, and so on, forming a patchwork quilt that is difficult to examine or communicate conveniently and comprehensively. This weakness can be turned into a strength by the assembly of a comprehensive list of the motivators which are available to managers for use within a given institution. This list, termed a **motivation framework**, presents all methods used by an organization to foster employee motivation. Importantly, it allows healthcare providers to view all motivators in a single presentation, permitting convenient reflection, evaluation, and, when necessary, revision of associated methods. Preparation also aids in ensuring that healthcare providers think broadly and creatively about motivation, compelling them to address options that are often overlooked when only patchwork attention is extended. A four-step assembly process is required for developing these frameworks.

3.6.1 Step 1: Craft a Series of Motivator Categories

Formulating a motivation framework begins by stipulating several broad motivator categories. Selection of categories is dependent on the preferences of given organizations, but the following categorization, with example motivators, represents an excellent typology: compensation (e.g., wages and salaries), benefits (e.g., health insurance, retirement, vacation, sick leave, tuition reimbursement, and related offerings), incentives and encouragements (e.g., reward systems, employee appreciation programs, celebratory events, special recognitions), environments (e.g., aesthetics, working conditions, technologies, employee parking, security), oversight and development (e.g., quality of leadership, mentorship opportunities, job design, general and specialized training, input and feedback opportunities), and community (e.g., teamwork opportunities, collegiality, respect, compliance). Reflecting on these broad categories and the general examples within them can help to stimulate creative thinking, aiding in formulating a comprehensive, unique array of motivators, tailored specifically for given healthcare providers, as called for in the ensuing step.

3.6.2 Step 2: Populate Each Motivator Category with Potential Options for Motivating Employees

The second step required to assemble a motivation framework involves populating each of the motivator categories identified in the prior step with potential options for motivating employees. Potential motivators should be informed by internal intelligence, acquired by consulting staff members regarding desired motivators, and by external intelligence, acquired by investigating motivators offered by competing entities in the marketplace. Health and medical providers also should investigate developments in the broader market, specifically endeavoring to identify any novel motivators that are emerging. New types of benefits, unique management techniques, fresh ideas regarding the structure of work, and the like offer opportunities to invigorate motivational arrays. As described earlier in the chapter, such novel motivators can even afford competitive advantages in many circumstances. Identifying these requires knowledge of emerging trends, necessitating ongoing **environmental scanning**, investigations of the environment aimed at identifying opportunities and threats, prevailing marketplace trends, and the like. Potential choices should be defined as specifically as possible, affording a series of thoroughly described options for consideration.

3.6.3 Step 3: Review the Options, Assess Feasibility, and Select Desired Motivators for Placement in the Motivation Framework

The third step involved in assembling a motivation framework involves reviewing options, assessing their feasibility, and determining the particular motivators which will be included in the motivation framework. Once selections have been made, they are compiled into a comprehensive list constituting the motivation framework. As referenced earlier, specificity is essential in presenting motivators. General portrayals offer limited practical value for managers, so they should be avoided. Under the category of "benefits," for example, instead of mentioning something generic like "paid vacation," present specifics, including the length of the vacation, eligibility, and anything that differentiates it from competitive offerings of the same. Under the "oversight and development" category, rather than generically saying "general and specialized training," actually define the given training opportunities, eligibility, and other meaningful characteristics. Such specificity moves what otherwise would be a forgettable list into a repertoire possessing considerable practical value, providing detailed descriptions of the array of motivators which managers can use to inspire their given workforces.

3.6.4 Step 4: Operationalize the Framework by Circulating It to Managers for Implementation in Their Given Work Units

With the motivation framework complete, efforts then turn to its operationalization via its circulation to managers for implementation in their given work units. Managers should become especially familiar with the framework, given their role in overseeing and encouraging subordinates. Tools, techniques, and incentives that are available yet remain untapped constitute wasted opportunities, so efforts to inform and enlighten managers regarding the use and application of the framework are essential. This framework can also serve as the foundation of managerial training programs centered on motivation, aiding managers in developing their motivation skill sets, permitting them to better understand and inspire employees. The contents of the framework also can supply an excellent source of information for recruitment advertisements, orientation sessions, and employee manuals, informing job candidates, new employees, and experienced personnel of the benefits associated with employment. With periodic reviews, including updates as needed, motivation frameworks can deliver significant value, aiding in ensuring that workforces remain enthusiastic.

3.7 Conducting Motivation Audits

Given the importance of maintaining a highly motivated workforce, it stands to reason that healthcare providers must develop proficiencies in determining the state of motivation within their given institutions. One mechanism which can shed significant light on motivation within healthcare establishments is known as a motivation audit. Formally defined, a **motivation audit** is an evaluation conducted to assess the state of motivation within an institution, permitting opportunities to maintain and potentially bolster noted strengths and remedy any discovered deficiencies. When conducted on a regular basis, these audits have the potential to vastly improve the degree of workforce motivation marshaled across the institution, as doing so ensures proactive management of this critical element of organizational life and institutional performance. Core steps for conducting motivation audits are as follows.

3.7.1 Step 1: Collect Evidence Indicating the State of Workforce Motivation

Motivation audits begin by collecting data which provides insights into the current state of workforce motivation. Several sources are particularly enlightening, namely, findings from employee performance evaluations, employee satisfaction surveys, and patient satisfaction surveys. Employee performance evaluation results offer keen insights regarding the degree of motivation expressed by workers, and, as such, this information should be comprehensively reviewed. Aggregate results supply excellent topline information, with high scores generally suggesting high levels of motivation and low scores pointing to low levels of motivation. Further insights can be gleaned by examining these results on facility, department, or similar bases.

Drilling down beyond aggregate results is also advised. If, for example, low-performance scores were noted within a particular department, the evaluations can be examined more closely to potentially identify causes. Comments supplied in performance evaluations can be especially enlightening, with these revealing specific details that can clarify whether performance was aided by a motivation success, impeded by a motivation problem, or impacted by some other factor.

Employee satisfaction survey results also offer fruitful insights into employee motivation and should be explored, accordingly. Employee satisfaction surveys directly query staff members about their employer, work settings, job satisfaction, morale, and so on. As such, they offer especially applicable details regarding the state of workforce motivation. This information is nicely complemented by details contained in patient satisfaction surveys which reveal customer perspectives about patient care and attention received. These very often include references associated with employee performance, motivation, and related facets, offering another excellent source of information for ascertaining the state of motivation in healthcare institutions. Such sources of information can be complemented by direct inquiries, including motivation-specific executive interviews, employee surveys, focus groups, and the like to further shed light on the state of workforce motivation.

3.7.2 Step 2: Analyze Collected Evidence to Assess the State of Workforce Motivation

After acquiring the data noted above, healthcare providers should carefully analyze it, looking for indications as to the particular state of motivation and its associated causes. Some findings will be obvious, but others likely will require a bit of detective work. Much depends on the quality and completeness of available data. The level of rigor is up to given healthcare providers, with this being determined by the degree of investment dedicated to given analyses. Operative questions include the following: Based on the evidence collected, would the state of motivation be considered to be high, medium, or low? What evidence suggests this rating? For any noted strengths of motivation, what appears to be the basis of those strengths? For any noted weaknesses, what appears to be the cause of those deficiencies? Does evidence suggest that the motivation framework of the institution is effective or ineffective? If effective, are any modifications to the framework suggested to bolster its potential to motivate? If ineffective, what modifications are needed to resolve its inadequacies? Ultimately, by addressing these and related questions, a picture of motivation should be revealed, complete with potential pathways for bolstering strengths and remedying any observed shortcomings.

3.7.3 Step 3: Prepare a Report Presenting Workforce Motivation Findings and Recommendations

The motivation audit concludes with the assembly of a comprehensive report detailing associated findings and noting recommendations. This report is then used by the given healthcare establishment to make decisions regarding its current approach to motivation and what, if any, changes are necessary to ensure that its employees address their work in an inspired, motivated fashion. Given the importance of motivation, it is best not to leave anything to chance. Formal attention, such as that afforded by a motivation audit, helps to ensure a workforce characterized by energy and enthusiasm.

WK Reflections: Sometimes Motivators Call for Subtraction Rather Than Addition

One of the greatest hardships facing most any employee within healthcare institutions is that of **workplace stress** or **job stress**, that is, the emotional tension or strain experienced by employees as a result of highly challenging circumstances and situations faced in their given work environments. Healthcare organizations are institutions characterized by high stress with this largely being due to the unique and highly complex nature of delivering health and medical services [1, 3, 7, 8]. In fact, high levels of workplace stress, if left unchecked, fuel the emergence of a profound **demotivator** (i.e., something which diminishes motivation), namely, employee burnout.

Burnout refers to a state of exhaustion felt by employees resulting from being bombarded by workplace stress over time, ultimately leaving them feeling overwhelmed, distressed, and demoralized. For those experiencing burnout, employee motivation would be considered to be at rock bottom. As such, burnout is a problem not only for impacted personnel but also for the healthcare organizations which employ them [1, 34, 35]. Proactivity by healthcare establishments to prevent employees from falling into states of burnout is highly encouraged, as waiting until after it sets in diminishes individual and institutional productivity. Reactive responses also entail the complex task of rejuvenation, which may or may not even be possible, as in cases where burned out employees simply resign.

It is perhaps most typical to view motivators to be things that healthcare organizations can add which offer attractive rewards or similar benefits to compel employee action. Such positive motivators, such as incentive pay and others which have been referenced at earlier points in the chapter, indeed come to the top of mind when considering opportunities to encourage and inspire workforces. But the concepts of workplace stress and burnout remind healthcare providers that, at least on occasion, motivators actually entail the elimination or subtraction of something. As it is well understood that workplace stress is chronically high in healthcare organizations, the items to be eliminated or at least reduced obviously would entail those things that are hastening stress. Note that, although this globally constitutes a subtractive process (i.e., the reduction or elimination of stress), remedies typically require additions of some sort, as described below. Still, thinking of motivators for their potential to eliminate or reduce negative aspects of work life can lead to creative solutions which might otherwise go unnoticed.

Willis Knighton Health has endeavored to create work environments which incorporate methods to diminish or outright eliminate **stressors** (i.e., sources of stress), reducing burdens on employees and freeing them to address their duties and responsibilities productively and positively. Through this elimination process, a powerful motivator emerged which ultimately aids in the prevention of employee burnout and the resulting demotivation that it causes. So how specifically does Willis Knighton Health reduce workplace stress? By offering amenities that reduce everyday burdens faced by employees. The institution, for example, is committed to ensuring appropriate staffing levels, reducing the likelihood that employees will carry overly burdensome workloads. Shuttle service is offered to employees who park their vehicles in more distant parking lots, removing the hardship of long walks to and from their particular work environments. Security guards patrol the totality of hospital campuses, reducing concerns of workplace violence, theft, vehicle burglaries, and the like, diminishing a common stressor impacting healthcare personnel. Through Willis Knighton Health's Spiritual Life Services Department, employees have access to chaplains who can help them cope with difficult circumstances in their personal and professional lives.

These and related mechanisms ultimately are the result of intensive efforts by Willis Knighton Health to dismantle common stressors, making organizational life more enjoyable for its employees. They also positively contribute to the institution's productive organizational culture, notably characterized by the system's "family feel," with this being described in particular detail in Chap. 8 and elsewhere in the text. Formulating motivators indeed requires deep thought and reflection. And in doing so, be certain to remember that sometimes motivators call for subtraction rather than addition, with this often generating helpful solutions that maximize the potential of healthcare organizations to motivate staff members.

3.8   Summary and Conclusions

The state of workforce motivation has a profound impact on the performance of health and medical institutions. If healthcare establishments can consistently field cadres of highly motivated employees, exceptional patient care and attention, as well as institutional prosperity, can be expected. Poorly motivated staffs will yield the reverse and can even threaten institutional viability. Given the extensive performance implications, the importance and essentiality of directing intensive efforts toward bolstering high levels of motivation in the workplace cannot be underemphasized. Investments in motivation certainly have the potential to pay generous dividends. Mastery of the knowledge and skills depicted in this chapter will afford health and medical providers with abilities to develop and maintain highly motivated workforces, affording an essential ingredient required for realizing exceptional performance in healthcare organizations.

Key Terms

- Acquired Needs Theory
- Adams' Equity Theory
- Alderfer's ERG Theory
- Burnout
- Cognitive Theories
- Content Theories of Motivation
- Demotivator
- Environmental Scanning
- Equity Theory
- ERG Theory
- Expectancy Theory
- Extrinsic Motivation
- Goal-Setting Theory
- Herzberg's Two-Factor Theory
- Hierarchy of Needs Theory
- Intrinsic Motivation
- Job Stress
- Locke's Goal-Setting Theory
- Maslow's Hierarchy of Needs Theory
- McClelland's Acquired Needs Theory
- Motivation
- Motivation Audit
- Motivation Framework
- Motivator
- Motivator-Hygiene Theory

- Need
- Needs Theories
- Needs-Based Theories
- Process Theories
- Stressor
- Two-Factor Theory
- Vroom's Expectancy Theory
- Want
- Workplace Stress

Exercises

1. In your own words, define the concept of motivation, and discuss its critical role in health and medicine.
2. Prepare a brief narrative distinguishing intrinsic motivation from extrinsic motivation. Reflect on your recent work experiences and supply an example of when you were motivated intrinsically and an example of when you were motivated extrinsically.
3. Define content theories of motivation, identify associated examples, and explain their impact on the knowledge base of motivation. Of the examples listed in the text, which content theory do you believe best describes motivation? Why?
4. Define process theories of motivation, identify associated examples, and explain their impact on the knowledge base of motivation. Of the examples listed in the text, which process theory do you believe best describes motivation? Why?
5. Compare and contrast Maslow's hierarchy of needs theory with Alderfer's ERG theory. Between the two, which theory do you prefer and why?
6. Compare and contrast Adams' equity theory with Locke's goal-setting theory. Between the two, which theory do you prefer and why?
7. Demonstrate your knowledge of Vroom's expectancy theory by supplying two recent examples, one where you were motivated by something and the other where you were not motivated by something. Through the lens of expectancy theory, describe both instances.
8. Try your hand at preparing a motivation framework for a hypothetical healthcare institution. Reflect on methods used by health and medical establishments to motivate employees, make associated selections, and formulate the framework. Prepare a brief narrative explaining the reasons for crafting your framework as presented.

References

1. Elrod, J. K. (2013). *Breadcrumbs to cheesecake*. R&R Publishers.
2. Shi, L., & Singh, D. A. (2023). *Essentials of the US health care system* (6th ed.). Jones and Bartlett.
3. McConnell, C. R. (2020). *Hospitals and health systems: What they are and how they work*. Jones and Bartlett.
4. Anderson, D. L. (2019). *Organization design: Creating strategic and agile organizations*. Sage.
5. Burton, R. M., Obel, B., & Hakonsson, D. D. (2020). *Organizational design: A step-by-step approach* (4th ed.). Cambridge University Press.
6. Flynn, W. J., Valentine, S. R., & Meglich, P. A. (2022). *Healthcare human resource management* (4th ed.). Cengage.
7. Ziebland, S., Coulter, A., Calabrese, J. D., & Locock, L. (Eds.). (2013). *Understanding and using health experiences: Improving patient care*. Oxford University Press.
8. Perez, O. J. (2009). *The patient experience: A guide to creating a meaningful patient experience in every healing encounter*. Florida Hospital Publishing.
9. Kotler, P., Stevens, R. J., & Shalowitz, J. (2021). *Strategic marketing for health care organizations: Building a customer-driven health system* (2nd ed.). Wiley.
10. Fortenberry, J. L., Jr. (2010). *Health care marketing: Tools and techniques* (3rd ed.). Jones and Bartlett.
11. Reeve, J. (2018). *Understanding motivation and emotion* (7th ed.). Wiley.
12. Deckers, L. (2018). *Motivation: Biological, psychological, and environmental* (5th ed.). Routledge.
13. Robbins, S. P., & Judge, T. A. (2019). *Organizational behavior* (18th ed.). Pearson.
14. Kanfer, R. (1995). Motivation. In N. Nicholson (Ed.), *Blackwell encyclopedic dictionary of organizational behavior*. Blackwell.
15. Kanfer, R. (1995). Motivation and performance. In N. Nicholson (Ed.), *Blackwell encyclopedic dictionary of organizational behavior*. Blackwell.
16. Griffin, R. W., Phillips, J. M., & Gully, S. M. (2020). *Organizational behavior: Managing people and organizations* (13th ed.). Cengage.
17. McShane, S. L., & Von Glinow, M. A. (2019). *Organizational behavior* (4th ed.). McGraw-Hill.
18. Hitt, M. A., Miller, C. C., Colella, A., & Triana, M. D. C. (2018). *Organizational behavior* (5th ed.). Wiley.
19. Barnett, T. (2000). Motivation and motivation theory. In M. M. Helms (Ed.), *Encyclopedia of management* (4th ed.). Gale Group.
20. Schermerhorn, J. R., Jr., Hunt, J. G., & Osborn, R. N. (1998). *Basic organizational behavior* (2nd ed.). Wiley.
21. Maslow, A. H., & Stephens, D. C. (2000). *The Maslow business reader*. Wiley.
22. Adler, S. (1995). ERG theory. In N. Nicholson (Ed.), *Blackwell encyclopedic dictionary of organizational behavior*. Blackwell.
23. Alderfer, C. P. (1972). *Existence, relatedness, and growth: Human needs in organizational settings*. The Free Press.
24. Wiersma, U. J. (1995). Motivator-hygiene theory. In N. Nicholson (Ed.), *Blackwell encyclopedic dictionary of organizational behavior*. Blackwell.
25. Herzberg, F. (2003). One more time: How do you motivate employees? *Harvard Business Review, 81*(1), 87–96.
26. McClelland, D. C. (1961). *The achieving society*. Van Nostrand Company.
27. McClelland, D. C. (1962). Business drive and national achievement. *Harvard Business Review, 40*(4), 99–112.
28. Vroom, V. H. (1964). *Work and motivation*. Wiley.
29. Greenberg, J. (1995). Equity theory. In N. Nicholson (Ed.), *Blackwell encyclopedic dictionary of organizational behavior*. Blackwell.

30. Adams, J. S. (1963). Toward an understanding of equity. *Journal of Abnormal and Social Psychology, 67,* 422–436.
31. Erez, M. (1995). Goal setting. In N. Nicholson (Ed.), *Blackwell encyclopedic dictionary of organizational behavior.* Blackwell.
32. Locke, E. A. (1968). Toward a theory of task motivation and incentives. *Organizational Behavior and Human Performance, 3*(2), 157–189.
33. Locke, E. A., & Latham, G. P. (1990). *A theory of goal setting and task performance.* Prentice Hall.
34. Halbesleben, J. (2023). *Preventing burnout and building engagement in the healthcare workplace* (2nd ed.). Health Administration Press.
35. Swensen, S. J., & Shanafelt, T. D. (2020). *Mayo Clinic strategies to reduce burnout: 12 actions to create the ideal workplace.* Oxford University Press.

Chapter 4
Communication in Health and Medicine

Learning Objectives
After examining this chapter, readers will have the ability to:

- Define communication and discuss its importance in health and medicine.
- Understand the mechanics of communication by describing its associated process.
- Realize common communication barriers experienced within healthcare institutions and describe methods for minimizing their impacts and effects.
- Appreciate the influence of body language and other nonverbal communicative expressions on verbal forms of communication.
- Define and discuss formal communication and informal communication, referencing also the grapevine and its impact in healthcare establishments.
- Understand directional flows of communication occurring within and outside of health and medical institutions.
- Discuss methods for fostering productive communication within healthcare establishments, permitting timely, accurate, and meaningful institutional interactions.

WK Reflections: Self-Awareness as a Communication Development Tool

Willis Knighton Health's vast institutional knowledge continually confirms the value of excellent communication skills and abilities for anyone serving in healthcare management roles. Communicating well is so important that the establishment actively seeks candidates who possess high communication proficiencies and a willingness to commit to continual improvement. Observations over many years have demonstrated that some individuals are natural communicators, thriving in their conveyance abilities almost

© The Editor(s) (if applicable) and The Author(s), under exclusive license to Springer
Nature Switzerland AG 2024
J. K. Elrod, J. L. Fortenberry, Jr., *Organizational Behavior and Management in Health and Medicine*, https://doi.org/10.1007/978-3-031-61823-9_4

effortlessly, while others must work diligently to overcome communication weaknesses. Those who are not naturally inclined communicators should not fret, however, as associated skills and abilities can be learned, advancing communication prowess. Regardless of the level of communicative acumen, proficiencies in communication must continually be shaped and honed throughout one's career. Communicative tools and techniques continue to evolve, necessitating that healthcare managers stay abreast of the latest developments, permitting beneficial methods to be incorporated into daily practice as needed or desired. Managers who do not actively and earnestly strive to develop communicative skills and abilities will see diminished performance, something which should compel all to work diligently to perfect their associated acumen.

Willis Knighton Health desires its managers to engage their given environments, and this naturally calls for them to demonstrate communication prowess. Consider the following scenario. A healthcare manager departs his office to have lunch in the hospital's cafeteria. While taking the brief walk through the hallway linking his office and the cafeteria, he encounters a housekeeping employee who is busy shining the floors. He says nothing to the employee, despite coming into direct contact with the individual. As he proceeds down the hallway, he passes by an elevator landing. There, he notices a patient looking down at a piece of paper, and then back and forth, showing clear indications of being lost. The healthcare manager thinks to himself that surely another employee will see the patient and offer a helping hand, and he continues his walk to the cafeteria. On entering the cafeteria and walking through the lunch line, the manager encounters numerous employees of the establishment but does little to interact with them. Despite the service experience being performed superbly by multiple dietary employees, not a single compliment is offered as he departs the checkout counter. He then passes by numerous employees and many patients and their loved ones in the dining room, acknowledging a few, but doing little to engage anyone meaningfully, finally taking his seat at a table alone where he eats his meal. In this scenario, the healthcare manager would be considered by Willis Knighton Health to be a poor communicator (and arguably a poor manager). This sort of scenario, however, is not terribly uncommon in hospitals far and wide. Any conscientious healthcare establishment must expect more of its managers.

Now consider another scenario, a modification of the first one which, this time, features a healthcare manager who exemplifies communication excellence. Here, the manager departs his office, and, on encountering the housekeeping employee shining the floors, he greets the employee and offers a compliment, being impressed by the staff member's results. Continuing down the hallway to the cafeteria, the healthcare manager notices the patient who, by all outward appearances, is conveying the need for assistance. Instead of walking by, he instead stops to ask the patient if he can be of assistance, gives her directions, and walks with her to her destination. The manager then makes his way to the cafeteria, greeting those he encounters in the lunch line and expressing appreciation to the dietary employees as they go about their work. In the dining room, he continues his excellent engagement efforts, greeting those he comes into contact with, even inviting several colleagues that he encountered to sit at his table, eating his meal in the company of fellow employees. This scenario illustrates that which Willis Knighton Health desires to see in its healthcare managers. In this scenario, the healthcare manager has proven to be a valuable asset of the establishment, courtesy of his efforts to communicate effectively. Ironically, the time taken by the healthcare manager in the second scenario would barely require more than that expended by the healthcare manager in the first scenario. Between the two efforts, the results could not be more differentiated, with the first scenario's manager offering practically nothing and the second scenario's manager delivering actual value.

This simple example illustrates quite a bit about effective communication. It requires one to be active, rather than passive, seeking opportunities to engage others, reading body language to help discern appropriate responses, and working diligently to deliver conveyances at the right time and proper place in the correct manner. Doing so should be considered to be a job requirement and healthcare establishments are well within their rights to demand this sort of performance from their managers. Of course, healthcare managers are not alone in this, as well-operated health and medical organizations seek to actively develop managerial communication skill sets via training programs, mentorships, evaluations, and the like. Still, each employee, himself or herself, has an obligation to deliver their best in all areas, including communication.

In the continual quest for communication excellence, healthcare managers would do well to maintain a robust level of self-awareness regarding their engagement efforts. Particularly, they should periodically reflect on their interactions with others and ask themselves if their efforts are delivering results and what, if anything, might be done to make improvements. Being honest with oneself is essential here, with healthcare managers candidly constructively criticizing themselves. Whenever weaknesses are revealed, action should be taken to eliminate the noted shortcomings. For example, if timidity, social reclusiveness, or similar characteristics are discovered, efforts should be taken to effect improvements. Similarly, if feelings of indifference are revealed, an immediate behavioral change must take place in order to improve communicative and managerial performance. Of course, if reflective exercises reveal positive communicative results, efforts should be continued, always keeping an eye on potential enhancement opportunities. Critical reflection indeed serves as a useful method for evaluating one's communication skills and abilities. These exercises foster self-awareness, helping healthcare managers see themselves in their given roles, permitting them to better understand and develop their engagement efforts.

4.1 Background

Health and medical organizations are involved in perhaps the most difficult, complex, and sensitive of missions of any institution [1]. Associated challenges occur on multiple fronts, largely due to the very nature of the product. The delivery of health services requires extensive coordination between and among personnel possessing vastly different backgrounds, skills, and abilities. Very often, the stakes are quite high, with life and limb hanging in the balance, requiring staff members to take quick and decisive actions in environments of perpetual stress [2–6]. This diverse array of personnel must interact with an equally diverse cadre of patients who face the pain of injury and illness in settings which are foreign, frightening, and bewildering to them [2, 7, 8]. Prominent third parties also are involved in the delivery of healthcare, notably including the loved ones of care recipients and the health insurance companies and other payers funding care provision [2, 9–12]. Each party involved in the process of healthcare delivery requires timely and accurate information, tailored specifically to their particular needs, all while complying with strict regulations regarding confidentiality [1, 2, 11]. Quite obviously, this places a premium on excellent communication.

Communication is one of the most important components of successful health and medical organizations. It is the glue that binds an institution [13], serving as the conduit linking the vast and diverse array of parties involved in the care experience together. Its associated power has led to communication being characterized as "the very essence of a social system or an organization" [14, p. 520]. As such, healthcare establishments must strive to master fundamentals of communication, ensuring associated competencies systemwide. As holders of oversight roles within healthcare institutions, managers quite obviously must possess communication prowess, given their responsibilities for guiding and directing others. But it is also critically important for those not holding managerial roles to have proficiencies in communication, especially as patient contact is possible for any staff member involved in health and medicine [1, 2, 15]. Unfortunately, even in well-operated healthcare institutions, breakdowns in communication can and do occur, with associated failures being ever-present threats. This requires vigilance on the part of healthcare providers to ensure that communication competencies proliferate within their given organizations [16, 17]. Indeed, health and medical institutions which foster excellence in communication can expect to benefit from those particular investments.

4.2 Defining Communication

Communication is defined as a process through which two or more parties exchange information, making use of mutually understood language, symbols, and other expressions to successfully convey meaning and understanding. It is derived from the Latin word *communicare*, a term which denotes sharing or imparting [18]. From both the contemporary definition and its term of origin, one can easily ascertain a central feature of communication, namely, that it involves the successful transfer of information between parties. It is not merely a volley of information cast upon others; reception and understanding also are required [19, 20]. This, of course, necessitates that parties are communicating in a manner comprehensible to each other. This might appear patently obvious at face value. Parties certainly would need to be able to speak and understand the particular language, gestures, or other mannerisms used in communication. But there are deeper considerations. Consider a physician discussing a medical diagnosis with a patient. Complex medical terminology, even when expressed to others in their native tongues, can immediately erect barriers to understanding, effectively blocking the successful transfer of knowledge. Seen in this light, successful communication requires a degree of discernment beyond simple face value assumptions.

In organizations, communication serves five major functions, namely, management, feedback, emotional sharing, persuasion, and information exchange [21]. Its **management function** pertains to the use of communication as a means of issuing directives and other commands from supervisor to subordinate, permitting work within an institution to be accomplished. Healthcare managers across all disciplines and foci use communication in this manner as part of daily organizational life. The **feedback function** of communication deals with the provision and receipt of constructive criticism and other forms of guidance between parties, allowing work approaches, level of performance, and more to be refined. Avenues such as annual employee performance evaluations held between nurse supervisors and their subordinate staff nurses offer excellent examples of the feedback function of communication. The **emotional sharing function** of communication pertains to its use as a mechanism for expressing feelings. This function is particularly pronounced in highly sensitive environments such as healthcare settings. For example, negative occurrences, ranging from coping with short staffing to experiencing the deaths of patients, can exact an immense emotional toll on staff members, with communication permitting one to share feelings, providing an outlet for relief. The **persuasion function** of communication pertains to its use as an instrument of motivation and encouragement. A hospital administrator praising the efforts of employees after receipt of a quality award, an imaging manager compelling a radiologic technologist to work the evening shift, and a dietary counselor shoring up the resolve of patients struggling with weight issues all constitute examples of the use of communication as a persuasive device. Lastly, the **information exchange function** of communication cuts to its core as the universal mechanism for sharing details between and among parties, notably facilitating decision-making and other critical administrative tasks occurring daily in health and medicine. Each of these functions is important and plays a critical role in healthcare operations [1, 21].

4.3   The Communication Process

In its most rudimentary form, the communication process involves two parties: a sender and a receiver. The **sender** is the initiator of the communication process, with his or her objective being to deliver a particular conveyance to a designated **receiver**, the intended target of a given communication. To do this, the sender crafts a **message**, that is, a particular dispatch containing the informational content desired to be conveyed to the receiver. This requires the sender to select a particular **channel** of communication, the medium used to route a message to its intended target. **Communication channels**, also referred to as **communication media**, are numerous, ranging from traditional forms (e.g., in-person meetings, posted letters) to technology-based variants (e.g., telephone conversations, email dialogues, text messaging, video conferencing). Selection generally is based on the objective of the communication, the content to be carried, and the channel's acceptability by both the sender and receiver. Once the channel is determined, the sender engages in **encoding** where the message is converted into a form suitable for delivery through the selected channel. Once the message has been sent, assuming success, it is received by the targeted recipient, with the receiver then engaging in **decoding** where he or she translates the content of the dispatch, ideally yielding an understanding of the message exactly as intended by the sender [10, 19, 20, 22].

If inclined to do so, the recipient may decide to forward **feedback**, a response in reply to a given message, requiring the recipient to select a channel, encode his or her desired dispatch, and forward it, accordingly, to the originating sender. The channel selected for routing feedback may or may not be the same one used for message delivery [10, 19, 20, 22]. Take, for example, a scenario where a hospital administrator sends an email to a staff physician to communicate that his request for additional equipment has been granted, prompting the physician to mail a handwritten "thank-you" card in response. Feedback is not always offered by message recipients, but especially in business contexts, it is very helpful and is known to enrich communication [23]. Its value is so pronounced that it is often requested and, in some cases, required of recipients, as stipulated in associated correspondence. Even in the absence of a feedback request or requirement, supplying such bolsters communication, providing assurances to the associated sender that the message was received and understood.

As the communication process occurs within the greater environment, message dissemination does not always occur as intended. This is due to disruptive influences, collectively referred to as **noise**, which can be interjected into the process, distorting messages or even outright eliminating receipt by intended targets. Noise is a **communication barrier**, an impediment that prevents the successful transmission of messages, and it can take many forms [10, 24]. Consider the following scenarios: a hospital administrator writes a letter but gets distracted and fails to post it in a timely fashion; a nurse receives instructions from a supervisor but exhaustion causes her to miss important details, prompting an error; a phlebotomist uses **jargon**—specialized terminology associated with particular occupational disciplines—when explaining the blood drawing process to a patient, generating immediate confusion. In these cases, for different reasons, message dissemination was unsuccessful due to noise entering and distorting the communication process.

Beyond things such as workplace distractions, physical and emotional stresses, and language miscues, communication barriers can be tied to poorly planned work environments. Noise, for example, can take its traditional form, namely that of loud, unwanted sounds. An ongoing renovation project in a hospital might produce excessive noise from construction equipment being utilized, hampering the ability of caregivers to dialogue properly with co-workers and patients. Even in the absence of such commotion, work environments might not be thoughtfully planned to facilitate communication. For example, technologies which aid communication may not be being utilized to their fullest. Perhaps phone conferencing is being used for meetings between the executive teams of two hospitals when video conferencing might be more suitable. Smartphones might have yet to be issued to critical administrators and caregivers who need to stay in constant contact. Even physical barriers, such as the overly distant placement of departments from one another, can impede communication. Careful scrutiny of environments is required to ensure that the design and features of workplaces facilitate communication excellence. Regardless of form, noise represents an ongoing threat to the productive exchange of information, necessitating efforts to minimize it, when and where possible [20, 25].

4.4   Verbal and Nonverbal Communication

Communication can occur verbally and nonverbally. **Verbal communication** is defined as a form of communication that makes use of written or spoken words to interact with others. The use of words is the defining characteristic of verbal communication, rather than the particular manner used to express those words [19, 20]. An offer letter sent to a newly hired physician, a vocally expressed directive issued by a pharmacy manager to a pharmacist, a medical appointment reminder texted by an admissions clerk to a patient, and a "state of the institution" address delivered by a CEO to hospital staff members all constitute forms of verbal communication.

Nonverbal communication is defined as communication that makes use of physical manifestations, such as eye contact, facial expressions, body posture, vocal tone, head movements, hand gestures, touch, spatial distance from addressee, and other behaviors, to convey meaning to others. **Body language** specifically refers to nonverbal communicative expressions conveyed via articulation of the human form. Even one's appearance (e.g., personal grooming, clothing) "speaks" nonverbally to others [26], giving indications of roles and responsibilities. While nonverbal communication does not rely on word use for the conveyance of meaning, it very often accompanies verbal communication, so much so that nonverbal expressions should be considered to be givens in face-to-face interactions. Nonverbal communication can be expressed consciously (e.g., a healthcare executive adopts an aggressive posture to express confidence as she addresses a new work group, a dietician humorously rolls her eyes on hearing a patient grumble about a prescribed low salt diet) or subconsciously (e.g., a patient's eyes brighten on receiving news of a good medical report from his physician, an LPN's shoulders shrug as she describes being passed over for a promotion).

For obvious reasons, one might be led to believe that the verbal communication component in a face-to-face interaction would have the greatest bearing on the impact of the given message. Research, however, suggests otherwise, with studies indicating that nonverbal elements play a greater role in message conveyance than do verbal elements [27]. Communication channels which combine both verbal and nonverbal elements (e.g., face-to-face interactions, video conferencing) are said to possess a higher degree of media richness than those of their more limited counterparts (e.g., telephone, letters, email). **Media richness** refers to the amount of detail that a particular communication channel is capable of conveying [28]. Generally, the more complex the communication, the richer the medium must be to properly convey the message, giving vehicles combining verbal and nonverbal expressions the edge whenever detailed discussions are required. Given the profound influence of nonverbal communication, including its potential to be evoked subconsciously, health and medical professionals must be keenly aware of their associated expressions. If conflict between verbal and nonverbal expressions occurs, message effectiveness will be diminished.

Aside from remaining self-aware, something discussed earlier in the chapter, additional steps to ensure consistency across verbal and nonverbal expressions are possible. One of the simplest involves arranging to be videoed while engaging in an exchange, permitting review and reflection from the perspective of the receiver. More advanced opportunities are available in the form of simulations featuring live actors, artificial intelligence, virtual reality, and other means which allow individuals to engage in exchanges with subjects (e.g., colleagues, patients) who react to various communications, including nonverbal ones, aiding in developing associated skill sets. These and related simulation opportunities are often used in schools of medicine, allied health, and other clinical programs to train students. They also have made their way into advanced workforce development programs in health systems, illustrating the importance of developing complementary verbal and nonverbal communicative abilities [29, 30].

WK Reflections: Strategizing Communication Beyond Words

When healthcare managers have critical meetings, it is not uncommon for them to rehearse their given presentations, whether it be to provide an update to department managers, accept an accolade for an accomplishment, negotiate a contract with a physician group, counsel an underperforming employee, or engage in similar interactions. In such preparations, the emphasis very typically is on the spoken word and perhaps the desired presentation materials accompanying the associated narrative. Very little energy, however, is directed toward addressing nonverbal communicative elements. This facet must be strategized, too, with the healthcare manager rehearsing the meeting in his or her mind to ascertain the best methods for positioning relevant parties to maximize communication impact.

Assume, for example, that a hospital president is meeting with the chief of staff of a physician group for purposes of exploring a strategic partnership between the establishments. Such a meeting could lead to numerous mutual benefits, so the hospital president prepares thoroughly for the meeting, ensuring that critical points necessary for conveyance and discussion are contained in his anticipated dialogue. Such preparation is a good start, but added value can be derived by envisioning and then arranging the best possible physical environment for conveying the necessary content. In this particular case, assuming the meeting will be taking place at the hospital, the executive likely would do well to avoid placing a desk between himself and the physician leader. Doing so has the potential to generate subconscious perceptions of superiority, harming an effective dialogue, particularly in situations where parties are seeking common ground. A better arrangement for the meeting would be for the hospital president to make use of a round table for the discussion, perhaps located in a sitting area within his office, sending a subconscious message of equality between parties. This philosophy draws on the timeless German proverb, "At a round table, every seat is the head place." It is a small but highly meaningful gesture that can aid in warming relationships. It also conveys respect and sends the message that the parties are peers. Such expressions certainly can set the stage for productive discussions [1].

Suppose, however, that the hospital president instead was preparing for a disciplinary session with a vice president who was failing to live up to expectations. In such situations, the establishment of authority is essential, calling for the hospital president to opt for the formality of the traditional executive desk arrangement. As equality, solidarity, and the like are not called for in these contexts, the sitting area table concept is unnecessary and almost certainly would be counterproductive. Here, conveyance of a strict supervisor-subordinate relationship is necessary for achieving the best results. This arrangement also works well in other contexts, including positive ones, such as in cases involving the delivery of instructions or the issuance of directives to others. This is especially useful when senior managers are conveying details to their junior counterparts, as this authority-conveying arrangement enhances attentiveness.

The scenarios presented above represent just a few of myriad situations where subtle physical arrangements can make a notable difference in one's success as a communicator. Certainly, there are many communicative situations where one does not possess the control required to structure these arrangements for optimal communication impact. But whenever options do exist for making such arrangements, healthcare managers should take advantage of the opportunity to enhance their interactions with given audiences. This begins by comprehensively strategizing about communications, ensuring that attention is directed toward not only verbal matters but also nonverbal matters, including physical arrangements, given their immense power to convey messages.

4.5 Formal and Informal Communication

Formal communication refers to messages which travel via official channels in organizations, generally in accordance with their established organizational hierarchies, but conveyances are not solely transmitted through these particular routes. They also are disseminated via unofficial channels, with these messages being referred to as **informal communication**. The informal communication network in an organization is referred to as the **grapevine**, and each organization has one. Its unique name derives from the manner of assembly of telegraph lines during the Civil War where such lines were strung through trees in highly complex and seemingly informal, unpredictable patterns resembling grapevines [31]. The grapevine operates far differently than its formal counterpart, being fueled largely by social relationships that develop between and among employees in organizations. Formal lines of authority mean nothing in the grapevine, as informal lines can run in any direction, dictated solely by employees and their associated communicative desires. Information which travels via the grapevine can be positive or negative, helpful or unhelpful, and accurate or inaccurate. The grapevine can carry innocent small talk (e.g., conversations about the latest movies, breaking news, how one's children are doing in school, etc.), rumors (e.g., forthcoming layoffs at the hospital, an expected merger with another healthcare establishment, proposed plans to increase nurse pay rates), gossip (e.g., sources of strife between nursing services and imaging departments, details about a physician's recent divorce), and virtually any other sort of communication. In many respects, the grapevine is a microcosm of how general communication operates in broad society.

The grapevine is especially prominent in healthcare institutions, as many operate around the clock, providing constant opportunities for dialogue within and across multiple shifts. Night and weekend shifts, in particular, offer fertile ground for the proliferation of the grapevine. Employees working those shifts often miss official engagements (e.g., CEO addresses, celebratory events) occurring during normal business hours, forcing them to learn about what transpired through unofficial channels. Healthcare managers can and should tap into the grapevine regularly as a means of staying abreast of developments. This can be accomplished by making inquiries directly with employees known to be influencers and opinion leaders, asking them about what they are hearing in the workplace and encouraging them to communicate any breaking developments [21]. Doing so will give managers opportunities to dispel any inaccuracies reported.

While the grapevine cannot be eliminated in health and medical institutions, it certainly can be less impactful if healthcare providers ensure that adequate information is supplied to staff members. When official communication is scarce and lacking, employees naturally will seek to fill associated gaps with speculation. Since gaps are going to be filled one way or another, it is best to preempt such by proactively supplying timely and accurate details about institutional operations and their associated impact. Unknowns can be acknowledged as such, coupled with commitments to inform employees once scenarios are better understood [21]. In seeking to keep employees abreast of developments, however, care must be taken to prevent **information overload**, the provision of so much information that employees cannot process it in a productive and meaningful manner. The flow of information should be regulated and monitored, seeking a balance that informs but does not burden personnel. Efforts to do so will undoubtedly pay dividends in enhanced employee morale and institutional productivity.

4.6 Directional Characteristics of Communication

Communication within organizations can be directed in downward, upward, horizontal, and diagonal fashions. It also can be directed externally [32]. Likely the first directional pathway that comes to mind when one thinks of communication in organizations, **downward communication**, essentially entails conveyances transmitted from those occupying higher-level positions in an institution's hierarchy to those occupying lower-level positions. A mission statement issued systemwide by a health system's president, a chief nursing officer's conveyance of details concerning revised recruitment incentives to nurse supervisors, and a hospital marketing director's issuance of website content updates to programmers all typify downward-pointed conveyances in healthcare establishments.

The reverse of downward communication, **upward communication**, is directed from those occupying lower-level positions in an organization's hierarchy to those in higher-level positions. Such communication is especially critical in health service environments, given extensive autonomy held by employees as they go about their assigned duties and responsibilities. By necessity, many assignments are conducted outside of the direct observation of supervisors, necessitating that employees apprise them of task outcomes, clinical issues, workplace observations, and myriad related matters, with these, of course, being transmitted upward in the hierarchy.

Downward and upward forms of communication essentially traverse the **scalar chain**, the formally devised **chain of command** extending from the very top authority within an organization to the lowest ranks of the establishment. As detailed in Chap. 1, dating all the way back to 1916, Henri Fayol, a French mining executive and engineer who issued the first complete theory of management [33], argued that formally devised lines of authority in organizations should be respected but cautioned that rigid adherence to such can be highly inefficient. He noted that sensible decisions must be made which honor the scalar chain but also ensure permissibility of certain communications between parties not directly connected in the chain for purposes of efficiency and productivity [34]. Fayol's call for a balanced approach resonated with business and industry and is now considered standard practice in modern institutions, with horizontal and diagonal communication complementing upward and downward communication as needed.

Horizontal communication occurs when individuals occupying similar levels within an institution's hierarchy interact directly with each other. Take, for example, the case of an administrator of a particular hospital in a multi-hospital health system who experiences a problem with patient parking, recalls that a fellow administrator at a sister hospital experienced a similar issue, and decides to contact this person directly for advice. Such horizontal communication offers efficiency that would not be possible with strict adherence to the chain of command, which would require the administrator to route his request for assistance to his peer administrator via his supervisor. A somewhat similar, efficiency-minded approach is that of **diagonal communication** which involves conveyances between parties who perform different functions in an organization and also occupy different levels within the establishment. This form of communication essentially cuts across the institutional hierarchy. It is likely the least used directional pathway [35]. An illustration of this would entail a situation where a hospital marketing director makes direct contact with a nursing supervisor for details concerning the preparation of a television advertisement featuring that particular nursing unit. In this scenario, the marketing director likely believed that the matter could be addressed most effectively through this particular action, as opposed to routing the communication horizontally through the director of nursing or upward through his supervisor. Efficiencies through horizontal and diagonal communications indeed can be realized, but discernment is needed to ensure that authority is not overstepped.

External communication refers to conveyances that are directed from inside an organization to parties situated outside of the establishment. Appointment reminders posted, emailed, or texted to patients serve as perhaps the most common example of external communications in the healthcare realm. Other examples include marketing initiatives, such as advertisements, direct mail, and other conveyances directed toward current and potential patients; recruitment initiatives designed to attract job seekers; utterances sent to third-party payers and other institutions involved in covering costs on behalf of patients; correspondence forwarded to regulatory bodies, such as state health departments; and press releases issued to news media organizations. These communications are as vital as those occurring within organizations. Care, of course, must be taken to ensure that conveyances directed externally are issued only by parties authorized to do so by their organizations, with content approved in advance of dissemination. An associated protocol regarding external communication is advised to bolster institutional control [9, 10].

4.7 Fostering Productive Organizational Communication

Healthcare establishments must be actively involved in developing communication acumen across all areas of operation. This requires establishing and maintaining systems that address communication matters of all kinds, ranging from infrastructure enhancements to managerial skills development, permitting active and effective engagement systemwide. The following sections present critical directives which collectively foster productive communication within healthcare organizations.

4.7.1   Develop a Communication-Friendly Organizational Structure

The foundation of productive communication in healthcare establishments rests with their given organizational structures. This is because, as indicated earlier, formal communication runs along the lines of the formal organizational structure. Communication flows beyond upward and downward directions must also be decided, notably including the degree of latitude permitted to employees to engage in horizontally and diagonally directed communications. External communication flows also should be addressed, with decisions revolving around who within the given healthcare establishment is authorized to engage in them and the associated protocols required for receiving approval for sending messages to outside parties. Each of these decisions is completely up to given healthcare institutions based on their communicative preferences. Whatever those preferences happen to be, healthcare establishments must ensure that the associated organizational structure is accommodative to these communicative desires.

4.7.2   Examine Work Environments and Remove Communication Barriers

Quite obviously, any barrier to communication, whether tangible or intangible, hampers the free flow of information between parties. As such, efforts should be taken to examine work environments, seeking to identify communication barriers, removing as many as possible in a bid to foster productive dialogues systemwide. As the physical design and layout of health and medical facilities have a profound bearing on exchanges, it is imperative for healthcare providers to be on guard for any design that restricts necessary engagements. This is especially important for new builds and renovations, as these represent opportunities to incorporate communication-friendly arrangements between and among departments and personnel. But even in situations of existing builds, opportunities for improving the communication potential of work environments might be possible. Something as simple as relocating a department, placing it closer in proximity to another with which it regularly interacts, can significantly facilitate communication. As discussed in Chap. 1, the location of managers in relation to their subordinates also plays a role in communication, particularly involving managerial oversight and guidance. Placement considerations and improvements can make all the difference in extracting additional performance.

4.7.3 Invest in Technologies that Facilitate Communication

Communication technologies have dramatically improved opportunities to productively dialogue with others. Healthcare providers must maintain an awareness of these technologies, permitting them to be incorporated into operations whenever it is advantageous to do so. When considering technologies for adoption, it is an excellent time to address the matter of **channel acceptability**, the identification of channels of communication deemed to be permissible for use by establishments and the types of communication that can be sent via those channels. If, for example, staff members are permitted to attend monthly department meetings via video conferencing rather than in person, this would call for investments in applicable computing technologies. Level of investment would be tied, at least to a degree, to frequency of use and quantity of users. Perhaps, though, video conferencing is deemed to be acceptable for use only by top executive ranks, but at the departmental level, only face-to-face, in-person conferencing is allowed. Or perhaps video conferencing can be used universally by all but never for highly sensitive matters, such as the termination of an employee. Such decisions associated with channel acceptability obviously would impact the depth and breadth of the required investment, effectively guiding healthcare establishments in their selections. Beyond such immediate decisions, as communication technologies are constantly evolving, healthcare providers must ensure that they stay abreast of the latest developments, helping to ensure that their communication technologies remain current.

4.7.4 Establish Communication Protocols

Hastening the free flow of information requires the establishment of broad guidelines concerning institutional communications. Much needs to be determined, including acceptable communication flows, permissible communication channels, and related institutional communication policy, conveying details to the workforce, accordingly. Notably, healthcare organizations must determine methods, manners, and timelines for keeping employees apprised of corporate and departmental actions. Recall that vigilance here can diminish the power of the grapevine, as supplying generous, but not overly burdensome, information leaves employees informed and satisfied rather than uninformed and guessing. A medical center might, for example, require its CEO to deliver a systemwide address to employees on a quarterly basis, apprising personnel of strategic initiatives, the health of the medical center, and more. Department managers might be required to hold formal, weekly meetings with subordinates to discuss department-specific initiatives, keeping employees apprised of the latest details. Its marketing department might be required to initiate website updates within 24 hours of receiving information from authorized parties. Employees who are assigned company smartphones might be required to actively monitor them and respond to calls and text messages within a designated time frame. Associated protocols, if well devised, support the continuous and reliable flow of productive information systemwide.

4.7.5 Establish Communication-Related Workforce Development Initiatives

Since the employees of healthcare establishments ultimately are charged with communicating on behalf of their given organizations, workforce development is essential. Managers, given their supervisory roles in healthcare institutions, must be provided assistance in developing their communicative skills, but such proficiencies also must be developed in the broader workforce, as every employee must interact effectively with others as they go about performing their assigned duties and responsibilities. Such skills can be developed through the provision of regular training opportunities on topics such as communicating accurately and respectfully, engaging in active listening, techniques for demonstrating empathy, and communicating effectively in stressful situations. These sessions, too, offer excellent opportunities to convey various communication protocols established by given healthcare institutions, noting acceptable communication flows, permissible channels, expectations, and the like, ensuring that staff members know what is and is not allowed. Such training is essential. It must be ongoing to ensure the continual development of communication skills and abilities in the workforce.

4.7.6 Monitor and Evaluate the State of Communication in the Workplace

Organizational communication must be assessed regularly, necessitating a plan for routine monitoring and evaluation. The plan for doing so need not be especially complex. It merely requires periodic reflections on communication performance, something which can easily be accomplished by periodically bringing up the subject during regularly scheduled executive meetings. These reflections, at least over time, will likely on occasion suggest the need for enhancements and improvements, demanding actions which will bolster the communication potential of given healthcare establishments. Especially complex queries or concerns, such as the evaluation of a new communication technology for potential deployment, can be addressed either through additional meetings of senior management or perhaps via a specially appointed committee. Regardless of the desired approach for the monitoring and evaluation of communication, healthcare establishments must ensure that responsible parties are engaging in proper oversight of this important organizational asset. By properly monitoring and evaluating institutional communication, healthcare providers can proactively address the communication infrastructure of their given organizations, helping them to maintain top performance.

WK Reflections: The Power of Handwritten Correspondence

In the modern era, healthcare establishments are treated to a dizzying array of communication options, courtesy of technological advancements that have dramatically enhanced the engagement capabilities of organizations. Communication options once considered to be unimaginable are now in the palms of everyone's hands in the form of smartphones which afford constant connectivity via telephone, video, text, and email. Messages, whether transmitted in print or electronically, can now be customized and sent to audiences with ease. Paperless options abound for virtually any process that comes to mind, expediting the completion of employee applications and patient paperwork, conveying appointment reminders to patients, providing opportunities for patients to complete patient satisfaction surveys, and the like, adding convenience never before experienced. The communication revolution will continue to evolve as new technologies continue to be developed, eventually finding their way into the work lives of employees across business and industry, including those serving in healthcare organizations.

As the healthcare industry continues to integrate new communication technologies into operations, motivated predominantly by desires to more impactfully engage parties, one should not neglect those traditional options that are decidedly low-tech. In some cases, the impact potential of little used, historic communicative techniques is higher than modern, cutting-edge solutions that maximize convenience but do so at the expense of the personal touch. The best example of this is the handwritten letter, something which has almost completely disappeared from business and industry, pushed aside in favor of easier, quicker communication options. It is the rarity of such that makes handwritten correspondence highly memorable to recipients. Further, handwritten letters take more effort to produce than do electronic variants, increasing the meaningfulness of the correspondence. These facets are very powerful, so much so that one could make a case that handwritten correspondence is the most impactful communication medium.

Given the demands of healthcare managers, widespread use of handwritten correspondence as a medium of communication would be unsustainable. The temporal requirements associated with preparation simply are too demanding. Further, at least in some cases, highly personal correspondence is not warranted, diminishing justifications for the labor required by handwritten efforts. But in situations where lasting impressions are desired (e.g., expressions of gratitude for helpful assistance and support, congratulatory notes celebrating meaningful accomplishments), handwritten correspondence offers a highly viable avenue.

To foster use of this communication option, healthcare managers are encouraged to keep in their desks a box of stationery, a quality writing instrument, and postage stamps. Having the tools needed for handwritten correspondence immediately at hand will facilitate preparation of such, as this makes for convenience and also helps to prevent procrastination. Depending on the impression desired, regular corporate letterheads and envelopes may be substituted for professional stationery. Handwritten notes, regardless of what they happen to be written on, will be read and remembered by recipients. Note also that little things make big differences. Metered postage, for example, might seem to be perfectly acceptable, but it should be avoided, as it depersonalizes handwritten correspondence. Postage stamps instead should be used. For added benefit, thematic stamps, which feature various subjects, can be selected, with these being more capable of capturing attention than traditional first-class postage stamps featuring the American flag. This is especially the case if the theme of the stamp is relevant (e.g., a healthcare-related stamp used on correspondence sent by a healthcare executive), offering an excellent finishing touch for handwritten correspondence.

Communication innovations will continue to be developed and introduced into the healthcare industry. The latest communicative tools and techniques certainly have a place in modern medicine and should be incorporated whenever they are deemed to be beneficial to given establishments. But in the rush to implement novel communication options, be certain not to neglect timeless selections, especially that of handwritten correspondence. As time and technology march on, the handwritten letter likely will become all the more a rarity, giving one even more reason to turn to this time-honored and highly memorable communication option when lasting impressions are wanted. As impactful communications are highly desired and sometimes absolute necessities, healthcare managers would do well to get into the practice of investing the time and effort required to pen letters by hand, with these having the potential to dramatically bolster communicative results.

4.8   Summary and Conclusions

Communication is an integral component of successful healthcare operations, necessitating intensive attention on the part of healthcare providers to develop and maintain thoughtfully planned mechanisms permitting productive dialogues to take place. It is especially important in healthcare environments, given the diverse backgrounds and roles of staff members, their exposure to equally diverse patient populations, and the overall sensitivity of health and medical operations. Healthcare establishments dedicating concerted efforts and investments toward communication will reap numerous benefits associated with the proliferation of efficient and effective interactions, fostering the accomplishment of institutional missions.

Key Terms

- Body Language
- Chain of Command
- Channel
- Channel Acceptability
- Communication
- Communication Barrier
- Communication Channel
- Communication Media
- Decoding
- Diagonal Communication
- Downward Communication
- Emotional Sharing Function of Communication
- Encoding
- External Communication
- Feedback
- Feedback Function of Communication
- Formal Communication
- Grapevine
- Horizontal Communication
- Informal Communication
- Information Exchange Function of Communication
- Information Overload
- Jargon
- Management Function of Communication
- Media Richness
- Message
- Noise
- Nonverbal Communication
- Persuasion Function of Communication
- Receiver
- Scalar Chain
- Sender
- Upward Communication
- Verbal Communication

Exercises

1. In your own words, describe the importance of communication in health and medical settings. Be sure to address its criticality from the perspective of both an employee and a patient.

2. Demonstrate your understanding of communication by diagramming and describing a recent exchange you have had with a colleague using the language of the formal communication process, identifying the sender, receiver, channel, and other process components, actions, and flows.
3. Think about communication channels and their various applications in health and medicine. Identify your top three channel preferences, and discuss the reasons behind your selections. Does your current employer communicate with you using your preferred channels or other channels less desired by you?
4. Reflect on the topic of communication barriers. Of the many types of barriers, which ones do you most often encounter in your work life? What steps, if any, have been taken to address them to permit the free flow of information? For any that remain unaddressed, what actions would you recommend to resolve them?
5. Jargon is used extensively in health and medicine. In your given occupational specialty, identify several examples used in daily practice. Assume that a person from outside of your work group visits and requests an overview of what you do. How would you go about simplifying jargon, permitting the visitor to understand your work?
6. Simulations, role-playing, and the like are very helpful for building communicative skills in health and medicine. A simple, related exercise involves videoing oneself while engaged in an exchange, permitting evaluation. Do so by arranging to have an associate capture a video of you engaging in a workplace interaction with a colleague. Review the video and evaluate your verbal and nonverbal expressions. What changes, if any, would you make?
7. Think about the directional flows of communication—downward, upward, horizontal, diagonal, and external—in health and medicine. When you are in the role of sender, how are most of your communications directed? From which direction are most communications received by you? What latitude are you offered to communicate with others outside of the formal chain of command? Do you consider the flow arrangement to be productive? Why or why not?
8. The grapevine is an ever-present feature in healthcare organizations. Reflect on your current employment opportunity and describe the grapevine and its operation within the institution. How would you characterize its impact on communication in the organization?

References

1. Elrod, J. K. (2013). *Breadcrumbs to cheesecake*. R&R Publishers.
2. McConnell, C. R. (2020). *Hospitals and health systems: What they are and how they work*. Jones and Bartlett.
3. Shi, L., & Singh, D. A. (2023). *Essentials of the US health care system* (6th ed.). Jones and Bartlett.
4. Marcinko, D. E., & Hetico, H. R. (2012). *Hospitals and health care organizations: Management strategies, operational techniques, tools, templates, and case studies*. CRC Press.

5. Flynn, W. J., Valentine, S. R., & Meglich, P. A. (2022). *Healthcare human resource management* (4th ed.). Cengage.
6. Ginter, P. M., Duncan, W. J., & Swayne, L. E. (2013). *Strategic management of health care organizations* (7th ed.). Jossey-Bass.
7. Ziebland, S., Coulter, A., Calabrese, J. D., & Locock, L. (Eds.). (2013). *Understanding and using health experiences: Improving patient care*. Oxford University Press.
8. Perez, O. J. (2009). *The patient experience: A guide to creating a meaningful patient experience in every healing encounter*. Florida Hospital Publishing.
9. Kotler, P., Stevens, R. J., & Shalowitz, J. (2021). *Strategic marketing for health care organizations: Building a customer-driven health system* (2nd ed.). Wiley.
10. Fortenberry, J. L., Jr. (2010). *Health care marketing: Tools and techniques* (3rd ed.). Jones and Bartlett.
11. Wilensky, S. E., & Teitelbaum, J. B. (2023). *Essentials of health policy and law* (5th ed.). Jones and Bartlett.
12. Reiter, K. L., & Song, P. H. (2021). *Gapenski's healthcare finance: An introduction to accounting and financial management* (7th ed.). Health Administration Press.
13. Griffin, R. W., Phillips, J. M., & Gully, S. M. (2020). *Organizational behavior: Managing people and organizations* (13th ed.). Cengage.
14. Katz, D., & Kahn, R. L. (2017). Communication: The flow of information. In C. D. Mortensen (Ed.), *Communication theory* (2nd ed., pp. 519–528). Routledge.
15. Elrod, J. K., & Fortenberry, J. L., Jr. (2018). Am I seeing things through the eyes of patients? An exercise in bolstering patient attentiveness and empathy. *BMC Health Services Research, 18*(Suppl 3), 41–44.
16. McCorry, L. L., & Mason, J. (2020). *Communication skills for the healthcare professional* (2nd ed.). Jones and Bartlett.
17. Schiavo, R. (2014). *Health communication: From theory to practice* (2nd ed.). Jossey-Bass.
18. Peters, J. D. (1999). *Speaking into the air: A history of the idea of communication*. University of Chicago Press.
19. Beebe, S. A., Beebe, S. J., & Ivy, D. K. (2021). *Communication: Principles for a lifetime* (8th ed.). Pearson.
20. Quintanilla, K. M., & Wahl, S. T. (2020). *Business and professional communication: Keys for workplace excellence* (4th ed.). Sage.
21. Robbins, S. P., & Judge, T. A. (2019). *Organizational behavior* (18th ed.). Pearson.
22. Edwards, A., Edwards, C., Wahl, S. T., & Myers, S. A. (2020). *The communication age: Connecting and engaging* (3rd ed.). Sage.
23. Clevenger, T., Jr., & Matthews, J. (2017). Feedback. In C. D. Mortensen (Ed.), *Communication theory* (2nd ed., pp. 78–87). Routledge.
24. Newman, A. (2017). *Business communication: In person, in print, online* (10th ed.). Cengage.
25. Adler, R. B., Maresh-Fuehrer, M., Elmhorst, J. M., & Lucas, K. (2023). *Communicating at work: Strategies for success in business and the professions* (13th ed.). McGraw-Hill.
26. Bowman, J. M. (2021). *Nonverbal communication: An applied approach*. Sage.
27. Mehrabian, A. (2017). Communication without words. In C. D. Mortensen (Ed.), *Communication theory* (2nd ed., pp. 278–286). Routledge.
28. Daft, R. L., & Lengel, R. H. (1986). Organizational information requirements, media richness and structural design. *Management Science, 32*(5), 554–571.
29. Nestel, D., Kelly, M., Jolly, B., & Watson, M. (Eds.). (2018). *Healthcare simulation education: Evidence, theory, and practice*. Wiley.
30. Levine, A. I., DeMaria, S., Jr., Schwartz, A. D., Sim, A. J., & (Eds.). (2013). *The comprehensive textbook of healthcare simulation*. Springer.
31. Trenholm, S. (2014). *Thinking through communication: An introduction to the study of human communication* (7th ed.). Pearson.

32. Konopaske, R., Ivancevich, J. M., & Matteson, M. T. (2018). *Organizational behavior and management* (11th ed.). McGraw-Hill.
33. Shafritz, J. M., Ott, J. S., & Jang, Y. S. (Eds.). (2016). *Classics of organization theory* (8th ed.). Cengage.
34. Fayol, H. (2016). General principles of management. In J. M. Shafritz, J. S. Ott, & Y. S. Jang (Eds.), *Classics of organization theory* (8th ed., pp. 53–65). Cengage.
35. Galbraith, J. R. (2014). *Designing organizations: Strategy, structure, and process at the business unit and enterprise levels* (3rd ed.). Jossey-Bass.

Chapter 5
Decision-Making in Health and Medicine

Learning Objectives

After examining this chapter, readers will have the ability to:

- Define decision-making and discuss its importance in health and medicine.
- Compare and contrast programmed decisions and nonprogrammed decisions and provide examples of each in healthcare establishments.
- Understand behavioral influences on decision-making and discuss their impact on decisions in health and medical institutions.
- Outline the rational decision-making process, discuss each of its steps, and reflect on its benefits and shortcomings in arriving at decisions in health and medicine.
- Define bounded rationality, distinguish it from rational decision-making, and indicate how it better portrays decision-making in actual practice.
- Discuss the concept of satisficing, indicate how it differs from the concept of maximizing, and discuss its impact on decision-making.

WK Reflections: Tackling Complex Decisions

In 2015, Willis Knighton Health had the opportunity to purchase Doctors' Hospital of Shreveport, once a cornerstone of healthcare in northwest Louisiana, but at the time, a shuttered and dilapidated building, representing the sad ending of a legacy which began in 1907. Having closed years earlier, inactivity and exposure had diminished the appearance, functionality, and safety of the formerly thriving establishment, but its solid structure and ideal location, overlooking the heart of downtown Shreveport, warranted a closer examination and evaluation [1]. What was Willis Knighton Health's response to this very interesting and unexpected opportunity? To answer that question required a stream of nearly countless decisions.

© The Editor(s) (if applicable) and The Author(s), under exclusive license to Springer Nature Switzerland AG 2024
J. K. Elrod, J. L. Fortenberry, Jr., *Organizational Behavior and Management in Health and Medicine*, https://doi.org/10.1007/978-3-031-61823-9_5

Even cursory reflection on such a scenario easily brings forth a daunting array of considerations. Some of the key inquiries necessary for Willis Knighton Health to address included the following: Does Willis Knighton Health have a need for the property? What services might be offered onsite? How would the new property impact existing properties in terms of resource availability, including technologies, staffing, and more? Is the location desirable, accessible to patients, and capable of advancing the institution's mission? Can the building be refurbished, or must it be demolished to make way for new construction? Is the price of the property acceptable? What expenditures will be required for renovation or new construction? What about design selections, ranging from architectural layout to color choices to facility signage and much more?

Clearly, whether to pursue the purchase of Doctors' Hospital represented a monumental decision-making exercise for Willis Knighton Health. Care must be taken in making any decision, but this is especially the case whenever decisions are complex, such as in this situation. This is because complex problems rarely involve a single decision. Instead, a daisy chain of decisions is required, with one decision typically begetting another. Vitally, earlier decisions form the foundation for later decisions. If poor decisions are made in formative stages, their impacts will be felt in subsequent decisions, potentially derailing intended pursuits. This places an even greater premium on making correct decisions, something that this chapter aims to address over its pages.

So what did Willis Knighton Health ultimately do? After intensive examination and evaluation, it purchased the building. Completing the two-year project in 2017, the facility was reintroduced as Willis Knighton Rehabilitation, a 150,000-square-foot building costing $26 million (acquisition plus renovations), a bargain price considering that equivalent new construction would have totaled $44.5 million. Modifications were extensive and even included reorientation of the building's main entrance to face the primary transit corridor leading to the facility, enhancing its roadside presence and improving access for patients. Beyond the $18.5 million savings achieved, Willis Knighton Health was afforded with one of Shreveport's most iconic locations, replacing a public eyesore with a virtually brand new institution, providing an impressive entryway into downtown. As a result, Willis Knighton Rehabilitation was welcomed by governmental officials and other stakeholders for its positive impact on the aesthetics and economics of the city of Shreveport [1].

Today, Willis Knighton Rehabilitation serves as a testament to perseverance in decision-making, demonstrating the positive outcomes that are possible through intensive reflection and informed choices, even in very complex scenarios. The opportunity to purchase Doctors' Hospital easily could have been rejected for countless reasons, but Willis Knighton Health was able to see beyond the tarnished appearance of the building and envision the facility as an all-new establishment, capable of bolstering its mission.

5.1 Background

Health and medical institutions exist in environments characterized by high complexity, intense rivalry, and constant change. In such environments, those charged with leading healthcare establishments face enduring challenges to steer operations productively toward fulfillment of their assigned missions. At any moment, circumstances calling for choices to be made can appear in any location and on any level within healthcare establishments [2–6]. Consider the following scenarios:

- The CEO of a medical center realizes that growth in patient volume has outstripped the capacity of the institution.
- A hospital marketing director learns that a new competitor is entering the market.
- A physician group receives an offer to be acquired by a health system.
- The manager of an imaging center learns about a new MRI unit with the potential to benefit patients.
- A nurse supervisor is informed that two nurses failed to show for work.
- A patient representative receives complaints from patients about limited parking.
- A medical clinic's IT manager discovers that a computer virus is wreaking havoc on information systems.
- A hospital's dietary manager discovers that a refrigeration unit is failing.

These and scores of similar scenarios are experienced each and every day within the halls of medicine. Although they typically are quite distinctive, being products of specific institutions and their particular environments, the one commonality that exists between and among them is that they each require decisions to be made. And not just any decision can be made; it must be a good decision, one that is of high quality and effected in a timely fashion [2, 7–9].

The stakes are high in the healthcare industry, given its operational sensitivities and competitive intensity. Missteps can be detrimental to institutions. An available opportunity that is not capitalized on fully or a threat that is overlooked or mishandled can have detrimental effects on the viability of healthcare establishments [2, 6, 10–12]. This places a premium on making good decisions, necessitating a thorough understanding of the fundamentals and practices of decision-making. This chapter directs attention to the vital area of decision-making in health and medicine, permitting healthcare providers opportunities to build associated prowess for the benefit of their institutions and patients.

5.2 Defining Decision-Making

Decision-making is the process of selecting a course of action from among available alternatives for purposes of addressing a particular matter or concern. It is one of the primary responsibilities held by managers, occupying a significant portion of their time, regardless of their level within institutional hierarchies. Nonmanagerial employees also are responsible for making many decisions, albeit at much more limited capacities than that of managers, illustrating the impact of decision-making across institutions. Decision-making can occur on virtually any front (e.g., strategic or tactical, clinical or administrative) and involve any degree of magnitude (e.g., simple or complex, departmental or systemwide, urgent or nonurgent). As the scenarios provided earlier illustrate, matters and concerns requiring decisions are constants of organizational life, and they are highly varied [2, 7, 13–15]. The task of "deciding" is just as pervasive in organizations as the task of "doing" [16]. Decision-making, in fact, is such an integral part of the practice of management that it has been suggested that management *is* decision-making [17].

A **decision** is the result of decision-making, reflecting the particular choice that was made. The alternative selected generally represents the best solution available under given circumstances, making a decision, in many respects, a matter of compromise. Decisions are based on a multitude of facts, values, conditions, and constraints [16]. Decisions ultimately drive healthcare organizations, with each choice effectively serving as a footstep which ideally is placed on a proper and productive pathway pointing toward the fulfillment of designated missions. Together, they determine the ultimate trajectory of the organization, with collections of good decisions generally yielding desirable outcomes and collections of bad decisions generally yielding undesirable outcomes. In some cases, however, even when most decisions have been prudent, a few bad choices—or even a single one—can be detrimental [18]. Consider the case where a hospital decides to merge with another yet finds that the organizational cultures are completely incompatible, leading to discontent that sees patient populations dwindle and failure loom. Healthcare providers must consistently make high-quality decisions in order to best position their establishments for success. And given that many parties are responsible for making decisions within health and medical institutions, decision-making skills and abilities must be widely distributed within healthcare establishments.

5.3 Types of Decisions

Many systems for categorizing decisions exist. Among these, the typology offered by Nobel laureate and administrative theorist Herbert Simon is perhaps the most widely circulated. Simon divided decisions into two types: programmed decisions and nonprogrammed decisions [19, 20]. This basic classification system aids in compartmentalizing the practice of decision-making and serves as an excellent starting point for developing associated knowledge.

When matters or concerns impacting institutions appear on a regular basis, it is very common for establishments to develop **decision rules** for handling them. Such rules permit matters which are encountered often to be addressed in a formulaic, planned fashion, with the resulting choices being termed **programmed decisions** [19–21]. Essentially, whenever a situation governed by a decision rule is encountered, a programmed decision appropriate for the given situation is prescribed, hastening decision-making and ensuring consistency in addressing routinely encountered matters and concerns. Programmed decisions are typically formulated for matters which are frequent, repetitive, and routine, with high degrees of certainty regarding associated cause-and-effect relationships [17]. Procedures for making these decisions are rigorously vetted and clearly defined. Due to their highly structured nature, programmed decisions can be made by managers throughout institutional hierarchies, as resulting decisions are guided by established rules and practices [21].

Programmed decisions in the healthcare industry are numerous. Certainly for clinical matters, such decisions are arguably more extensive than that witnessed in other industries, given the regimented practices associated with the delivery of health and medicine [2, 22]. Procedures for handling a patient's admission into a hospital's emergency department, for example, are highly structured, predetermined practices, guiding a range of decisions, formulated based on routine situations encountered. Credentialing physicians, ordering medical equipment and supplies, recruiting and selecting employees, scheduling advertising and other forms of promotion, cleaning and sanitizing patient rooms, and discharging patients from their care experiences all constitute occurrences happening with such regularity that standard protocols for making associated choices exist. Programmed decisions indeed are well understood by the employees charged with carrying them out [17, 20, 21]. They may or may not be reduced to writing in the form of an operations manual or similar publication. Even if not formally documented, though, decision rules associated with routine matters encountered are common knowledge to staff members, transferred between and among employees through socialization, on-the-job training, and similar methods.

Sometimes matters and concerns experienced by organizations fall outside of the routine, necessitating what are known as **nonprogrammed decisions**. In these cases, there are no established decision rules governing how to go about addressing the given issues. When these situations are encountered, problem-solving is required. **Problem-solving** is a particular form of decision-making called upon when situations encountered are unique, requiring alternatives to be formulated and evaluated without the aid of decision rules [20, 21]. The particular situations could be rarely or never before experienced, or they could be of very high importance or extreme complexity. As such, special treatment is warranted. Nonprogrammed decisions are typically called for when encountering novel, unstructured problems, with high degrees of uncertainty regarding associated cause-and-effect relationships. Creativity, intuition, and judgment are vital for resolving associated matters and concerns [17, 21]. Given their unique properties, nonprogrammed decisions are the domain of those occupying upper management [21].

The impact of the COVID-19 pandemic on healthcare institutions serves as one of the best examples to illustrate nonprogrammed decisions. Given the novel characteristics of the virus, healthcare providers had very little to go on during the early stages of the pandemic, forcing them to improvise in initial days, weeks, and months. Operations also were upended, with healthcare providers being notably forced to cancel elective procedures, generating scores of issues for which they did not have a playbook. In time, procedures for handling COVID-19 patients and related operational matters emerged, resulting largely from trial-and-error and the sharing of best practices, and associated decisions began to enter the realm of the routine. Nonroutine matters, however, typically are not as profound as the COVID-19 pandemic but instead occur from time to time over the course of organizational life. Receiving an acquisition offer from a competitor, introducing a new service line, constructing a new medical campus, purchasing expensive medical technologies, and the like are not everyday occurrences, and, as such, are not typically covered by decision rules, necessitating the problem-solving orientation required when making nonprogrammed decisions.

5.4 Individual and Group Decision-Making

Decision-making very often is viewed to be an individual effort, and, many times, that is the case. Programmed decisions typically are handled at the individual level, as decision rules guide associated choices. In many respects, these decisions could be said to be the product of a group, albeit with the group interjecting itself through rules developed prior to the actual decision being made by a sole individual. In the case of nonprogrammed decisions, however, decision-making often resides in the hands of active, real-time groups, typically composed of individuals occupying upper management ranks, as the novelty and complexity of the circumstances faced require insights from multiple, experienced parties [17]. The process of decision-making is essentially the same whether conducted by individuals or groups. This is because groups typically operate in concert, permitting them to be treated as a unit, allowing the group decision-making process to parallel the individual one [23].

Although groups often operate as unified collections of people, group members usually do not shed their individuality but instead direct it collectively toward resolving the problem at hand [23]. Groups typically take more time than individuals to make a decision, but the result of collective efforts tends to be better than that afforded by singular efforts. This is due to multiple minds being directed in unison toward the matter or concern [17]. While decision outcomes can be enhanced by groups, care must be taken to avoid traps that effectively see groups operate as individuals. One particular occurrence is known as **groupthink**, a phenomenon where group members opt to go along with a particular course of action in an effort to maintain consensus rather than engage in sufficient debate to thoroughly vet the pathway under consideration. When this occurs, the benefits that groups are capable of deriving through their diverse perspectives are diminished, reducing the potential of group decision-making. Such hindrances can be avoided, however, by following common practices designed to foster productive group communications, such as encouraging active participation and issuing assurances that all opinions are valued. Safeguards such as decision oversight and decision-making protocols also can be put into place by organizations, ensuring that decision-making remains orderly and free of distortion [24–30].

5.5   Behavioral Influences on Decision-Making

Decision-making is heavily influenced by a number of behavioral qualities, including intuition, judgment, ethics, risk orientation, and creativity. **Intuition** is defined as the ability to instinctively understand something without the application of conscious reasoning [25]. Whenever one makes a decision based on a "gut feeling," the individual effectively is using intuition in decision-making. It often is called for in situations when time constraints prohibit detailed analyses of options, forcing quick decisions. Intuition also is frequently used in situations of high uncertainty and extreme complexity [17]. Intuition often complements, and sometimes even overtakes, logic when making decisions.

Judgment refers to the ability to draw sound conclusions after assessing and evaluating a particular matter or concern. For obvious reasons, excellent judgment is a foundational requirement of good decision-making. Every step of the decision-making process requires discernment, making judgment essential. Just like intuition, judgment is the product of knowledge and experience. In abundance, and with common sense fully deployed, it has the potential to amplify decision-making and resulting decision outcomes [17].

Ethics are moral principles, values, and beliefs which govern the actions and behaviors of individuals, with associated mindsets providing them with guidance regarding what is good or bad and right or wrong. Human life necessitates that one exercises judgment on an ongoing basis, comparing alternative courses of action when facing particular situations and scenarios and deciding on proper pathways to pursue. Through one's sense of ethics, these decisions are made [31, 32]. Applied in organizational settings, ethics are sometimes termed **business ethics** or **managerial ethics**, acknowledging the institutional context of associated judgments and decisions [33, 34]. Expectations are higher than ever for healthcare organizations to operate in a manner guided by a high sense of ethics, following moral standards, as defined by society. Importantly, the ethics of decision-makers must be aligned with those of their employing organizations, ensuring that proper choices conforming with institutional wishes and desires are made.

Another characteristic that must be aligned between decision-makers and their respective organizations is that of risk orientation. **Risk orientation** is defined as the degree of risk an individual or institution is comfortable accepting [17]. A classic example to illustrate risk orientation concerns the approaches of newly established and seasoned healthcare organizations. Those that are newly established typically assume a very entrepreneurial orientation which involves taking chances. Risk assumption is on the high side. This is contrasted with mature healthcare institutions which, already having established their reputations, operate in a more risk-averse manner. As all decisions carry risk, one's risk orientation will influence resulting choices. Risk assumption, up to a point, can be beneficial, but there are limits which, if breached, can lead to catastrophe. Derailment can be seen in behavioral propensities such as **escalation of commitment** which occurs when an individual continues to direct resources to a particular course of action even after its failure becomes obvious and imminent [17, 35]. Assumption of risk is a slippery slope which must be kept in check.

Creativity is defined as the ability to address problems in a novel, imaginative fashion. This involves "outside of the box" thinking that sidesteps status quo approaches in favor of new ones with the potential to yield better decisions and resulting outcomes. Creativity sometimes can be difficult to generate, prompting methods to stimulate fresh perspectives, insights, and approaches. One of the most common techniques for such is that of **brainstorming**, group discussions aimed at generating ideas or solving problems. Ideas brought forth during brainstorming sessions typically beget more ideas as discussions proceed and multiple parties interject their thoughts and opinions, vastly increasing the prospects of generating useful perspectives that can benefit decision-making. A variant of brainstorming, known as the **nominal group technique** (**NGT**), also can be tapped. With this method, members of a decision group prepare individual responses to a moderator's questions on a topic of concern, after which they are shared collectively and ranked by the group. This approach prevents a common problem that can occur in brainstorming where discussions are dominated by one or several members. It also prevents some members from avoiding participation, as insights are required from all, leading to enriched perspectives that can enlighten decision-making [24, 35, 36].

Insights from outsiders also can be helpful for fostering creativity. One method that permits this is known as the **Delphi technique**. With this technique, a panel of experts is surveyed, typically through multiple rounds which permit a running dialogue between the decision-makers and the expert panel, for insights regarding a particular decision matter. The external perspectives breathe life into what ordinarily would be limited to an internal discussion, potentially offering new and different perspectives shedding light on topics of inquiry. Ultimately, the insights provided by the expert panel help decision-makers shape and hone their approach for addressing the decision at hand [21, 24]. Perhaps more simply, external ideas can be acquired by scheduling **expert consultations**, meetings with thought leaders for purposes of soliciting advice or insights regarding a topic of concern. Decision-makers would simply schedule a meeting with a recognized authority on the decision matter at hand and inquire about how he or she would address the matter. If desired, this expert opinion could be complemented by other consultations, giving decision-makers a range of perspectives from multiple, independent sources. Such external, expert perspectives offer great potential for generating creative approaches which might otherwise never come to light through internal discussions alone, improving decision-making, resulting decisions, and associated outcomes.

5.6 Rational Decision-Making

Decision-making, in its ideal state, follows a coherent and comprehensive process designed to maximize outcomes through the examination and evaluation of all available alternatives [35]. This particular approach is known as **rational**

decision-making. It is characterized by its adherence to a logical process, pursued through an objective lens, influenced by complete information [21]. The rational decision-making approach is most applicable to nonprogrammed decisions, as decision rules are not available which otherwise would provide guidance, as in the case of programmed decisions. Without such rules, the entirety of the decision-making process is needed to make sense of things and select an appropriate course of action [17].

The rational decision-making process consists of six sequential steps. Decision-makers must define the problem, develop comprehensive alternatives, evaluate alternatives, select the best alternative (i.e., make the decision), implement the decision, and evaluate outcomes. In its purest, most rigorously defined form, rational decision-making is unrealistic, given that it requires perfect information, complete objectivity, and strict adherence to logic. These things are beyond the capacity of human ability and reason. Due to inherent limitations, humans never have more than a fragmentary knowledge of the events and circumstances surrounding a course of action [16]. Most modern theories of rational decision-making, however, incorporate modifications that relax the assumptions which characterize the pure conception of rationality [23]. Regardless, there is value in understanding the rational approach for its orderly treatment of the decision-making process. Following such a process, even factoring in the prospect of human imperfections, can help decision-makers realize better outcomes than would be possible without the benefit of a systematic approach. The steps of the rational decision-making process are profiled in following sections.

5.6.1 Step 1: Define the Problem

The rational decision-making process begins when a problem is identified, indicating a discrepancy between a desired state and current reality [17]. A solution is needed to close this gap, moving an institution from where it is today to where it wants to be tomorrow [24]. Gaps appear regularly in healthcare establishments. Some scenarios are quite common: patient growth exceeds capacity, a physician announces his retirement, patients demand a new service, signage throughout the facility is inadequate, and patient satisfaction scores are not high enough. These and similar examples each indicate problems which must be addressed by healthcare providers, prompting decision-making pursuits. In the course of defining problems, organizations must seek to understand applicable matters and concerns accurately and comprehensively, with this placing a premium on quality information [21]. Great care must be taken, as errors introduced here will have a domino effect on all other steps, potentially leading to decisions which do not close gaps. A complete understanding of the problem should be sought, informing subsequent steps and setting the course for problem resolution.

5.6.2   Step 2: Develop Comprehensive Alternatives

After defining the problem, a comprehensive list of **alternatives**—potential solutions for the problem experienced—must be identified, with this step effectively constituting a search process [16, 17]. The alternatives available to address a given problem typically are numerous, with some being more feasible than others. At this stage, the goal is to populate a thorough and complete list of alternatives viewed to be capable of successfully addressing the problem at hand [25]. Suppose a hospital experiences rapid growth, so much so that its current location can no longer accommodate patient volume, necessitating expansion of its capacity. Potential alternatives might include expanding the size of the current facility, building a new facility to complement the existing one, pursuing an adaptive reuse option by purchasing an existing building and renovating it to complement the existing one, and similar avenues permitting patient volume to be accommodated.

On deeper exploration of these broad pathways, further alternatives typically will come to light, which often is the case as the search process advances. The prospect of building a new facility to complement the existing one, for example, would alone entail significant considerations regarding things such as location, capacity, and service mix. Even merely expanding the current facility would beget many questions, including determining the proper scale, architectural design and layout, and much more. During this particular step, broad and deep perspectives are needed, requiring decision-makers to tap intensively into their own education and experience and also solicit insights from others within and outside of their given institutions to build comprehensive options [21].

5.6.3   Step 3: Evaluate Alternatives

With a range of alternatives presented, the next step of the rational decision-making process involves examining the options discovered. Alternatives differ in terms of the consequences flowing from them, and these consequences must be clearly understood in order for an optimal decision to be made [16]. Each alternative should be examined to ascertain its potential for closing the gap between actual and desired states, resolving the associated problem [21]. This step involves significant fact-finding work to acquire sufficient information to permit proper vetting of potential solutions. Items of analysis commonly include the efficacy, costs, benefits, and risks associated with each noted pathway. Decision-makers must endeavor to understand the consequences associated with each alternative [16].

In the case of the hospital in need of expansion, as presented earlier, the range of options derived certainly will require intelligence from architects, engineers, commercial real estate specialists, and industrial planners, complementing the education and experience of the hospital's management team. The resulting pool of knowledge will allow the hospital's staff to fully flesh out each alternative. Determining the viability of options accurately is essential, as failures here can lead to inappropriate selections being made, destroying the benefits that otherwise could be gained from the decision-making process. By the end of this step, a complete array of alternatives, coupled with comprehensive results from their associated evaluations, should be available for review and reflection.

5.6.4 Step 4: Select the Best Alternative (i.e., Make the Decision)

Selection of the best alternative entails making the actual decision, and as such, it often is considered to be the most crucial step of the rational decision-making process [17]. This step requires the identification of the pathway deemed by objective analyses to deliver the top result, resolving the defined problem more effectively than competing alternatives. Essentially, the consequences associated with each option are compared, with a selection following [16]. The goal of rational decision-making is to **maximize**, that is, choose the best alternative possible [23]. In addition to stipulating a choice, this step represents an opportune time to make contingency plans, given that comprehensive analyses and evaluations of multiple alternatives have just been completed. Designating a course of action on which to fall back in the event that a selection does not have its intended impact makes sense [21]. Doing so is a risk-averse move that can conserve resources if problems are not resolved as planned.

Making the actual choice, as this step requires, would seem to be a simple, straightforward assignment, but it can prove to be difficult, especially in some circumstances. For example, selection can be complicated in scenarios where two or more options appear to be equivalently optimal [21]. The hospital portrayed earlier might discover that expansion of its current campus appears to be equivalently attractive to an adaptive reuse alternative involving the renovation and repurposement of an existing building located nearby. In such cases, additional information should be sought in an effort to break the tie, revealing the superior choice. The hospital might, for example, find that the adaptive reuse alternative offers future growth opportunities beyond those afforded by the expansion of its current site, giving that particular option an edge.

Sometimes it is discovered that a single alternative will not fully resolve the problem, warranting consideration of a combined approach involving the selection of multiple alternatives to fully close gaps [21]. In the hospital scenario, patient growth might be so remarkable that the establishment decides to pursue both the expansion of its current site and the adaptive reuse option of renovation and repurposement of an existing building to wholly meet patient volume demands. Despite the best of intentions, occasionally decision-makers will find that none of the alternatives are found to properly address the problem. In such cases, retracement of one or more steps of the decision-making process or even its entire reinitiation is warranted in order to resolve matters. Essentially, if a selection is not clear, decision-makers must go back to the drawing board to identify more suitable options.

5.6.5 Step 5: Implement the Decision

Implementation follows selection of the best alternative, with this step effectively operationalizing the decision. Quality of implementation is paramount, as even if the decision is optimal, poor enaction can be detrimental to its success [17]. Sound implementation involves excellent resource utilization and management prowess [21]. The more complex the decision, the more essential the need for oversight in its operationalization. Continuing the hospital example as presented earlier, the expansion of capacity, regardless of form, would involve significant resource outlays and likely require a fairly lengthy timeline for completion. Such characteristics have the potential to complicate the implementation process, prompting high levels of managerial attention. Great care must be taken to ensure a prudent and effective rollout of the selected choice.

5.6.6 Step 6: Evaluate Outcomes

The final step in the rational decision-making process involves the evaluation of outcomes, notably entailing determining whether the gap between current and desired states has been narrowed or ideally eliminated [25]. Consequences of decisions can be revealed quickly or take quite some time, depending on the nature of the matter addressed and prevailing environmental circumstances. Managers cannot assume that on making decisions, outcomes will be as intended and desired, warranting careful scrutiny [17]. Post-decision surprises, which can be pleasant or unpleasant, are part of decision-making. Also possible is that of post-decision regret, as it is very typical for the consequences of decisions to reveal that better choices could have been made if outcomes could have been better envisioned [23]. Once outcomes are known, it is helpful to reflect on them in the context of the decision-making process for insights which can aid future decision-making pursuits.

In the case of the running hospital example, the operative inquiry during this step involves determining if the choice made successfully accommodated the burgeoning patient volume which prompted the decision-making pursuit. If it is discovered that the selected alternative did not work as well as intended or not at all, steps must be taken to resolve the matter [24]. This could involve making minor adjustments to better operationalize the selected option, it could entail comprehensive revisions to the selected approach, or call for the abandonment of the decision altogether. If especially negative outcomes are experienced, contingency plans, if available, could be put into place, or the decision-making process could be initiated once again, aided by knowledge gained from the first round. If, however, the selected choice proves to be successful, the rational decision-making process draws to a close.

5.7 Bounded Rationality

Modern perspectives of decision-making largely consider the rational decision-making approach to be unrealistic, failing to reflect the way that decisions actually are made. Pure versions of rational choice simply do not make for credible portraits of decision-making in practice. Human ability and reasoning are limited, thus limiting rationality in decision-making [23]. Knowledge is fragmentary, restricting acquisition of a complete understanding of the consequences of each available choice. Further, only a fraction of the available alternatives capable of addressing a problem are considered in real-world decision-making. As such, even an approximation to objective rationality is difficult to imagine. Decision-making in real-world applications therefore is the product of **bounded rationality**, rationality which is limited and imperfect [16, 23].

Bounded rationality is known as a **behavioral approach to decision-making**, as it acknowledges the role of human behavior in the decision-making process, notably factoring in real-world managerial actions, activities, and constraints [21]. It is also known as **administrative decision-making**, as it reflects the decision-making approach of the executive or manager as used in actual practice. Bounded rationality does not seek maximization in decision-making but instead opts to **satisfice**, pursuing an avenue that is satisfactory or "good enough," rather than one deemed to be the best possible. Satisficing permits choice to occur without the need to examine all possible alternatives. Essentially, once a fitting alternative is discovered, the further search for alternatives ceases and the decision is made [23]. In the running hospital example, decision-makers would be said to be satisficing if, in their quest to find a solution capable of addressing burgeoning patient volume, they examined the prospect of expanding the current building, discovered that the option would satisfactorily accommodate capacity, and made the selection without investigating additional alternatives. The acceptable, "good enough" choice—expanding the current building—would be pursued, despite the prospect of identifying a superior course of action through more detailed efforts to formulate and examine alternatives.

The decision-making process under bounded rationality is similar to that of rational decision-making with several key differences acknowledging human limitations, incorporating the practice of satisficing. Under bounded rationality, decision-makers define the problem, seek an alternative believed to be capable of satisfactorily addressing the problem, evaluate the alternative to ensure merit, select the alternative (i.e., make the decision), implement the decision, and evaluate outcomes. Bounded rationality and satisficing infuse realism into the rational decision-making process, acknowledging the limitations on rationality courtesy of the human condition [16, 20]. It does not suggest a reckless, uninformed approach. Decision-makers, regardless of situation faced, should strive to make the best possible decision, being informed as much as reasonably possible, as they go about making choices [26]. Bounded rationality simply acknowledges human limitations and, as such, better represents the manner in which decisions actually are made in practice [16, 20].

WK Reflections: Attacking Decisions

As referenced earlier in the chapter, vetting of prospective decisions is a very important activity. Many techniques for doing so exist, with most centering on some sort of evaluative reflection designed to ensure that a prudent selection is made before moving forward with a given decision. One particularly useful and memorable method for vetting prospective decisions is to attack them. As the technique's descriptor suggests, it involves attacking the decision under evaluation by lobbing arguments against its implementation, criticizing its pursuit, tearing away at its underlying assumptions, and engaging in like activities for purposes of revealing any weaknesses or vulnerabilities that might suggest a better course of action for addressing the matter at hand. The concept of attacking oneself has been used in other contexts, such as marketing, with the approach typically being conducted for purposes of revealing opportunities for improvement [11, 37]. The strategy ultimately is used in the same fashion in decision-making to test the merit of anticipated decisions.

Several outcomes are possible when attacking decisions. If the attacks successfully undermine the planned course of action, the intended decision can simply be discarded in favor of something else. Attacks also can reveal the need for minor modifications to be made to decisions under evaluation, improving their prospects for viability when implemented. And, of course, attacks also can indicate that particular courses of action indeed are ready for implementation in their current state. In Willis Knighton Health's experience, attacks rarely have suggested discarding given decisions, due largely to great care being taken whenever decisions are at hand, with such care serving as somewhat of an ongoing vetting process. Attacks, however, have on occasion indicated the need for slight modifications to decisions which ultimately amplified their ability to deliver desired results. And due to intensive efforts and good fortune, Willis Knighton Health has witnessed many of its decisions survive attacks without any need for modification.

Recall also the earlier guidance referencing the need for contingency plans to be developed whenever making decisions. Quite handily, the strategy of attacking decisions offers an ideal opportunity for decision-makers to incorporate this into the decision-making process, as the attack provides a brief pause on the eve of implementation to consider what might be done if things do not go according to plan. What happens if given decisions go awry? Formulating options can be most helpful. When Willis Knighton Health made the decision to purchase Doctors' Hospital, as described earlier in the chapter, the results of the decision attack suggested viability. However, the activity of attacking the decision also gave executives the opportunity to plan alternatives should the building prove to be unsuitable for healthcare operations, with conversion into a hotel or an apartment building representing the chief contingency plan. Fortunately, fallbacks were not necessary, as the decision went according to plan, resulting in Willis Knighton Rehabilitation. Still, it was nice having a safety valve, something that is most helpful whenever facing uncertainty.

Attacking decisions requires honesty and courage, as at the final stage when a decision essentially has been made but not yet enacted, preferences often are deeply entrenched in the hearts and minds of decision-makers. Criticisms at this late stage can be quite difficult to evoke, but for those brave enough to launch associated attacks, an invaluable, vetting experience is afforded. Healthcare institutions desirous of a useful capstone assessment for decisions certainly should consider the strategy of attacking their anticipated choices.

5.8 Summary and Conclusions

Decision-making is the process of selecting a course of action from among available alternatives for purposes of addressing a particular matter or concern. It is one of the primary responsibilities held by managers, occupying a significant portion of their time, regardless of their level within institutional hierarchies. Decisions have the potential to profoundly impact health and medical establishments. This impact can be positive, in cases where good decisions are made, or negative, in cases where bad decisions are made. Given the competitive nature of the healthcare industry, constantly changing environments, and sensitivities associated with delivering health and medicine, healthcare providers must be extremely careful to avoid missteps associated with poor choices. As such, they must strive to consistently make good decisions that collectively plot clear and expedient pathways toward mission fulfillment. Improved decision-making begins with acquiring a thorough understanding of the concept. Associated knowledge can help to guide healthcare managers as they go about making decisions on behalf of their given establishments, bolstering their potential to make choices which advance operations and foster excellence in the delivery of health and medicine.

Key Terms

- Administrative Decision-Making
- Alternatives
- Behavioral Approach to Decision-Making
- Bounded Rationality
- Brainstorming
- Business Ethics
- Creativity
- Decision
- Decision-Making
- Decision Rules
- Delphi Technique
- Escalation of Commitment
- Ethics
- Expert Consultations
- Groupthink
- Intuition
- Judgment
- Managerial Ethics
- Maximize
- Nominal Group Technique (NGT)
- Nonprogrammed Decision
- Problem-Solving
- Programmed Decision
- Rational Decision-Making
- Risk Orientation
- Satisfice

Exercises

1. In your own words, define decision-making, and discuss why it is vital in health and medical institutions.
2. Compare and contrast programmed decisions and nonprogrammed decisions. Reflect on your recent work experiences, and provide an example of a programmed decision and a nonprogrammed decision.
3. Outline the rational decision-making process and profile each of its steps. Describe why the process does not reflect decision-making as it is practiced in real-world settings in health and medicine.
4. Define bounded rationality, distinguish it from rational decision-making, and indicate how it better portrays decision-making in actual practice. What steps would you suggest to improve decision-making in light of the fact that rationality is limited?

5. Describe a situation where you satisficed and indicate what circumstances led you to take this course of action rather than attempt to maximize.
6. Provide a brief overview of individual and group decision-making. Although both types are required in healthcare organizations, do you prefer to make decisions alone or with the aid of others? Why?
7. Define the concept of intuition and discuss its role in decision-making. How might intuition help decision-making, and how might it harm decision-making? What advice would you offer for keeping the use of intuition in check, ensuring that it helps rather than harms decision-making?
8. Discuss methods for bolstering creativity in the decision-making processes of healthcare organizations. Which technique do you most prefer and why?

References

1. Elrod, J. K., & Fortenberry, J. L., Jr. (2017). Adaptive reuse in the healthcare industry: Repurposing abandoned buildings to serve medical missions. *BMC Health Services Research, 17*(Suppl 1), 5–14.
2. Elrod, J. K. (2013). *Breadcrumbs to cheesecake*. R&R Publishers.
3. Shi, L., & Singh, D. A. (2023). *Essentials of the US health care system* (6th ed.). Jones and Bartlett.
4. Walston, S. L., & Johnson, K. L. (2021). *Healthcare in the United States: Clinical, financial, and operational dimensions*. Health Administration Press.
5. McConnell, C. R. (2020). *Hospitals and health systems: What they are and how they work.* Jones and Bartlett.
6. Ginter, P. M., Duncan, W. J., & Swayne, L. E. (2013). *Strategic management of health care organizations* (7th ed.). Jossey-Bass.
7. Robbins, S. P., & Judge, T. A. (2019). *Organizational behavior* (18th ed.). Pearson.
8. Krogerus, M., & Tschappeler, R. (2012). *The decision book: Fifty models for strategic thinking.* W. W. Norton.
9. Bazerman, M. H., & Moore, D. A. (2013). *Judgment in managerial decision making* (8th ed.). Wiley.
10. Kotler, P., Stevens, R. J., & Shalowitz, J. (2021). *Strategic marketing for health care organizations: Building a customer-driven health system* (2nd ed.). Wiley.
11. Fortenberry, J. L., Jr. (2010). *Health care marketing: Tools and techniques* (3rd ed.). Jones and Bartlett.
12. Hillestad, S. G., & Berkowitz, E. N. (2020). *Health care market strategy: From planning to action* (5th ed.). Jones and Bartlett.
13. Buchanan, L., & O'Connell, A. (2006). A brief history of decision making. *Harvard Business Review, 84*(1), 32–41.
14. Garvin, D. A., & Roberto, M. A. (2001). What you don't know about making decisions. *Harvard Business Review, 79*(8), 108–116.
15. Davenport, T. H. (2009). Make better decisions. *Harvard Business Review, 87*(11), 117–123.
16. Simon, H. A. (1997). *Administrative behavior: A study of decision-making processes in administrative organizations* (4th ed.). The Free Press.
17. Konopaske, R., Ivancevich, J. M., & Matteson, M. T. (2018). *Organizational behavior and management* (11th ed.). McGraw-Hill.
18. Hammond, J. S., Keeney, R. L., & Raiffa, H. (2006). The hidden traps in decision making. *Harvard Business Review, 84*(1), 118–126.

19. Shafritz, J. M., Ott, J. S., & Jang, Y. S. (Eds.). (2016). *Classics of organization theory* (8th ed.). Cengage.
20. Simon, H. A. (1977). *The new science of management decision* (Rev. ed.). Prentice Hall.
21. Griffin, R. W., Phillips, J. M., & Gully, S. M. (2020). *Organizational behavior: Managing people and organizations* (13th ed.). Cengage.
22. Pfeffer, J., & Sutton, R. I. (2006). Evidence-based management. *Harvard Business Review, 84*(1), 62–74.
23. March, J. G. (1994). *A primer on decision making: How decisions happen.* The Free Press.
24. Hitt, M. A., Miller, C. C., Colella, A., & Triana, M. D. C. (2018). *Organizational behavior* (5th ed.). Wiley.
25. McShane, S. L., & Von Glinow, M. A. (2019). *Organizational behavior* (4th ed.). McGraw-Hill.
26. Bazerman, M. H., & Chugh, D. (2006). Decisions without blinders. *Harvard Business Review, 84*(1), 88–97.
27. Janis, I. L. (2016). Groupthink: The desperate drive for consensus at any cost. In J. M. Shafritz, J. S. Ott, & Y. S. Jang (Eds.), *Classics of organization theory* (8th ed., pp. 161–168). Cengage.
28. Janis, I. L. (1982). *Groupthink: Psychological studies of policy decisions and fiascoes* (2nd ed.). Cengage.
29. Campbell, A., Whitehead, J., & Finkelstein, S. (2009). Why good leaders make bad decisions. *Harvard Business Review, 87*(2), 60–66.
30. Charan, R. (2006). Conquering a culture of indecision. *Harvard Business Review, 84*(1), 108–117.
31. Daft, R. L. (2022). *Management* (14th ed.). Cengage.
32. Ferrell, O. C., Fraedrich, J., & Ferrell, L. (2019). *Business ethics: Ethical decision making and cases* (12th ed.). Cengage.
33. Collins, D. (2019). *Business ethics: Best practices for designing and managing ethical organizations* (2nd ed.). Sage.
34. Griffin, R. W. (2022). *Management* (13th ed.). Cengage.
35. Colquitt, J. A., Lepine, J. A., & Wesson, M. J. (2019). *Organizational behavior: Improving performance and commitment in the workplace* (6th ed.). McGraw-Hill.
36. Kinicki, A., & Fugate, M. (2018). *Organizational behavior: A practical, problem-solving approach* (2nd ed.). McGraw-Hill.
37. Ries, A., & Trout, J. (1986). *Marketing warfare.* McGraw-Hill.

Chapter 6
Strategy in Health and Medicine

Learning Objectives

After examining this chapter, readers will have the ability to:

- Define strategy, understand its role in advancing institutional goals and objectives, and realize its impact on activities and operations across healthcare establishments.
- Define competitive advantage, indicate why healthcare institutions must pursue them, and discuss the role of strategy in their acquisition.
- Define mission statement, vision statement, and values statement, understand the roles played by each, and discuss methods for their assembly in health and medicine.
- Compare and contrast macroenvironments and microenvironments, identify common tools and techniques for their assessment and evaluation, and discuss how they respectively impact healthcare organizations.
- Outline the strategy process, discuss each of its three stages, and describe why its mastery is vital for success in the healthcare industry.
- Compare and contrast intended strategies and emergent strategies, and discuss the pathways and circumstances which lead to their appearance in healthcare establishments.
- Discuss the concept of strategic thinking, outline its key benefits, and describe avenues which can be used by healthcare managers to develop their abilities in this important area.

J. K. Elrod, J. L. Fortenberry, Jr., *Organizational Behavior and Management in Health and Medicine*, https://doi.org/10.1007/978-3-031-61823-9_6

WK Reflections: Improving Strategy by Keeping Patients at the Top of Mind

When one reflects on the concept of strategy, images of business-oriented practices and processes invariably come to mind. Formulating mission statements for healthcare establishments, determining their overall direction, selecting medical service arrays to be offered, formulating plans to capture market share, orchestrating plans to ensure the delivery of high-quality patient experiences, monitoring the environment in order to identify opportunities and threats, and the like are all common pursuits falling under the auspices of strategy. These types of endeavors clearly fall in the realm of business. Of course, strategy pursuits are required of any organization, even those focused on delivering health and medicine, with associated decisions and actions dramatically impacting the current and future viability of given establishments. But special care must be taken by healthcare managers as they go about addressing matters of strategy.

Sometimes, when dealing with the pressing concerns associated with strategy, sensitivity to patients and their associated wants and needs can be lost, being crowded out by bottom-line matters and similar concerns impacting healthcare organizations. This can occur intentionally when managers simply do not respect the delicate nature of health services delivery, situations which must be rectified immediately by healthcare establishments. But very often, waning sensitivity to patients happens unintentionally, being driven by the rigors of daily organizational life where multiple issues are constantly competing for the attention of managers, resulting in distractions, fatigue, and lost focus. Strategy matters are especially burdensome, as they involve concerns of the highest magnitude in health and medical establishments, handled predominantly by the top executives of healthcare institutions. Pressures abound, as would be expected in any complex organizational setting, and these pressures, if not kept in check, can see a detachment between the strategist and the patient. This, in turn, sets the stage for suboptimal decisions that fail to keep patients at the forefront of thought and action [1, 2].

While the business of healthcare must be addressed in health and medical organizations, such concerns should never cause healthcare managers to lose sight of the ultimate reason their organizations exist, namely, to serve patients and serve them well. In fact, it could be argued that it is all the more important to keep patients at the top of mind during the strategy process, as matters of strategy are far-reaching, often impacting healthcare organizations in their entirety. But how are those involved in strategy to do this, given the typical pressures associated with handling the strategic affairs of healthcare institutions? The answer rests with managers developing a conscious awareness of the need to focus on patients as they address matters of strategy within their healthcare organizations. Achieving this vital perspective ultimately is up to those holding responsibilities for managing strategy, but healthcare organizations, too, bear responsibility in developing and perpetuating such an essential mindset within their given institutions [1, 2].

Willis Knighton Health addressed this complex matter in a rather simple but highly effective fashion, by actively encouraging its executives to see themselves and their actions from the perspective of patients. Specifically, they are encouraged to reflect on their actions in real time, asking themselves the following question: "Am I seeing things through the eyes of patients?" On the surface, such an inquiry might seem to be profoundly rudimentary, but one must remember that distractions are ever-present in organizational life and can cause even the most dedicated employee to lose focus. Sometimes the focus can become too intense, causing the big picture to be missed, with results missing the mark in similar fashion to that of waning or lost focus. A simple reminder to keep patients at the forefront of one's mind, conveyed routinely during employee orientations, department meetings, special events, and other opportunities, often is just enough to help staff members remain patient-centered as they go about performing their work [1].

Notably, maintaining a patient-focused perspective has the potential to improve strategy. When making strategy, opportunities to maximize institutional gains often are discovered, but are they fitting for given healthcare organizations to pursue? Many times, they are not because in some shape, form, or fashion, they generate negative impacts, sometimes at the expense of patients [2]. Consider the scenario faced by a large health system's dietary director who happened to be pursuing a strategy of fleshing out efficiency at every reasonable opportunity. On reviewing a recent proposal from a food vendor, the director noticed that cost savings could be achieved but also observed that the quality of ingredients appeared to be inferior to that of current offerings. Testing of the proposed food items was conducted, ultimately revealing that the taste was not comparable to products already in use. Although budgetary savings could have been enjoyed, the gains achieved financially were outweighed by the potential loss of patient satisfaction, leading the director to reject the more budget-friendly food proposal, despite his quest for efficiency. Business metrics aside, what decision was called for when viewing the matter through the eyes of patients? The answer is quite obvious, with this simple example nicely illustrating how a patient-focused mindset can shape and influence strategy.

Of course, situations sometimes demand that healthcare providers make painful choices, but even in those difficult circumstances, maintaining a genuine understanding of patients and their particular viewpoints can improve decision-making, potentially reducing whatever pain might be necessary. Ultimately, regardless of the environmental issues and circumstances faced by healthcare institutions, strategy can be improved when one places patients at the forefront of thought and action. The simple "Am I seeing things through the eyes of patients?" inquiry can help to ensure that those immersed in healthcare strategy do not inadvertently get caught up in business complexities and become blind to those they have been charged to serve.

6.1 Background

Healthcare establishments operate in what many consider to be the most complex of industries. Hardships indeed are ever-present in health and medical organizations, but this does not deter dedicated providers from accepting these challenges with great enthusiasm, realizing the important role that their establishments play in the lives of patients. Navigating this tumultuous environment requires intensive attention and intricate precision, especially for those occupying top managerial positions, as they ultimately are responsible for the performance of their respective establishments [2–4]. Operations associated with the delivery of patient care are complex in and of themselves, but this is all the more the case when one factors in the constant threat posed by competitors in the marketplace, ever-changing policies which impact operations, perennial staffing challenges which must be overcome in order to properly address patients, and much more [5–8]. Given the hardships and uncertainties which typify the environments in which health and medical institutions operate, healthcare providers must be astutely aware of their designated missions and associated aspirations and be capable of directing operations in a manner leading to success on all fronts [3, 6, 9].

In many respects, healthcare institutions could be said to be on a journey; they each are seeking to reach a particular destination. Destinations vary greatly between and among institutions as their associated desires, practices, and pursuits are unique. One healthcare organization might, for example, seek to achieve a position of market leadership. Another might desire to be recognized as a beacon of hope for the medically underserved. Still another might wish to become the undisputed authority in a particular area of medicine in the given marketplace. Regardless of destination, healthcare providers must possess advancement capabilities, notably including skills to successfully traverse any and all obstacles encountered. Perhaps most importantly, a roadmap leading to the desired destination must be in hand with reasonable assurances that it indeed will accurately lead the institution to its target [2, 3, 6, 9]. These and related endeavors all fall under the domain of strategy. While not traditionally considered to be a topic of organizational behavior and management, strategy guides many of the components of the discipline. As such, an associated understanding is vital for anyone engaged in organizational behavior and management.

6.2 Defining Strategy

Strategy is defined as a directed course of action which seeks to identify, pursue, and achieve a desired outcome, usually involving the securing of one or more competitive advantages. It typically is long-range in focus and dictates the overall direction of organizations for enduring periods of time [10]. Essentially, strategy stipulates a particular destination and supplies the roadmap for reaching that destination. It involves making decisions regarding what to do and what not to do [2, 6, 11]. Strategy is an essential component of any substantive pursuit within health and medicine. It is demanded in myriad situations, such as when a hospital desires to become the market leader, when a medical clinic wishes to expand its service array, or when a nursing home seeks to improve the service experiences of residents. Success on such fronts requires significant strategic focus and attention, directing efforts especially toward preparation and development, oversight and guidance, and assessment and evaluation, with these pursuits being known as **strategic planning**, **strategic management**, and **strategic analysis**, respectively [10, 12].

Competitive advantage—any attribute or quality possessed by an establishment which gives it an edge over its competitors—is a frequent goal of strategy [3]. Common competitive advantages in health and medicine include market-leading technologies, highly renowned physicians, the most service locations in a particular region, and the quickest admission times. Competitive advantages also can be more subtle but equally differentiating. Things like convenient parking, highly accessible service locations, attractive buildings and grounds, and similar qualities also can serve as competitive advantages. Regardless of type or magnitude of competitive advantage, strategy is required for their acquisition and maintenance [3, 12].

Tactics are action steps which aid in the accomplishment of strategy [6, 10, 13]. The hospital desirous of market leadership might use tactics such as increased advertising expenditures, construction of new facilities in the marketplace, and expansion of services to attract more patients. The medical clinic seeking to bolster services might rely on tactics such as the renovation of buildings to accommodate the delivery of new services, the hiring of physicians and other personnel capable of providing the new offerings, and the purchase of equipment and other technologies permitting the services to be offered. The nursing home desirous of enhancing the experiences of residents might rely on tactics such as upgrading the quality of food provided by dietary services, improving the recreational activities offered onsite, and introducing concierge services, such as personal shopping, dry cleaning, and other convenience features for residents.

Strategy has been a vital pursuit since time immemorial, specifically emerging from ancient military science. This is illustrated perhaps best by *The Art of War* by Sun Tzu, an epic work dating to the fifth century BC which profiled battle planning and provided insights for waging war. Much later, *On War* by Clausewitz, published in 1832, advanced the science of war by profiling strategy and its role in and impact on military conquests [14–16]. These works and many like them paved the way for the development of theory associated with strategy and its application, with this eventually being applied in modern times to business and industry, including operations focused on the delivery of health and medicine. The notion that strategy used in contemporary healthcare establishments originated from the science of war is not so farfetched when one considers the competitive nature of the healthcare industry. In markets far and wide, healthcare establishments vie against rivals, seeking to attract and retain patients. In many respects, this requires institutions to fight for their very survival, as weaknesses and miscalculations will quickly be capitalized on by rivals [3, 9, 17]. Much as military commanders must strategize for victory, so too must healthcare providers. The strategy tools and techniques originally developed for making war have proven to be highly adaptable to competitive healthcare environments. They now are a staple of most any healthcare organization.

6.3   Mission, Vision, and Values

An organization's mission, vision, and values constitute pillars of its strategy. Its **mission** essentially outlines the organization's purpose or reason for being, its **vision** denotes what the establishment desires to become, and its **values** present the mindsets and beliefs which drive its operation. Established at the onset of an organization's life, these facets collectively serve as mechanisms for strategic guidance. An organization's mission, vision, and values typically are enduring, continuing as originally envisioned, or being refined gradually as circumstances and situations change. Major changes in these foundational tenets generally occur in response to monumental events, such as entry into new areas of operation, merger and acquisition activities, and similar pivotal occurrences. Given their lasting qualities and the role that they play in guiding institutions, much care and thought must go into their development. Furthermore, as mission, vision, and values provide a basis for all strategy activities, accuracy is critical as they will be used to determine strategic priorities, select strategies from available alternatives, decide how workplaces and processes will be structured to pursue directives, and render evaluations of associated performance [10, 12, 18].

While an organization's mission, vision, and values are intangible, they enter the realm of tangibility through their presentation in statement form, with these depictions serving to remind employees and other stakeholders of operational approaches and philosophies. These statements frequently are featured in annual reports and employee handbooks, presented on institutional websites, and posted throughout healthcare facilities. They essentially become cultural artifacts as tangible conveyers which express the underlying values and beliefs associated with an organization's culture [19, 20]. Sometimes excerpts of these statements are even placed on business cards, employee badges, or in similar novel locations, aiding in their circulation to employees and others. Broad conveyance is highly desired to make full use of these statements as guidance mechanisms. Definitions, characteristics, and tips for assembling mission, vision, and values statements are presented in following sections.

6.3.1   Mission Statements

A **mission statement** is a document which succinctly stipulates the purpose of an organization. It is used to convey strategic priorities and other institutional characteristics. It is presented in a positive and inspiring fashion to inform and educate employees and other stakeholders about the organization and its aims. Mission statements must be balanced—not too general, not too specific. If they are overly general, they will not be able to provide direction. If they are overly specific, they will be confining, limiting institutional potential. Although variation in length of statement is quite common, organizations should strive to craft mission statements using no more than 100 words. From comprehensive mission statements, organizations often will select a summary mission statement, typically limited to a single phrase or sentence, to facilitate memory and recall by employees. This assists them in keeping mission statements at the top of their minds as they go about conducting their duties and responsibilities. This also can be helpful in situations where recall is tested, for example, when employees are queried by the site teams of healthcare accrediting bodies regarding their knowledge and understanding of their establishment's mission, further motivating succinct statements. Although mission statements are enduring documents, they are not unchangeable. Whenever circumstances warrant, they can and should be modified [10, 12].

Components commonly featured in high-quality mission statements include (1) a profile of the organization and how it is distinguished from others; (2) an overview of the product offerings provided by the organization; (3) a description of the establishment's current and prospective customers; (4) identification of the geographic markets served by the organization; (5) the organization's philosophy of operation, referencing values and beliefs embraced by the establishment; (6) distinctive competencies which afford competitive advantages; and (7) identification of employees and other stakeholders, noting their value in achieving the organization's mission [5]. In assembling these components, when possible, healthcare providers should seek input broadly from across their given organizations, as doing so will aid in assembling an accurate mission statement and also facilitate buy-in from those given the privilege of making contributions to its development.

6.3.2 Vision Statements

A **vision statement** is a document which succinctly presents the aspirations of an organization. It essentially communicates that which an organization intends to become at some point in the future. It nicely complements the mission statement by presenting a vision of tomorrow. The aspirations expressed in vision statements must be achievable but challenging. As with mission statements, vision statements are very brief. Since the content conveyed by vision statements is less than that of mission statements, vision statements are typically shorter, with full versions often being merely a single phrase or single sentence [4, 10, 12]. The approach to writing vision statements is simple and direct. A newly established hospital might, for example, seek "To become the community's leading provider of high-quality medical care." As a start-up in an area featuring existing competitors, market leadership would not currently be held by the hospital, making its achievement a desired future state. Similarly, an eye center which has been competing for years against other area ophthalmology practices using essentially parallel technologies might desire to leapfrog rivals by endeavoring to feature the most advanced technologies available in the vicinity. In keeping with this aspiration, the eye center might adopt the following vision statement: "To establish ourselves as the premier provider of ophthalmologic technology and innovation in the region." This vision might see the practice slowly begin to acquire novel capabilities over time, permitting realization of leadership on this front at some point in the future. As with mission statements, when possible, organization-wide input should be solicited when formulating vision statements, improving resulting efforts.

6.3.3   Values Statements

A **values statement** is a document which succinctly presents the core standards, ideals, and principles that guide and direct an organization's pursuit of its designated mission and vision. Organizations tend to have only a small handful of core values, typically between three and five. As such, values statements are usually very brief, often being presented as a single sentence or a list depicting the values which guide the organization in all aspects of operation [4, 6, 10, 18]. A federally qualified health center (FQHC) dedicated to serving all individuals, regardless of their ability to pay, might embrace a values statement such as the following: "In our quest to serve the underserved, we are motivated by several key values: respect, commitment, competence, compassion, and love." Similarly, an urgent care clinic might select a values statement such as the following: "Our approach to addressing your health is motivated by three core values: convenience, speed, and precision." In each of these values statements, the given establishments might opt to define the noted values, offering a brief description of their meaning and how they are demonstrated in their daily operations.

The labor associated with compiling values statements is usually less than that required for assembling mission and vision statements. This is because through the process of developing mission and vision statements—tasks typically preceding values statement development—guiding values invariably will be revealed. Assuming comprehensive efforts were directed toward mission and vision development, assembly of values statements merely entails retrieval of motivating values and compilation of such in a succinct manner. The key to selecting values involves identifying those that are meaningful and relevant to the organization and its operation. Quite obviously, significant reflection is required to identify a values framework which represents a good fit for a given establishment. Associated efforts, however, will pay dividends over time. Values are very stable in organizational life, making values statements quite enduring [4, 6, 10, 18].

6.4   Environmental Analysis

Successful strategy pursuits are heavily dependent on the depth and breadth of understanding of one's environment. As such, those involved in strategy direct significant time and attention toward environmental analysis. **Environmental analysis** goes by many names, including **environmental surveillance** and **environmental**

scanning. It essentially refers to the activity of studying the environment for purposes of identifying opportunities and threats, permitting them to be proactively addressed by an organization. This activity is inherently tied to strategy, as an organization's environment dictates what is and is not possible. This is understandable as environmental influences impact operations, and this, in turn, impacts strategy. Environmental influences can arise from both within and outside of healthcare establishments, necessitating proactive surveillance on both fronts.

Various tools are used by healthcare providers to monitor their environments, with the PEST analysis and SWOT analysis being called upon extensively [3, 21, 22]. A related, popular environmental analysis tool, focusing specifically on competitor analysis, is known as the five forces analysis [3, 23, 24]. Another commonly deployed tool, known as blue ocean strategy, aids managers in viewing opportunities in their environments comprehensively, specifically encouraging the pursuit of novel pathways filled with potential [3, 25–27]. Many more exist. The information captured in these analyses often is placed into what is known as a **dashboard**, a strategic resource which combines various sources of information into a single presentation, permitting a comprehensive portrayal which can aid in planning, decision-making, and other strategic aims [28–30]. Dashboards increasingly are electronic, making use of computerization, but some still rely on manual systems, with, for example, strategists summarizing findings on a dedicated whiteboard or similar display placed in a boardroom, permitting executives to examine associated content. Regardless of format of presentation, the resulting depiction should be considered to be a "living document" as it must be updated regularly in tandem with the constantly changing environment. Ultimately, dashboards are most helpful in revealing "big picture" perspectives only available by combining details gleaned from multiple environmental analyses. Brief profiles of several of the more popular tools of environmental analysis are presented in following sections.

6.4.1 The PEST Analysis

The **external environment** or **macroenvironment** refers to forces emerging from outside of an organization which have the potential to influence the given establishment and its operation. These forces can be divided into four categories—political, economic, social, and technological—with their associated assessment being known as the **PEST analysis**. **Political forces** refer to all aspects associated with the legal and political framework of a society. Policy changes issued by Medicare and Medicaid insurance programs and regulatory oversight by state licensure boards, health departments, and other entities serve as excellent examples of this force. **Economic forces** refer to all aspects associated with the economy of a society, including matters concerning economic health (e.g., income, unemployment, inflation, rising or falling demand) and the state of marketplace competition (e.g., competitors entering or departing markets, service lines introduced or eliminated by rivals). **Social forces** refer to all aspects associated with a society's demographic composition (e.g., age, gender, race, family status, education) and system of values and beliefs (e.g., dietary habits, state of physical fitness, prevalence of drug, or alcohol addiction), with these carrying obvious implications for healthcare establishments and the services they provide. **Technological forces** refer to all aspects associated with the state of innovation in a society, with associated developments (e.g., revolutionary surgical techniques, innovative pharmaceuticals) having the potential to impact healthcare providers and their service arrays. Completing the PEST analysis simply involves (1) actively monitoring the environment for any developments on political, economic, social, and technological fronts, (2) discerning how noted developments might potentially impact one's healthcare establishment, and (3) compiling observations in a list which can aid in determining opportunities and threats and inform associated strategy [3, 21, 22].

6.4.2 The SWOT Analysis

The **internal environment** or **microenvironment** refers to forces emerging from within an organization which have the potential to influence the given establishment and its operation. Internal forces are numerous, they can be positive or negative, and they can involve virtually any element inside the walls of a particular institution. Organizations often monitor these forces by preparing a **SWOT analysis**. Also known as a **situation analysis** because it depicts the state of affairs of an organization, the SWOT analysis identifies institutional strengths, weaknesses, opportunities, and threats. Strengths and weaknesses pertain to internal environmental factors, while opportunities and threats relate to external ones, affording the SWOT analysis with the capability of portraying an organization's microenvironment in the context of its macroenvironment [3].

   Strengths are positive features of an organization, such as outstanding quality, rising market share, excellent management, superior technology, and the like. **Weaknesses** are negative features of an organization, such as poor customer service, inconvenient access to care, outdated technology, weak infrastructure, and similar elements. **Opportunities** are events and circumstances in the environment that have the potential to be exploited by an institution for gains. Examples include newly discovered product uses, substantial market growth, newly developed technologies, favorable government legislation, and so on. **Threats** are events and circumstances in the environment that have the potential to negatively impact an organization. Examples include new competitors, adverse government legislation, changing customer preferences, and competitors equipped with superior technologies. Given their transferability, details from the PEST analysis can be used to expedite completion of the opportunities and threats components of the SWOT analysis. Completing the SWOT analysis involves (1) actively monitoring a given organization and its surroundings to identify strengths, weaknesses, opportunities, and threats, (2) discerning the impact potential of observations, and (3) compiling observations in a list to aid and inform strategy [3].

6.4.3 The Five Forces Analysis

A useful complement to broad-based environmental analyses, such as the SWOT analysis and PEST analysis, is the **five forces analysis**. Developed by renowned strategy scholar Michael Porter, this particular model directs attention toward the competitive environment. This is an especially helpful strategic tool for health and medical organizations, as the healthcare industry is characterized by intense competition and rivalry, necessitating acquisition of competitive intelligence. Almost any strategic pursuit must take into consideration competition, anticipating, for example, the potential steps that might be taken by rivals if a particular course of action is pursued. This, of course, requires identification of competitors, permitting them to be studied and monitored. While this might seem like a simple task, very often, healthcare organizations fail to properly define their competitive field, identifying obvious competitors while neglecting to recognize others. This overly narrow perspective of competition is dangerous in that unidentified rivals can operate without detection, representing a strategic vulnerability for the uninformed establishment. The five forces analysis provides guidance to ensure that the complete competitive field is identified [3, 23, 24].

According to the five forces analysis, the nature of competition in any industry is based on five forces, namely, existing competitors, potential entrants, substitutes, suppliers, and buyers. **Existing competitors**—the head-to-head rivals of an organization delivering similar or identical products to similar or identical customer groups—are the most obvious and widely recognized competitive force [3, 23, 24]. An orthopedic medical practice, for example, would view other establishments currently offering orthopedic medical services to constitute existing competitors in the market.

Potential entrants are those establishments which are not currently offering competing products in the market but might do so in the future. The orthopedic medical practice mentioned earlier would not currently view a multispecialty medical clinic which currently does not provide orthopedic services as a rival, but that could quickly change if it decided to add an orthopedic line. As the prospect of new rivals entering markets is largely unknown, healthcare organizations must rely on environmental surveillance techniques and intuition for ascertaining associated threat potential. The sooner a new rival's intentions to enter a given market are known, the better [3, 23, 24].

Substitutes are products which are different from particular offerings but largely, and sometimes completely, address the same wants and needs [3, 23, 24]. The services of a chiropractor, for example, could be viewed as a substitute for the services of an orthopedic surgeon. Similarly, over-the-counter pain medications which relieve sore backs, joints, and the like also could be viewed as substitutes for orthopedic medicine. The quality and comprehensiveness of a substitute may or may not be equivalent to that provided by the orthopedic medical practice. That, however, does not remove the threat potential, as some individuals will opt to pursue those avenues rather than the ones provided by the orthopedic clinic.

Suppliers provide the components required for health and medical organizations to offer their products to customers. Carrying forward the orthopedic medical practice example, associated suppliers would entail vendors providing myriad items, including diagnostic imaging equipment, surgery scalpels, hospital beds, patient information systems, and much more. These raw materials are required in order for the establishment to offer medical services and dependence on such poses a significant threat. Suppliers, for example, might raise their prices, lower the quality of the components that they provide, or even go out of business, creating significant hardships for those institutions which rely on them. Supplier power is increased when they are few in number, when few substitutes exist, and when given establishments are not key customers [3, 23, 24].

Buyers are the customers of given establishments, with their patronage ultimately determining institutional survival, growth, and prosperity. The orthopedic medical practice's customers would obviously include its patients but also any patient-enabling party, including insurance companies and other third-party payers. Buyers—customers—hold significant bargaining power over organizations, as without them, operations cease [3, 23, 24].

Operationalizing the five forces analysis requires healthcare organizations to (1) determine the product to be evaluated (e.g., orthopedic medical services, nursing home services, home health services) and (2) prepare a diagram, identifying existing competitors, potential entrants, substitutes, suppliers, and buyers. If comprehensive investigative efforts are directed toward assembly of this diagram, healthcare providers will be afforded with an overview of their complete competitive field. Such competitive intelligence greatly complements the information gleaned from other environmental analyses, assisting healthcare providers in establishing strategic priorities [3].

6.4.4   Blue Ocean Strategy

Blue ocean strategy was developed by W. Chan Kim and Renee Mauborgne to aid managers in viewing their environments in a manner to understand and recognize productive opportunities for their given organizations to pursue. They created memorable descriptors to characterize options based on their potential, labeling them red oceans and blue oceans. **Red oceans**—an analogy referencing the bloody red seas that appear in the wake of shark attacks—represent pathways with little to no potential. Red oceans are the product of traditional thinking where organizations typically "follow the herd," pursuing the same basic things in the same basic ways as their peers, limiting opportunity [3, 25–27]. Consider the following scenario where three hospitals compete against each other in a given city with a stable population. If each facility offers essentially equivalent services, targets the same population, and follows industry norms in doing so, upside potential is limited as new demand is not being created. Limited growth prospects and keen competition effectively bloody the seas as rivals vie against each other for dominance. As such, the hospitals would be said to be operating in a red ocean. Though the market may be viable, capable of supporting the three hospitals, as the market is currently being addressed, the potential for greater gains is low to nonexistent.

By contrast, **blue oceans**—an analogy referencing open, clear blue water in the seas—represent avenues burgeoning with potential. Blue oceans typically are revealed by thinking "outside of the box," often via the discovery and deployment of innovations and other novel approaches that yield value for given organizations [3, 25, 26]. Continuing the example expressed earlier, assume that one of the three hospitals looked out into the marketplace and noticed high growth occurring in a suburb located a distance away from the city. The suburb had yet to be served by any healthcare establishment, necessitating that residents commute many miles for their health needs. Recognizing the opportunity, the hospital decided to launch a satellite clinic in the suburb, capturing the associated demand and advancing institutional growth and prosperity. Essentially, the hospital discovered a blue ocean and pursued it, accordingly.

Blue oceans exist anywhere that opportunity is plentiful and they can appear on any front [3, 25, 26]. Uncontested market space, such as that described in the hospital example, represents a classic blue ocean, but many more exist. The provision of value-added services also can yield blue oceans, such as when a physician differentiates his practice from others in a given community by offering house calls to better serve patients. Price advantages and similar incentives also can generate blue oceans, such as when a pharmacy chooses to offer free home delivery services to help customers save money. Innovative techniques, too, can produce blue oceans, such as when a medical center devises a novel incentive program to more successfully attract and retain nurses. In each of these cases, someone was inquisitive enough to seek out opportunities that few, if any, institutions were pursuing at the time, affording blue oceans. On discovery of a blue ocean, innovative thinking must not cease, however, as novel ideas are often copied by rivals over time, necessitating the continual quest for blue water.

Blue ocean strategy naturally requires advanced environmental analysis skills and abilities, coupled with a willingness to actively seek novel approaches that go against the grain of traditional thought within given industries and markets. Critically, it relies heavily on strategic thinking, a topic discussed in detail later in the chapter. Blue ocean strategy's greatest strength arguably is that it serves as a helpful, memorable reminder to look off the beaten path for opportunities [3]. As understanding available options is essential for plotting the course of healthcare institutions, blue ocean strategy usefully complements other environmental analyses.

6.5   The Strategy Process

The accomplishment of strategy occurs in many ways in healthcare organizations. Some avenues are highly formalized, while others are more informal. Regardless of approach, whenever good strategy is made, it usually emerges via a process involving three sequential stages: strategy formulation, strategy implementation, and strategy evaluation [10]. The last stage of the process effectively serves as an assessment which, in turn, influences future strategy efforts. The strategy process is administered by those in the highest levels of organizations, making strategy skills increasingly important as one scales the organizational hierarchy. Although it is dominated by top-level executives, the strategy process also relies heavily on those occupying lower levels who provide critical assistance and insights across pursuits [10–12]. The three stages of the strategy process are explained as follows.

6.5.1   Stage 1: Strategy Formulation

Strategy formulation constitutes the first stage of the strategy process. Here, organizations carefully craft strategy by analyzing their environments and their capabilities, stipulating their desires, and developing goals and objectives which are anticipated to hasten achieving those desires. As its definition suggests, strategy formulation requires a wealth of foundational information, requiring attention on several fronts, including (1) developing an understanding of internal and external environments, aided by conducting applicable environmental analyses; (2) assessing the current state of the entity in focus, essentially addressing "Where are we now?" types of questions; (3) envisioning the desired state of the entity in focus, addressing "Where do we want to be?" types of questions; and (4) comparing the current state with the desired state, addressing "What do we need to do to get from where we are now to where we want to be?" types of questions. By the conclusion of the strategy formulation stage, healthcare organizations should have in their possession a series of goals and objectives which are deemed to be achievable and capable of seeing the establishment realize its desired state. A road map of sorts is revealed at this point [10–12, 31–33].

6.5.2   Stage 2: Strategy Implementation

Strategy implementation, also referred to as **strategy execution**, follows strategy formulation, making it the second stage of the strategy process. The strategy implementation stage specifically calls for the enactment of the strategy devised during the formulation stage. It is considered to be the most difficult stage, given natural challenges associated with putting often complex directives into practice. This stage necessitates discipline and dedication from parties across organizations [9]. When organizations demonstrate proficiencies in strategy implementation, they are often said to be skilled at **executional excellence** [13]. This is vital as the best developed strategies are meaningless if they are not carried out successfully [10, 13]. As such, healthcare establishments must be especially vigilant when operationalizing formulated plans, as doing so will enhance the likelihood of a satisfactory return on investment for all of the labor and other resources demanded by the strategy process.

Several foundational assets are required in virtually any implementation scenario. Mandatory resources include (1) top leadership support and commitment, (2) financial resources sufficient for funding strategy endeavors, (3) competent personnel charged with effecting given initiatives, and (4) formal processes permitting the effective operationalization of associated initiatives. With these resources in place, the stage is set to implement strategy proficiently. The specific activities required of strategy implementation are dependent on the nature of the goals and objectives devised during the strategy formulation stage. This, of course, will be institution-specific as strategy roadmaps will vary widely between and among organizations. Importantly, each party involved in strategy implementation must examine formulated directives, ascertain what is demanded of them, determine how best to accomplish their associated responsibilities, and follow through by successfully delivering the requirements demanded. During this stage, skills at motivating employees are especially important [2, 10]. While tools and techniques are essential components of implementation, people ultimately are responsible for effecting strategy, and they must be compelled to do so, making motivation a key requirement for success.

6.5.3   Stage 3: Strategy Evaluation

The final stage of the strategy process is known as **strategy evaluation**. It involves the assessment of strategies following their implementation to ascertain the degree of success achieved. For strategy matters which have run their course and achieved success, this particular stage represents a conclusion. Many strategy matters, however, are enduring, requiring years of work to achieve (e.g., a new hospital seeking to become the market leader amidst a pool of powerful rivals) or perhaps are structured in a manner to represent continued quests (e.g., a medical center dedicated to technology leadership). In such cases, the importance of evaluation is profound as it is the primary mechanism for keeping healthcare organizations on course, producing knowledge which either confirms proper direction or reveals the need for corrective actions to remedy misdirection. The basic formula for conducting strategy evaluations entails comparing results experienced against those desired, taking corrective steps when necessary to achieve stipulated aims [10, 12]. As strategies typically extend over lengthy periods of time, evaluations usually are conducted at periodic intervals. For highly critical strategy matters, such as those faced by hospitals during the COVID-19 pandemic, strategy evaluation often occurs on a continual basis, affording essentially real-time progress reports, with these being most helpful, especially in situations of crisis.

Evaluation indeed is necessary in strategy. Despite enormous expenditures of time, money, and other resources directed toward formulating and implementing strategy, experience often indicates the need for alterations to be made. Due to immense environmental complexities, virtually any component of strategy, when put into actual practice, can be discovered to be in need of a modification to improve associated performance and better deliver desired results [10–13]. Tactics, for example, might prove to be insufficient for achieving a designated aim. Particular strategy deliverables assigned to one department might be found to be better suited for another. Stipulated goals could be revealed to offer little toward actual accomplishment of a given mission and vision. Healthcare providers could even discover that their overall strategies are not meeting the mark, necessitating associated reengineering.

In a perfect world, **intended strategies**, those initial strategies formulated to address a challenge and achieve a desired result, would deliver everything wanted without any need for modification or adjustment. This, however, is unrealistic. Instead, strategies are frequently modified to accommodate situational changes, resulting in what are known as **emergent strategies** [34, 35]. Without proper strategy evaluation activities, such alterations could not be made as given establishments would not possess knowledge revealing the need for modification. Whether strategies deliver desired results in their initial incarnations or emerge through experience matters not. What matters is simply that a strategy permitting desires to be realized is identified and pursued with vigor, something facilitated by the evaluative process.

6.6 Strategic Thinking

One of the most essential skills required of healthcare managers involved in the strategy process is the ability to think strategically. **Strategic thinking** permits strategists to view their given organizations in an integrated, connected fashion—seeing the whole and its parts—as they go about using intuition, logic, and creativity to discover productive avenues that will lead to mission fulfillment and vision attainment. Strategic thinkers are adept at synthesizing information from many different sources (e.g., one's personal experiences, insights from colleagues, clues from the environment), ultimately affording them with a working approach for addressing an issue or matter of concern. This mindset is essential for "connecting the dots," linking bits and pieces of data together to make sense of things, revealing the big picture [36, 37]. Deep conceptualization indeed is essential for good strategy, and, as such, healthcare managers must work to develop their skills in this area.

The process of becoming a strategic thinker can best be understood by examining the characteristics of those who have mastered the ability. The most prolific strategic thinkers are known as **visionaries**, individuals who possess an uncanny ability to examine their environments and identify avenues and opportunities which can be exploited for gains of some sort [2, 37, 38]. Visionaries typically are highly educated, very experienced, driven by a vigorous work ethic, and extremely inquisitive. This collection of characteristics has great potential to develop one's intuition and judgment, ultimately permitting those involved in healthcare strategy to make excellent calls whenever issues present themselves in given organizations.

The qualities that define visionaries and support their strategic thinking abilities are obtainable by most anyone willing to make proper investments of time and effort. One specifically must work to advance his or her education to broaden knowledge regarding the operation of healthcare institutions. Additionally, progressively responsible work experience must be acquired over time, permitting individuals to build practical skills that complement those gained in the classroom. Furthermore, one must develop and maintain a very intensive work ethic which affords exposure to work environments and an intensive understanding of jobs and their requirements in the context of institutional missions. One also must develop a mindset of inquiry, examining his or her environment, questioning observations, and pondering meaning in an unending quest for knowledge, understanding, and opportunity. Patience, of course, is required, as these qualities take time to develop and ultimately converge, advancing one's capacity to think strategically, potentially even leading to recognition as a visionary. When this is accomplished, healthcare managers become defined assets of their given organizations as they are capable of operating proficiently at the strategic level to advance institutional aims.

6.7 The Strategic Plan

Across the pages of this chapter, key components of the practice of strategy in healthcare establishments were presented. When arranged in an orderly fashion, these components can be used to form a **strategic plan**, a formal document, typically long-range in focus, which describes an organization comprehensively, noting its mission and vision, historical development, strengths and weaknesses, environmental characteristics, and more, outlining its strategic goals and objectives and methods for their achievement. Strategic plans are staples in healthcare establishments, being very familiar to most anyone serving in managerial capacities across given organizations. Preparation is typically a laborious task, calling on multiple perspectives and consuming many hours of effort. As one logically might surmise, many variations of assembly exist.

A basic outline for assembling a healthcare organization's strategic plan is presented in Box 6.1. This outline, when populated with robust details, is capable of supplying most any healthcare organization with a roadmap for achieving aspirations. Of course, the value of any strategic plan rests with the quality of the information used in its preparation. This is well-known in healthcare organizations, motivating extensive efforts to perfect associated strategic plans. Diligence indeed is required, but it must be kept in check. It is not terribly uncommon to observe enthusiasm for strategic planning being so pronounced that the means overtakes the end. This should never be allowed. Maintaining at top of mind the patient-focused perspective communicated at the chapter's introduction can help to ensure that one's focus is never blurred while formulating given strategic plans, reminding strategists that outcomes beneficial to the healthcare organization and its patients are the prevailing motivation of the strategic planning process.

Box 6.1: A Basic Outline for a Healthcare Organization's Strategic Plan

(1) Title page
(2) Table of contents
(3) Executive summary
(4) Overview of the institution

    (a) History
    (b) Mission statement
    (c) Vision statement
    (d) Values statement

(5) Analysis of the environment

    (a) The internal environment
    (b) The external environment

(6) Goals and objectives

    (a) Current state
    (b) Desired state
    (c) Closing gaps between current and desired states

        (i) Formulation and identification of goals and objectives
        (ii) Justifications for pursuing goals and objectives

(7) Implementation requirements and projected timeline
(8) Evaluation methods and projected timeline
(9) Conclusion

Another cautionary note regarding the strategic plan is that, with its preparation, some can be led to believe that strategy is all set. The fact of the matter is that the strategic plan is merely a formal guide that helps to coordinate and direct strategic actions leading an organization from its current state to a desired state. It is prospective, detailing the best guesses of institutional experts as to the steps necessary to lead an establishment to a better place. Certainty of outcome is not guaranteed, especially given the tumultuous environment characterizing healthcare organizations. A substantive change on virtually any front can relegate once sensible aims into impossibilities, necessitating immediate modification. As such, as alluded to earlier, altering associated strategy should be expected, as circumstances warranting change are highly likely to occur over the course of a strategic plan. Strategy is an ongoing activity, requiring constant attention. The strategic plan is an important component for properly addressing strategy within healthcare establishments.

6.8   Summary and Conclusions

Few elements of organizational life are as impactful as strategy on institutional operations. Complexities associated with the healthcare industry and the ever-changing environments of health and medical institutions demand that providers carefully plot courses aimed at reaching desired destinations. Without an understanding of where an establishment is going, coupled with a roadmap for actually getting there, organizational pursuits are nothing more than exercises in futility. Through strategy, healthcare providers are afforded with critical tools and techniques permitting them to guide their institutions through often tumultuous circumstances and situations to successfully achieve their missions and realize their associated aspirations. Behind every successful healthcare organization, one will find capable strategists responsible for guiding and directing their given institutions to points of prosperity.

Key Terms

- Blue Ocean Strategy
- Blue Oceans
- Buyers
- Competitive Advantage
- Dashboard
- Economic Forces
- Emergent Strategy
- Environmental Analysis
- Environmental Scanning
- Environmental Surveillance
- Executional Excellence
- Existing Competitors
- External Environment
- Five Forces Analysis
- Intended Strategy
- Internal Environment
- Macroenvironment
- Microenvironment
- Mission
- Mission Statement
- Opportunities
- PEST Analysis
- Political Forces
- Potential Entrants
- Red Oceans

- Situation Analysis
- Social Forces
- Strategic Analysis
- Strategic Management
- Strategic Plan
- Strategic Planning
- Strategic Thinking
- Strategy
- Strategy Evaluation
- Strategy Execution
- Strategy Formulation
- Strategy Implementation
- Strengths
- Substitutes
- Suppliers
- SWOT Analysis
- Tactics
- Technological Forces
- Threats
- Values
- Values Statement
- Vision
- Vision Statement
- Visionary
- Weaknesses

Exercises

1. In your own words, define strategy and discuss its role and importance in health and medicine.
2. Define competitive advantage, indicate why healthcare institutions must pursue them, and discuss the role of strategy in their acquisition. Reflecting on recent work experiences, profile a competitive advantage that you observed, and discuss how it benefited your employer.
3. Outline the strategy process and profile each of its steps. Describe why mastery of this process is vital for success in the healthcare industry.
4. Define mission statement, vision statement, and values statement, discuss the role played by each, and discuss methods for their assembly in health and medicine. Take the opportunity to enhance your understanding by reviewing the statements maintained by your current employer. Are the statements assembled in keeping with the guidelines depicted in this chapter? Are they current and suitable for the establishment? Are any missing or otherwise unavailable? What changes, if any, would you make and why?

5. Visit a range of websites of healthcare institutions which are unfamiliar to you, specifically seeking to identify and review their mission, vision, and values statements. From those you were able to locate and examine, identify the ones which most appealed to you, and indicate the reasons why you found them to be compelling.

6. Compare and contrast macroenvironments and microenvironments, identify common techniques for their assessment, and discuss how they respectively impact healthcare operations. Reflect on a recent employment experience and describe the macroenvironment and the microenvironment of the organization. How would you rate your employer's proficiencies at monitoring its environments? What improvements could be made to enhance its environmental scanning abilities?

7. Strategy implementation requires a series of foundational assets necessary for achieving executional excellence. Identify these resource requirements. How proficient has your employer been in providing these resources for its associated strategy pursuits? Explain your perspectives in detail.

8. Compare and contrast intended strategies and emergent strategies. Reflect on your recent work experiences, and provide an example of a strategy that worked as intended, leading to its continuation. Then, provide an example of a strategy that did not work as intended, necessitating modifications yielding an emergent strategy. Did the emergent strategy deliver the desired results?

References

1. Elrod, J. K., & Fortenberry, J. L., Jr. (2018). Am I seeing things through the eyes of patients? An exercise in bolstering patient attentiveness and empathy. *BMC Health Services Research, 18*(Suppl 3), 41–44.
2. Elrod, J. K. (2013). *Breadcrumbs to cheesecake*. R&R Publishers.
3. Fortenberry, J. L., Jr. (2010). *Health care marketing: Tools and techniques* (3rd ed.). Jones and Bartlett.
4. Ginter, P. M., Duncan, W. J., & Swayne, L. E. (2013). *Strategic management of health care organizations* (7th ed.). Jossey-Bass.
5. McConnell, C. R. (2020). *Hospitals and health systems: What they are and how they work.* Jones and Bartlett.
6. Hillestad, S. G., & Berkowitz, E. N. (2020). *Health care market strategy: From planning to action* (5th ed.). Jones and Bartlett.
7. Wilensky, S. E., & Teitelbaum, J. B. (2023). *Essentials of health policy and law* (5th ed.). Jones and Bartlett.
8. Flynn, W. J., Valentine, S. R., & Meglich, P. A. (2022). *Healthcare human resource management* (4th ed.). Cengage.
9. Kotler, P., Stevens, R. J., & Shalowitz, J. (2021). *Strategic marketing for health care organizations: Building a customer-driven health system* (2nd ed.). Wiley.
10. David, F. R,, David, F. R., & David, M. E. (2020). *Strategic management: A competitive advantage approach* (17th ed.). Pearson.
11. Rumelt, R. P. (2011). *Good strategy, bad strategy: The difference and why it matters.* Currency.

12. Luke, R. D., Walston, S. L., & Plummer, P. M. (2004). *Healthcare strategy: In pursuit of competitive advantage*. Health Administration Press.
13. Berry, L. L. (1999). *Discovering the soul of service: The nine drivers of sustainable business success*. The Free Press.
14. Shafritz, J. M., Ott, J. S., & Jang, Y. S. (Eds.). (2016). *Classics of organization theory* (8th ed.). Cengage.
15. Freedman, L. (2015). *Strategy: A history*. Oxford University Press.
16. Creveld, M. V. (2015). *A history of strategy: From Sun Tzu to William S. Lind*. Castalia House.
17. Berkowitz, E. N. (2022). *Essentials of health care marketing* (5th ed.). Jones and Bartlett.
18. Collins, J. C., & Porras, J. I. (1996). Building your company's vision. *Harvard Business Review, 74*(5), 65–77.
19. Schein, E. H., & Schein, P. A. (2019). *The corporate culture survival guide* (3rd ed.). Wiley.
20. Deal, T. E., & Kennedy, A. A. (2000). *Corporate cultures: The rites and rituals of corporate life*. Basic Books.
21. Elrod, J. K., & Fortenberry, J. L., Jr. (2017). Peering beyond the walls of healthcare institutions: A catalyst for innovation. *BMC Health Services Research, 17*(Suppl 1), 35–38.
22. Elrod, J. K., & Fortenberry, J. L., Jr. (2018). Catalyzing marketing innovation and competitive advantage in the healthcare industry: The value of thinking like an outsider. *BMC Health Services Research, 18*(Suppl 3), 45–48.
23. Porter, M. E. (2008). The five competitive forces that shape strategy. *Harvard Business Review, 86*(1), 78–93.
24. Porter, M. E. (1998). *Competitive strategy: Techniques for analyzing industries and competitors*. The Free Press.
25. Kim, W. C., & Mauborgne, R. (2004). Blue ocean strategy. *Harvard Business Review, 82*(10), 76–84.
26. Kim, W. C., & Mauborgne, R. (2005). *Blue ocean strategy: How to create uncontested market space and make the competition irrelevant*. Harvard Business School Press.
27. Kim, W. C., & Mauborgne, R. (2015). Red ocean traps. *Harvard Business Review, 93*(3), 68–73.
28. Wexler, S., Shaffer, J., & Cotgreave, A. (2017). *The big book of dashboards: Visualizing your data using real-world business scenarios*. Wiley.
29. Eckerson, W. W. (2010). *Performance dashboards: Measuring, monitoring, and managing your business* (2nd ed.). Wiley.
30. Kusleika, D. (2021). *Data visualization with Excel dashboards and reports*. Wiley.
31. Kaplan, R. S., & Norton, D. P. (1996). *The balanced scorecard: Translating strategy into action*. Harvard Business School Press.
32. Kaplan, R. S., & Norton, D. P. (1996). Using the balanced scorecard as a strategic management system. *Harvard Business Review, 74*(1), 75–85.
33. Kaplan, R. S., & Norton, D. P. (2004). *Strategy maps: Converting intangible assets into tangible outcomes*. Harvard Business School Press.
34. Mintzberg, H. (1987). Crafting strategy. *Harvard Business Review, 65*(4), 66–75.
35. Mintzberg, H. (1989). *Mintzberg on management: Inside our strange world of organizations*. The Free Press.
36. Mintzberg, H. (1994). *The rise and fall of strategic planning: Reconceiving roles for planning, plans, planners*. The Free Press.
37. Mintzberg, H. (1994). The fall and rise of strategic planning. *Harvard Business Review, 72*(1), 107–114.
38. Nanus, B. (1992). *Visionary leadership: Creating a compelling sense of direction for your organization*. Jossey-Bass.

Chapter 7
Ethics and Social Responsibility in Health and Medicine

Learning Objectives

After examining this chapter, readers will have the ability to:

- Define ethics, understand its prominent role in organizational prosperity, and discuss its importance in health and medical establishments.
- Discuss the benefits of operating ethically, note how ethical operations influence the reputations of healthcare institutions, and reflect on how ethical practices impact employees and other stakeholders in health and medicine.
- Realize the frequency of ethical dilemmas faced by healthcare employees, understand the various influences which impact employee responses to these dilemmas, and identify methods for ensuring that employees address ethical scenarios in an institutionally sanctioned fashion.
- Identify and describe methods which can be used by healthcare establishments to maintain high ethical standards of operation, including codes of conduct, ethical staffing practices, ethical training programs, and systems of accountability and control.
- Define the concept of social responsibility, identify its role in positioning health and medical establishments as ethical institutions, and discuss practices that healthcare institutions can use to demonstrate that they are operating in a socially responsible manner.

© The Editor(s) (if applicable) and The Author(s), under exclusive license to Springer
Nature Switzerland AG 2024
J. K. Elrod, J. L. Fortenberry, Jr., *Organizational Behavior and Management in Health and Medicine*, https://doi.org/10.1007/978-3-031-61823-9_7

WK Reflections: The Pervasiveness of Ethics in Health and Medicine

Shreveport, Louisiana-based Willis Knighton Health is comprised of five hospitals, an all-inclusive retirement community, and scores of general and specialty medical clinics. Through intensive efforts over many years, the institution acquired the prominent position of market leader in northwest Louisiana. This achievement resulted from well-devised, intensive strategic management activities taking place over its history. The lofty position currently occupied by Willis Knighton Health stands in stark contrast to that of its former self, namely, a single-site facility—Willis Knighton North (formerly known as Willis-Knighton Medical Center)—dedicated to serving the population of west Shreveport, an area situated in the shadow of the downtown business district and city center. This geographically narrow mission persisted virtually unchanged for decades, initiated on the institution's establishment in 1924. In the 1970s, however, growth ambitions prompted a major course alteration, with executives embracing an expanded perspective, envisioning the organization as a regional healthcare provider.

Realizing this vision first required executives to shore up the sole campus of the institution, investing significantly to bolster patient care and attention. By the early 1980s, associated investments led to a burgeoning patient population, with loyalty reaching its highest point to date. These successes afforded the institution with options for expansion. In considering alternatives, executives noticed that the population of south Shreveport was growing rapidly, yet not a single hospital was offering services in the area. This represented an obvious opportunity for the institution to pursue. But what would become of its original site? At the time, growth prospects in west Shreveport were far less attractive than those of south Shreveport or even that of neighboring Bossier City which was slowly becoming a population center. As hospitals are very costly endeavors, significant research was required to plot optimal steps.

An economic case certainly could be made for shuttering the institution's existing, sole site, relocating operations to a new building in an area with better prospects for future growth. Decisions, however, carry more than economic implications. Among scores of considerations in such complex scenarios, ethics also must be taken into account, and that is exactly what occurred. On careful reflection and detailed examination, executives came to the conclusion that closing the west Shreveport campus would place an undue burden on the population in the area. Located in Shreveport's most urban setting, Willis Knighton North was immersed within poverty-stricken neighborhoods whose residents relied on the establishment for convenient access to healthcare. As such, executives believed that closure of this facility would effectively strand these patients. Such a practice was viewed to be incompatible with the institution's operational philosophy as a not-for-profit, charitable enterprise. To this day, the practice of closing facilities which would leave patients with no convenient care options is shunned by the institution.

Ultimately, Willis Knighton North continued serving the population of west Shreveport as it introduced its second facility in south Shreveport, becoming a multi-hospital system in 1983. Over time, additional facilities followed, further increasing the number of campuses in Shreveport, adding one in neighboring Bossier City, and introducing dozens of medical clinics, yielding the comprehensive system that exists today. Interestingly, the west Shreveport campus remains the main campus of Willis Knighton Health, receiving the greatest investments and effectively serving as the hub of the institution's hub-and-spoke network [1, 2], something described in full in Chap. 9.

Reflecting on the institution's growth and development over the past several decades, it is ironic that Willis Knighton Health's sense of ethics ultimately guided the establishment to full geographic coverage, with the majority of residents in the twin cities of Shreveport and Bossier City being located no more than eight minutes away from a Willis Knighton Health hospital. Had the institution embraced a reduced sense of ethics that valued bottom-line business fundamentals over patient wants and needs, the west Shreveport campus likely would have been closed, leaving a noted geographic gap that might have been difficult or impossible to refill at a later date. Competitors, for example, could have claimed the area, making reentry problematic. Prime locations also could have been acquired by other businesses that moved into the area further hindering reentry prospects. But by following a moral compass which viewed it to be wrong to withdraw from served markets, especially those featuring hardshipped populations, such difficulties and concerns never materialized.

Ethics-related considerations underlie scores of decisions faced by those serving in health and medical organizations. While the ethical concern regarding Willis Knighton Health's expansion pathway is a particularly prominent example situated firmly in the top management realm, everyone, regardless of their location in the chain of command, faces ethical dilemmas daily. These must be resolved in a suitable manner in order for healthcare institutions to survive and thrive as patient care providers. As perspectives of what is good or bad and right or wrong ultimately drive behaviors, healthcare establishments must ensure that their employees understand associated institutional mindsets and embrace them, accordingly. The pervasiveness of ethical dilemmas across healthcare organizations demands an equally pervasive response to combat unethical thoughts and actions and ensure institution-wide integrity.

7.1 Background

Health and medical services are highly complex and intensely personal, and, as such, great care must be taken by healthcare establishments in their provision. These services, of course, must be delivered with precision by competent personnel who appreciate and respect patients, treating them with care and compassion [1–3]. Even the slightest lapse of concentration can spell disaster for care recipients. But due to the sensitive nature of the offerings provided by healthcare organizations, attention must be extended beyond merely the delivery of quality services. The information provided in medical histories, details on the nature of injuries and illnesses, emotional responses of patients to diagnoses, and the like represent the ultimate of sensitive information and must be protected without fail, both for reasons of patient confidence and legal compliance [4, 5]. Deeper operational matters, seldom observed by patients, also must be addressed with integrity. Healthcare establishments must, for example, treat employees, vendors, and other parties respectfully and fairly; manage financial matters in a trustworthy, honorable fashion; fulfill any and all obligations to the communities in which they operate in a comprehensive and timely manner; and conduct themselves in a way that builds stakeholder confidence [2, 6, 7]. In essence, healthcare establishments must exemplify integrity in all aspects of operation.

The necessity for institutions, regardless of their type or mission, to operate with integrity is nothing new. Arguably, this has been a required component of any conscientious establishment dating back to the earliest forms of organization. The need, however, is magnified in healthcare establishments, given the deeply personal nature of the services that they provide and their noteworthy status as anchors within the communities in which they operate. Concerns regarding the integrity of organizations, building trust with customers and greater communities, operating respectfully and honestly in all areas of practice, and the like fall under the ethics component of organizational behavior and management. Closely related to this, and increasingly important in the modern era, is the topic of social responsibility which challenges organizations to operate in a manner which extends benefits to the societies in which they are based [8–10]. These topics are explored in detail over the course of this chapter.

7.2 Defining Ethics

Ethics are moral principles, values, and beliefs which govern the actions and behaviors of individuals, with associated mindsets providing them with guidance regarding what is good or bad and right or wrong. One's sense of ethics has a profound impact on how that individual sees and interacts with the world, influencing virtually every element of the person's life. Human life necessitates that one exercises judgment on an ongoing basis, comparing alternative courses of action when facing particular situations and scenarios and deciding on proper pathways to pursue. Through one's sense of ethics, these decisions are made [11, 12]. Applied in organizational settings, ethics are sometimes termed **business ethics** or **managerial ethics**, acknowledging the institutional context of associated judgments and decisions [13, 14]. Business or managerial ethics are distinguished from **medical ethics**, which concerns medical decision-making and related clinical judgments [15, 16], with this highly specialized ethical application being beyond the focus of this chapter.

The moral principles, values, and beliefs which guide ethical determinations within an organization are collectively referred to as the **moral code** or **moral framework** of the institution. Moral codes frequently are formalized by health and medical enterprises in published **codes of conduct** which stipulate the ethical positions of given organizations, providing guidance for employees and assurances for patients and other parties as to the moral stance taken by establishments, with these additionally often echoing the consequences of noncompliance. Many of these elements also appear in **values statements**—documents which succinctly present the core standards, ideals, and principles that guide and direct an organization's pursuit of its designated mission and vision—with these being discussed in detail in Chap. 6. Moral codes are not universal; they can and often do vary between and among healthcare organizations depending on the nature of the services offered by them, priorities influenced by underlying organizational cultures, and the preferences of institutional leaders. Actions which comply with governing moral codes are considered to be ethical (i.e., good or right); actions which violate operative moral codes are considered to be unethical (i.e., bad or wrong) [13, 17].

While moral codes and resulting codes of conduct vary between and among healthcare organizations, values traditionally associated with ethical operation—altruism, compassion, honesty, integrity, fairness, justice, and the like—appear with regularity in them. Values presented on paper, however, have limited utility and benefit. They must be **operationalized**—translated into actual practice—bringing life to associated moral frameworks. The operationalization of such in daily work life involves things such as showing support whenever employees encounter hardships, communicating openly and honestly in all interactions, being impartial with respect to distributing rewards and benefits, refraining from engaging in counterproductive organizational politics, reporting violations (e.g., harassment, theft) which undermine ethical operation, and ensuring that actions are consistent with prevailing codes of conduct [18–20]. When employees express the ethical mindsets embraced by given healthcare establishments, they are capable of inspiring confidence and trust, aiding them in their interactions with others.

7.3 Benefits of Operating Ethically

Operating ethically affords numerous benefits with perhaps the most universal one being peace of mind, allowing those working within healthcare establishments to focus their energies completely on their assigned duties and responsibilities, free from the chaos, discontent, and strife that pervades unethical environments. This comprehensive benefit sets the stage for healthcare institutions to realize related benefits commonly associated with ethical operation, including improved efficiency and effectiveness, heightened institutional performance and prosperity, and enhanced employee morale and well-being. Ethical operation also serves as an enhancer of **reputation**, bolstering the opinions, perspectives, and beliefs held by others regarding given organizations [21, 22]. These benefits positively impact not only the employees of healthcare establishments but also the entirety of institutional **stakeholders**—parties which have vested interests in the operation and performance of given organizations—with some of the most prominent ones being patients, vendors, board members, oversight agencies, and the citizenry of the communities in which healthcare establishments are based [14, 23]. Given the associated benefits of ethical operation, healthcare organizations should endeavor to carefully steer their employees to embrace and demonstrate ethical behaviors, making integrity and related ethical facets central components of their respective organizational cultures, perpetuating upright and proper behaviors, attitudes, and mindsets.

Ethics have always been important in business and industry, as conducting operations with honesty and integrity have always had value. The need to operate in an ethical manner, however, is all the more important today. Demands for accountability have increased in recent years, as customers, employees, and other parties dependent on institutions seek and expect respectful treatment and prudent corporate stewardship. Now more than ever, **transparency**—being open and honest in all matters of institutional operation—is an essential ingredient for successful organizational management, especially in light of prominent ethical failures which have captured headlines in recent years [24–27]. Such incidents have a tendency to erode public confidence in all institutions, increasing associated skepticism and creating heightened needs for establishments to embrace and demonstrate principled operations. Healthcare organizations bear a particularly heavy burden in this, as these institutions generally are more heavily scrutinized, given their critical role as community assets entrusted with attending to the health and medical needs of the populace. Safety factors associated with the delivery of patient care and the extremely sensitive nature of healthcare service provision add additional urgency for these operations to be ethically sound [2, 6].

7.4   Ethical Dilemmas

At face value, the task of distinguishing good from bad and right from wrong appears to be a fairly simple endeavor, and many times it is. Consider the following scenarios: an accountant in a hospital misrepresents financial information, a nurse with knowledge of a patient's medical diagnosis shares that information with an unauthorized party, the marketing director of a medical clinic creates a misleading advertising campaign, and a dietary aid in a medical center's cafeteria falsifies her time sheet. Such instances clearly are well outside the bounds of ethical behavior, with most any reasonable individual being able to determine that these are unethical actions. The noted scenarios even carry legal consequences, making associated determinations quite simple. However, when situations are not so clear, occupying gray areas which cloud obvious decision pathways, they present **ethical dilemmas**, something that is especially pronounced when scenarios under scrutiny are not explicitly against the law. While the rule of law certainly can be helpful in determining whether an action is or is not ethical, this is not foolproof, as many actions which do not constitute violations of law indeed are unethical [28, 29]. An imaging department director's decision to park his personal vehicle in a patient-designated parking area technically would not be an illegal act, but it would be viewed to be unethical—and almost certainly represent a workplace policy violation.

Ethical dilemmas are not at all uncommon in health and medicine, playing out each and every day across a wide variety of areas [2, 30]. Scenarios faced are practically endless and range from items of little consequence to items of great consequence, as illustrated by the following examples. Is it appropriate for a billing manager to check her personal social media accounts while she is "on the clock?" Can a maintenance technician repair his personal vehicle in the service bay of a hospital's maintenance garage? Is it proper for a housekeeping employee to keep a 20-dollar bill that he found in the hallway of the medical center he is responsible for cleaning? Is it acceptable for a nurse manager to force a staff nurse to fill a critical coverage gap in the work schedule? Can a laboratory manager accept a food basket gifted by a representative of a laboratory supply company? What level of constructive criticism can be forwarded by a manager to a subordinate without it entering the realm of harassment? How should a hospital billing manager handle the account of a patient who experienced a personal tragedy and cannot afford to pay his bill? What should a patient representative do when she encounters a patient's family members and notices that they are starving but cannot afford food?

Regardless of the ethical dilemma faced, opinions likely will differ between and among individuals as to what does and does not constitute an acceptable course of action. Healthcare organizations, however, cannot tolerate such variation as this leads to inconsistencies in operation. Instead, they must take steps to ensure that all employees respond in an institutionally sanctioned manner to any dilemma encountered. The variation inherent in employee responses to ethical dilemmas stems from their many influences. Individuals enter employment with extensive personal histories that shape their views for distinguishing good from bad and right from wrong, impacting how they address situations and circumstances that they encounter [31, 32]. One's family and friends, their educational experiences, their religious views, and the like are common influences of what are referred to as **individual ethics**. More broadly, people are exposed to and influenced by **societal ethics**, perspectives on topics of fairness, justice, individual rights, and similar ethical mindsets as embraced by the societies in which individuals reside, with these being derived from applicable laws, customs, and practices [21].

The basic ethical operation framework provided by individual and societal ethics is made more specific when one enters employment, with the ethics perspectives of both given professions and specific organizations having perhaps the most noteworthy impact on how individuals respond to ethical dilemmas. **Occupational ethics** refer to the standards embraced by the members of a profession, trade, or craft regarding appropriate conduct in their work lives. This has a significant bearing on those in the healthcare industry, given extensive specializations across many different types of professions, with each possessing its own guidelines regarding standards of practice. Licensure and certification bodies also extensively control and regulate what can and cannot be done by those holding associated credentials, further shoring up influences stemming from one's occupation. Individuals also are influenced by the ethical guidelines of their employers. These **organizational ethics** stipulate the particular standards which are embraced by given institutions and required of those working within them, with these typically being presented in codes of conduct, conveyed robustly at employee orientations, and reinforced during department meetings, employee training sessions, and similar events [21].

As one moves from individual to societal to occupational to organizational ethics, specificity of application to work environments obviously becomes more pronounced. Shaping each employee's sense of ethics to equate with the framework espoused by given employers is essential for operational consistency. It also provides the pathway for resolving any ethical dilemma faced. Employees need only consult organizational policy or, if still in doubt, confer with their given supervisors to ascertain the correct, institutionally approved pathways to take in order to bring resolution to the dilemmas encountered. To permit this to become a reality, though, healthcare establishments must make proper investments, with the establishment of comprehensive ethics programs being absolutely essential.

7.5 Ethics Programs and Their Associated Components

Maintaining work environments characterized by high ethical standards requires that health and medical organizations establish comprehensive ethics programs. Given the differentiated backgrounds of employees within healthcare establishments and the various influences that form their perspectives of right and wrong and good and bad, healthcare establishments cannot assume that employees will simply "do the right thing" when encountering ethical dilemmas, as they likely will have varying ideas of what constitutes correct pathways. Consistent ethical operation requires institutional direction, informing employees of proper, organizationally sanctioned approaches for addressing and resolving any ethical dilemma encountered. Several components are required in any comprehensive ethics program, namely, a formal code of conduct, staffing practices which emphasize ethics, ethics training programs, and systems of accountability and control which foster ethical behaviors.

7.5.1 Codes of Conduct

A **code of conduct**—defined earlier as a formal document presenting an institution's moral code, outlining and describing the ethical tenets embraced by the given organization—is an essential component of an ethics program. Sometimes referred to as a **code of ethics** or **code of ethical conduct**, this document presents an organization's position on matters of ethics, and as such, it should be considered to be the centerpiece of an ethics program [17, 25]. A code of conduct ideally should be formulated when a healthcare organization is founded, being updated as circumstances and situations warrant. Early formulation permits the core benefits of ethical codes to be realized from the very start of operations, setting the stage for integrity to be promoted and realized throughout the institution. A code of conduct is useful both for educational purposes, informing employees of the expectations demanded of them by their employers, and for public relations purposes, informing stakeholders of the ethical stance of given health and medical organizations. The ultimate value of a code of conduct, however, rests with employee adherence to its tenets, as operationalization, described earlier, is essential for purposes of bringing life to the qualities expressed in associated codes. When establishments prioritize ethical codes, regularly reinforce their importance, and penalize those who violate associated rules, a code of conduct serves as an effective foundation for building and maintaining a successful ethics program [2, 25, 30].

7.5.2 Ethical Staffing Practices

Staffing practices, centering on recruitment and selection activities, are vital in healthcare establishments for many reasons, offering opportunities for them to determine if the qualifications of job candidates match the requirements of given employment opportunities. As past performance is the best predictor of future performance, staffing managers seeking an environment characterized by ethical behavior should be especially vigilant in conducting job interviews, ensuring that they include assessments of candidate integrity. Inquiries specifically querying individuals about ethical dilemmas faced and how they were addressed can be particularly enlightening. Presenting "What if?" scenarios also can help to determine the ethical mindsets and perspectives of prospects. Of course, background checks must be conducted, with these necessarily being thorough. Findings should be evaluated through an ethical lens, building as clear a picture as possible of a candidate's past history and potential for operating ethically in the future [25]. Efforts here should be especially pronounced when evaluating job candidates for management positions, given their oversight duties and responsibilities and associated opportunities to influence and impact scores of staff members. **Moral managers**—individuals who emphasize ethical behavior as they go about engaging in the practice of management—are particularly desirable personnel [17]. They should be vigorously sought by healthcare establishments in order to shore up and advance the ethical integrity of the workforce.

7.5.3   Ethics Training Programs

Ethics training programs constitute another critical component of a comprehensive institutional ethics offering. These educational opportunities typically are multifaceted, addressing a wide variety of ethical issues and concerns, and they are ongoing, ensuring that ethics knowledge remains current. New employee orientation and onboarding sessions routinely feature modules on institutional ethics, notably introducing codes of conduct and more, with new employees typically being required to acknowledge their understanding of content conveyed. These early exposures are reinforced through a variety of methods, with mandatory annual training in ethics being a common requirement, serving to remind employees of the ethical framework of their given employers and their associated responsibilities as agents of their healthcare organizations. Reinforcement opportunities are not limited to formal events operated by institutional human resource departments. They also are threaded by managers into departmental meetings and other interactions with staff members, further emphasizing the ethics positions of healthcare providers. While ethics training programs offer no guarantees that employees will behave ethically, they provide essential educational information that, if conveyed routinely, will remain at the forefront of employees' minds as they go about conducting their assigned duties and responsibilities, increasing the likelihood that they will choose to operate in a manner compliant with institutional policy. These programs also demonstrate that institutions are serious about operating ethically, investing in learning opportunities to guide staff members, accordingly [17, 25, 29].

7.5.4   Systems of Accountability and Control

Systems of accountability and control are vital elements of ethics programs, as they help to ensure that employees follow standards of ethical operation by monitoring compliance and issuing penalties for noncompliance. The range of accountability and control mechanisms is wide and selection typically depends on the nature of the workplace and its associated task requirements. Common mechanisms with broad applicability include things such as video surveillance and computer surveillance which can deter unethical behaviors simply by virtue of employees being aware that they are being monitored. Many employment activities, especially those involving the handling of financial resources, are well suited for auditing, offering a protective mechanism against theft and related unethical behaviors. Performance evaluations, too, provide opportunities to evaluate the ethical behaviors of employees and issue rewards or penalties in accordance with merit demonstrated. Regardless of the methods used to monitor actions and behaviors, mechanisms must be devised which permit suspected ethical violations to be reported, allowing authorities to investigate the associated claims. Individuals reporting claims of misconduct, often referred to as **whistleblowers**, should be protected, assuming their claims are made in good faith [17, 25, 29]. Employees confirmed to have committed ethical failures should be penalized in a manner fitting the violation, up to and including the termination of their employment. In cases where violations are believed to constitute crimes, law enforcement must also be notified for purposes of ensuring ethical integrity.

While the referenced mechanisms of ethical accountability and control are often among the first to come to mind when considering defenses against unethical behavior, they certainly should not crowd out one of the most essential vehicles for ensuring integrity and forthright actions and behaviors: managerial oversight and guidance. As conveyed earlier, many ethical dilemmas faced by the employees of healthcare establishments have no easy answers. Codes of conduct and training sessions cannot possibly cover all of the potential scenarios that one might face in the workplace, leaving gaps which can prove problematic if not handled properly. Employees can best fill these gaps via consultations with their given supervisors, requesting their assistance in addressing vexing ethical dilemmas encountered. Managerial oversight indeed bolsters employee compliance across all areas of operation, including those associated with ethical duties and responsibilities. As such, managers serve as excellent accountability and control mechanisms for fostering ethical behaviors and actions [2, 23, 25, 26], nicely complementing the ethical structures featured in health and medical establishments.

7.6 Defining Social Responsibility

A concept that is closely related to ethics is known as **social responsibility**, an institutional philosophy and practice which challenges an organization to operate in a manner that extends benefits to the societies in which the establishment is based. For socially responsible organizations, motivations go beyond focusing on institutional concerns, incorporating also concerns for their given communities [14, 22]. Socially responsible practices, in essence, represent a form of **organizational altruism**, as they involve engaging in pursuits which are beyond the scope of the core mission of institutions. Socially responsible practices are optional pursuits, not required by law or economics [25]. They also serve as excellent ways of demonstrating proper **stewardship**, showing stakeholders that institutions are carrying out operations and using the resources earned and entrusted to them in a responsible, selfless manner, making them assets in their given communities.

Acting in a socially responsible fashion serves as perhaps the greatest exemplification of operating ethically, as healthcare organizations expand their pools of concern beyond patients and employees to include the well-being of their given communities. As social responsibility is an optional practice, however, healthcare institutions vary in their level of commitment to these practices. Four stances on social responsibility are possible, with these forming a continuum ranging from least to most dedicated to the practice. An **obstructionist stance** is one where organizations choose to do as little as possible to positively impact their communities, with this generally equating with refraining from socially responsible initiatives altogether. A **defensive stance** is a minimalistic approach, with establishments opting to do only what is absolutely required of them to maintain their reputations, with perhaps some attention being directed toward social responsibility but only for self-serving purposes. An **accommodative stance** sees organizations begin to genuinely embrace social responsibility where they opt to pursue associated practices on a limited basis. A **proactive stance** represents the most robust approach to social responsibility where organizations aggressively pursue these endeavors in an effort to become valued assets of the communities in which they reside [14, 21]. Healthcare institutions should strive to at least hold an accommodative stance and, ideally, a proactive stance, permitting them to maximize their contributions in their environments.

The methods used to demonstrate social responsibility are highly varied. Socially responsible endeavors often center on performing charitable acts. A hospital's decision to establish an indigent clinic in a medically underserved neighborhood and a medical clinic's decision to establish a college scholarship fund for underprivileged high school graduates serve as excellent examples of such initiatives [33]. Social responsibility themes also commonly focus on environmental stewardship [34, 35]. A medical center's commitment to use recycled products at every available opportunity and a mobile physical therapy clinic's decision to make use of electric vehicles rather than those relying on internal combustion engines represent good examples of environmentally conscious social responsibility pursuits. Acts of social responsibility, however, have no set boundaries. Essentially anything that a healthcare institution wishes to do to improve their given communities, whatever that might be, falls under the umbrella of social responsibility. Selection is dependent on the desires of institutional leaders. Creative thought is particularly useful in formulating social responsibility initiatives, often yielding meaningful and memorable altruistic pursuits and pathways. Highly creative and unique social responsibility endeavors are particularly inspiring and laden with potential, providing mutual benefits for healthcare establishments and their constituencies, making associated pursuits worthwhile.

7.7 Benefits of Social Responsibility

Reflecting on the examples provided earlier, it can rightfully be assumed that social responsibility initiatives carry costs for the healthcare organizations which offer them, with commitments of time, money, and other resources climbing as initiatives become more robust. As these are selfless endeavors, motivated by the desires of health and medical establishments to "give back" to their communities, associated resource outlays are not forwarded with the intention of achieving a particular return on investment. Instead, they are goodwill gestures designed to benefit the communities of given healthcare organizations by improving the environment, helping the needy, bolstering education, or effecting similar advancements that help those living in the sphere of influence of these establishments. This does not mean, however, that healthcare establishments engaging in social responsibility do not benefit from their investments. An improved community ultimately is the goal of social responsibility, and, as such, generous healthcare institutions, as members of their given communities, share in this benefit. And for such investments, they might even see associated rewards multiply. Social responsibility expressed by one institution in a community often is infectious, compelling neighboring institutions to take up the mantle, engaging in acts of selflessness, further improving given communities and benefiting all parties residing within them [14].

Beyond matters of community benefit, altruistic, socially responsible endeavors powerfully influence stakeholders, with this improving the prospects of them looking favorably upon the healthcare organizations engaged in such. Employees, for example, often feel a greater affinity for their socially responsible employers, viewing them to not be solely focused on reaping the benefits derived from their labor. This can improve employee retention, and it also can help attract job candidates desirous of working for healthcare organizations which demonstrate selflessness in their operation. This, too, can improve employee morale. Patients can be similarly inspired by social responsibility initiatives, with their confidence in healthcare providers being heightened by seeing evidence of selfless service in their communities. This also can encourage prospective patients to direct their patronage toward given healthcare providers. The reputational enhancements afforded by social responsibility additionally can prompt governmental entities to look favorably upon the healthcare establishments which provide these investments, potentially aiding organizations in successfully traversing any policy barriers faced. Ultimately, the goodwill generated by social responsibility has a profound and positive impact on the reputations of healthcare establishments, furthering their positions as ethical institutions, making for a compelling reason to incorporate various initiatives into operations.

WK Reflections: Tithing the Bottom Line

Willis Knighton Health has been engaged in prominent social responsibility initiatives for decades. Of all of the establishment's charitable endeavors, the institution's Tithing the Bottom Line program is the most notable and comprehensive. This program takes a portion of annual earnings (i.e., the bottom line) and donates (i.e., tithes) it to charitable endeavors supportive of the establishment's mission and deemed to be of benefit to the community [2, 36]. The program's unique "Tithing the Bottom Line" descriptor is a reference to tithing in the context of Christianity where parishioners voluntarily contribute or tithe a portion of their income to support their church. Such a design facilitates program continuity as the level of investment changes in tandem with the finances of the institution. More prosperous times permit more robust giving; leaner times reduce the amount. This design offers flexibility that is not possible in scenarios involving a set contribution which might not be able to be accommodated consistently over time, given the possibility of economic downturns, frequent health policy changes that can impact financial reimbursements, and similar events and occurrences beyond the control of healthcare institutions.

The Tithing the Bottom Line program was designed to be a purely charitable initiative. In healthcare organizations, charity care and bad debts expenses together constitute uncompensated care. While the two are very different, they are often intermingled due to operational and reporting complexities. Charity care is forwarded with no expectation of payment; bad debt expenses emerge from services rendered with payment expected but not received [37, 38]. Contributions forwarded by Willis Knighton Health's tithing program are separate and distinct from bad debt expenses incurred by the institution. The funds are forwarded to worthy causes within the community with no expectation of remuneration.

Willis Knighton Health's Tithing the Bottom Line program has awarded millions of dollars to support charitable healthcare, education, and humanitarian initiatives, with award recipients and associated amounts being determined by a dedicated committee. Funding has been provided to support various poverty care initiatives, such as free pharmacies serving the underprivileged. Area universities have benefited by receiving funding to establish professorships and offer scholarships in health and medical-related departments and programs, aiding them in their ability to supply a robust healthcare workforce. Support also has been richly extended to organizations endeavoring to bolster the housing and nutrition needs of the poor in the community. These and related investments have had a positive impact on Shreveport and the greater region of northwest Louisiana.

While the community has benefited greatly from the Tithing the Bottom Line program, so, too, has Willis Knighton Health. Contributions have generated and continue to generate significant publicity which, in turn, helps to promote the institution. This publicity also demonstrates the establishment's willingness to invest in its community which generates significant goodwill. This has had a profound, positive impact on the institution and its reputation, garnering robust stakeholder support and loyalty. Numerous mutual benefits abound, something that well-planned and implemented social responsibility initiatives are known to provide.

The Tithing the Bottom Line program is Willis Knighton Health's cornerstone social responsibility initiative. Importantly and uniquely, it provides a framework for evaluating causes of importance in communities and determining which will be funded and at what level. Replication of this type of initiative requires a few basic steps. Institutions must (1) determine the program's focus and objectives; (2) designate the funding methodology, notably including the percent contribution and distribution timeline; (3) stipulate eligibility criteria and selection methods for awards; (4) devise mechanisms to notify award recipients; and (5) determine methods for evaluating program performance. The Tithing the Bottom Line program illustrates the value of "outside of the box" thinking regarding social responsibility and the contributions forwarded by institutions.

7.8   Summary and Conclusions

As health and medical organizations are collections of individuals entrusted with carrying out associated operations, great care must be taken to ensure that each employee acts in an ethical fashion. This requires vigilance on the part of healthcare establishments, necessitating the development of a formal code of conduct, staffing practices which emphasize ethics, ethics training programs, and systems of accountability and control which foster ethical behaviors. Such efforts educate and enlighten staff members regarding what is right, what is wrong, what is good, and what is bad, aiding them in making proper decisions as they go about completing their assigned duties and responsibilities. Entrusting employees to operate in an ethical fashion without supplying direct and comprehensive guidance is a formula for disaster, as individuals are products of their own respective histories, leading to different views of what does and does not constitute an ethically appropriate action. As such, proper investments must be directed toward instilling within employees the ethical mindsets espoused by healthcare providers, leading to consistent behaviors, especially when ethical dilemmas present themselves. Ideally, investments in ethical operation should be extended to also include investments in socially responsible initiatives, permitting healthcare establishments to reach their highest ethical state, generating numerous mutual benefits that positively impact communities in their entirety.

Key Terms

- Accommodative Stance
- Business Ethics
- Code of Conduct
- Code of Ethical Conduct
- Code of Ethics
- Defensive Stance
- Ethical Dilemma
- Ethics
- Individual Ethics
- Managerial Ethics
- Medical Ethics
- Moral Code
- Moral Framework
- Moral Manager
- Obstructionist Stance
- Occupational Ethics
- Operationalize
- Organizational Altruism
- Organizational Ethics
- Proactive Stance
- Reputation
- Social Responsibility
- Societal Ethics
- Stakeholder
- Stewardship
- Transparency
- Values Statement
- Whistleblower

Exercises

1. In your own words, define ethics, share insights regarding its prominent role in organizational prosperity, and discuss its importance in health and medical establishments.
2. Prepare a brief essay summarizing the benefits of operating ethically. After doing so, reflect on why ethical operation is particularly vital in health and medical institutions.
3. In your own words, define stakeholders, and discuss how they impact healthcare organizations. Then, select a local healthcare establishment and investigate its stakeholders, identifying these groups as precisely as possible. Of the stakehold-

ers identified, indicate the top three groups you view to be most critical to the healthcare establishment, and describe how ethical operation impacts those groups. Be sure to justify your selections.

4. Define ethical dilemma, and, reflecting on your recent work experiences, describe in detail an ethical dilemma that you faced. Outline the process that you used to resolve the dilemma and identify the associated outcome. Looking back at the process you used to resolve the matter, would you change anything? Why or why not?

5. Healthcare organizations use a variety of tools and techniques to maintain high ethical standards. What methods does your current employer use? Do you see any room for improvement? If so, identify these improvements and indicate why they are needed. If not, describe in detail why improvements are not needed.

6. The moral manager is a prized asset in healthcare organizations. Conduct a personal assessment of your professional life, and describe your development as a moral manager. Are you currently fully exemplifying moral management, or is more work required for you to reach this state? Going forward, how do you plan to advance your development as a moral manager?

7. Assume that you have observed an unethical activity in your current workplace and you have made the decision to report the violation, effectively becoming a whistleblower. Reflect on what steps you will need to take in order to report the matter, what mechanisms your organization provides for such, what risks are involved in doing so, what protections are offered to employees reporting concerns in good faith, and similar considerations. After sharing your perspectives, indicate how this exercise has enhanced your understanding of the concerns and challenges faced by whistleblowers when they decide to report ethical violations.

8. Define the concept of social responsibility, and describe its role in positioning health and medical establishments as ethical institutions. Assume that you have been tasked with identifying three social responsibility initiatives to be offered by your employer, with these being in addition to any that are currently being offered. What would they be and why would you make the noted selections?

References

1. Elrod, J. K., & Fortenberry, J. L., Jr. (2018). Am I seeing things through the eyes of patients? An exercise in bolstering patient attentiveness and empathy. *BMC Health Services Research, 18*(Suppl 3), 41–44.
2. Elrod, J. K. (2013). *Breadcrumbs to cheesecake*. R&R Publishers.
3. Donohue, R., & Klasko, S. K. (2021). *Patient no longer: Why healthcare must deliver the care experience that consumers want and expect*. Health Administration Press.
4. Hoffman, S. (2022). Privacy and security: Protecting patients' health information. *New England Journal of Medicine, 387*(21), 1913–1916.
5. Pozgar, G. D. (2020). *Legal and ethical issues for health professionals* (5th ed.). Jones and Bartlett.
6. Shi, L., & Singh, D. A. (2023). *Essentials of the US health care system* (6th ed.). Jones and Bartlett.

7. McConnell, C. R. (2020). *Hospitals and health systems: What they are and how they work.* Jones and Bartlett.
8. McShane, S. L., & Von Glinow, M. A. (2019). *Organizational behavior* (4th ed.). McGraw-Hill.
9. Hitt, M. A., Miller, C. C., Colella, A., & Triana, M. D. C. (2018). *Organizational behavior* (5th ed.). Wiley.
10. Chandler, D. (2023). *Strategic corporate social responsibility: Sustainable value creation* (6th ed.). Sage.
11. Daft, R. L. (2022). *Management* (14th ed.). Cengage.
12. Ferrell, O. C., Fraedrich, J., & Ferrell, L. (2019). *Business ethics: Ethical decision making and cases* (12th ed.). Cengage.
13. Collins, D. (2019). *Business ethics: Best practices for designing and managing ethical organizations* (2nd ed.). Sage.
14. Griffin, R. W. (2022). *Management* (13th ed.). Cengage.
15. Wilkinson, D., Herring, J., & Savulescu, J. (2020). *Medical ethics and law: A curriculum for the 21st century* (3rd ed.). Elsevier.
16. Desai, M. K., & Kapadia, J. D. (2022). Medical professionalism and ethics. *Journal of Pharmacology and Pharmacotherapeutics, 13*(2), 113–118.
17. Schermerhorn, J. R., Jr., & Bachrach, D. G. (2015). *Management* (13th ed.). Wiley.
18. Yukl, G., Mahsud, R., Hassan, S., & Prussia, G. E. (2013). An improved measure of ethical leadership. *Journal of Leadership and Organizational Studies, 20*(1), 38–48.
19. Brown, M. E., Trevino, L. K., & Harrison, D. A. (2005). Ethical leadership: A social learning perspective for construct development and testing. *Organizational Behavior and Human Decision Processes, 97*(2), 117–134.
20. Trevino, L. K., & Brown, M. E. (2004). Managing to be ethical: Debunking five business ethics myths. *Academy of Management Executive, 18*(2), 69–81.
21. Jones, G. R., & George, J. M. (2022). *Contemporary management* (12th ed.). McGraw-Hill.
22. Trevino, L. K., & Nelson, K. A. (2021). *Managing business ethics: Straight talk about how to do it right* (8th ed.). Wiley.
23. Kinicki, A., & Soignet, D. B. (2022). *Management: A practical introduction* (10th ed.). McGraw-Hill.
24. Suddaby, R., & Panwar, R. (2022). On the complexity of managing transparency. *California Management Review, 65*(1), 5–18.
25. Robbins, S. P., & Coulter, M. (2021). *Management* (15th ed.). Pearson.
26. Stanwick, P. A., & Stanwick, S. D. (2016). *Understanding business ethics* (3rd ed.). Sage.
27. Hougaard, R., & Carter, J. (2022). Clarity is kindness: Why transparency at work matters. *Personal Excellence, 27*(3), 32–34.
28. Hartman, L. P., DesJardins, J., & MacDonald, C. (2021). *Business ethics: Decision making for personal integrity and social responsibility* (5th ed.). McGraw-Hill.
29. Marcus, A. A., & Hargrave, T. J. (2021). *Managing business ethics: Making ethical decisions.* Sage.
30. Morrison, E. E. (2020). *Ethics in health administration: A practical approach for decision makers* (4th ed.). Jones and Bartlett.
31. Flynn, W. J., Valentine, S. R., & Meglich, P. A. (2022). *Healthcare human resource management* (4th ed.). Cengage.
32. Konopaske, R., Ivancevich, J. M., & Matteson, M. T. (2018). *Organizational behavior and management* (11th ed.). McGraw-Hill.
33. Elrod, J. K., & Fortenberry, J. L., Jr. (2017). Bridging access gaps experienced by the underserved: The need for healthcare providers to look within for answers. *BMC Health Services Research, 17*(Suppl 4), 37–41.
34. Elrod, J. K., & Fortenberry, J. L., Jr. (2017). Adaptive reuse in the healthcare industry: Repurposing abandoned buildings to serve medical missions. *BMC Health Services Research, 17*(Suppl 1), 5–14.

35. Elrod, J. K., & Fortenberry, J. L., Jr. (2017). Advancing indigent healthcare services through adaptive reuse: Repurposing abandoned buildings as medical clinics for disadvantaged populations. *BMC Health Services Research, 17*(Suppl 4), 5–14.
36. Elrod, J. K., & Fortenberry, J. L., Jr. (2017). Tithing programs: Pathways for enhancing and improving the health status of the underprivileged. *BMC Health Services Research, 17*(Suppl 4), 15–22.
37. Valdovinos, E., Le, S., & Hsia, R. Y. (2015). In California, not-for-profit hospitals spent more operating expenses on charity care than for-profit hospitals spent. *Health Affairs, 34*(8), 1296–1303.
38. Morrisey, M. A., Wedig, G. J., & Hassan, M. (1996). Do nonprofit hospitals pay their way? *Health Affairs, 15*(4), 132–144.

Chapter 8
Organizational Culture in Health and Medicine

Learning Objectives

After examining this chapter, readers will have the ability to:

- Understand the concept of organizational culture, its various components, and its critical role in healthcare institutions.
- Discuss the differences between dominant organizational cultures and countercultures.
- Recognize the role of subcultures, identify their various types, and discuss their associated impact on organizational culture.
- Understand methods for developing and managing productive organizational cultures in healthcare establishments.
- Realize the value of culture audits and understand techniques for their implementation in health and medicine.
- Understand methods for closing culture gaps in healthcare institutions by engaging in culture change initiatives.

WK Reflections: Multiple Sites, One Willis Knighton Health

In the 1970s, when Willis Knighton Health decided to embark on an ambitious expansion plan which eventually led to market leadership, scores of decisions and associated actions were required as new campuses were added to its initial single-site location—Willis Knighton North (formerly known as Willis-Knighton Medical Center)—in west Shreveport, Louisiana. Many of the necessary pursuits concerned issues readily apparent to most anyone, including preparation of market analyses, selection of attractive sites, formulation of

J. K. Elrod, J. L. Fortenberry, Jr., *Organizational Behavior and Management in Health and Medicine*, https://doi.org/10.1007/978-3-031-61823-9_8

service arrays, acquisition of engineering and architectural expertise, construction of facilities, hiring and training of personnel, and the like. An often overlooked but equally important concern also was at the forefront of thought: ensuring that Willis Knighton Health's philosophy of operation, notably including its highly regarded patient experience, remained intact, even as its footprint across the region expanded.

Executives were particularly desirous of achieving consistency so pronounced between and among sites that patients familiar with one Willis Knighton Health facility would feel perfectly at home whenever they visited another one. To state it most simply, Willis Knighton Health sought to extend the organizational culture established at its original campus to its other sites as they came online, creating a universal look and feel, leading to a consistent patient experience regardless of facility selected. This required proactive, concerted planning on the part of executives to develop and put into place a range of components designed to evoke the desired culture at each new site established.

As would be expected, especially in complex organizations, numerous elements were required to perpetuate the health system's culture. Chief among these included the application of sound operational tenets as portrayed in Willis Knighton Health's mission, vision, and values statements; a capable organizational structure which ensured operational consistency across sites; the employment of managers dedicated to the corporate culture, permitting it to spread throughout given establishments; designing and appointing facilities in like fashion, affording equivalent form and function; educating employees about the health system's organizational culture through orientation and other socialization activities; and holding systemwide events which bring the Willis Knighton Health family together to foster learning, celebrate successes, and engage in similar pursuits.

Through these and related investments, the successful transfer of organizational culture was realized, occurring on numerous occasions over the years whenever new establishments were added to Willis Knighton Health's range of operations. Today, the system entails nearly 1300 beds across 5 hospital campuses and 1 retirement community, complemented by numerous general and specialty medical clinics located throughout northwest Louisiana. Culture transfer activities, however, have not ceased. The system continues to grow, necessitating continued efforts to extend Willis Knighton Health's productive organizational culture to new operations as they emerge to ensure consistency across the entire enterprise.

By dedicating significant time and attention toward developing and extending its organizational culture, Willis Knighton Health was able to grow its footprint across the region without compromising the highly desired characteristics and qualities that historically have defined the institution. Despite operating multiple sites, there really is only one Willis Knighton Health, and it is comprised of the entire collection of its establishments [1]. As the organizational culture of an institution bleeds into virtually every aspect of its operation, vigilance is required in any developmental pursuit. While challenging, achieving and advancing a productive organizational culture is entirely possible, with the end result being a consistent, reliable patient experience, complete with all of the benefits that this affords.

8.1 Background

Within health and medical establishments, the diversity of occupations is epic. From lower-level support roles (e.g., housekeepers, dietary aides) through to arguably the most advanced positions available anywhere (e.g., medical specialists), the range of employment opportunities housed within single entities is staggering and unique among industries. Driving this extensive diversity of occupations is an equally varied array of individuals possessing credentials spanning the continuum of educational offerings, from high school equivalencies or less to elite post-graduate medical qualifications. Salaries, too, mirror this diversity, with healthcare institutions routinely offering minimum wage rates through to vast sums based on one's education, ability, role, and market value [2, 3]. Beyond highly unique task, education, and income differentiators, healthcare establishments deal with the usual and customary diversity which characterizes any work environment, spanning the range of demographic variables (e.g., age, gender, race, nationality), psychographic qualities (e.g., social class, personality), and behavioral attributes (e.g., attitudes, loyalties, outlooks) [4–6]. All in all, such profoundly diverse work environments create challenges associated with directing staff members in a coordinated and unified fashion to fulfill designated missions.

Successfully managing organizational environments featuring the diversity characterizing health and medical institutions requires extensive efforts to foster shared mindsets which permit all to value and desire mission achievement [7]. In pursuit of such, direct measures are often the first to come to mind. Things like hiring right, providing proper guidance and direction, incentivizing desired performance, penalizing noncompliance, and related actions are part of the fabric of healthcare organizations and aid in directing personnel in prescribed manners. But a more powerful, all-encompassing mechanism exists—namely, organizational culture—which, if managed properly, has the potential to compel those working in healthcare establishments to embrace institutional missions and successfully pursue patient care endeavors in a unified fashion [1, 8]. This, in turn, positively impacts and influences patients and their perspectives of given health and medical institutions, generating high satisfaction, loyal patronage, burgeoning word-of-mouth referrals, and enduring prosperity [1, 9]. This particular chapter explores the concept of organizational culture and offers guidance for harnessing its power in healthcare establishments.

8.2   Defining Organizational Culture

Formally defined, an **organizational culture** is a mindset, expressed through and influenced by tangible and intangible means, which characterizes an institution and its operation. More simply, it could be described as a philosophy of operation embraced by an organization and expressed through both visual and nonvisual means. An organizational culture is institution specific [8, 10]. It is an exclusive feature of an organization, just as a fingerprint is to a particular human being. In addition to being unique to an institution, an organizational culture is shared (i.e., embraced by broad groups of employees), pervasive (i.e., prevalent across institutions), enduring (i.e., lasting over time in organizations), and implicit (i.e., understood by those operating in organizations) [11]. Its transfer from employee to employee occurs notably through **socialization** [7, 12], a process through which individuals come to realize and understand the expectations of a group, permitting them to adjust their behaviors in a manner to foster acclimation and approval. New employee orientations, onboarding sessions, mentoring, and related socialization activities commonly provided within healthcare establishments offer outstanding culture conveyance opportunities.

Organizational cultures exist in all establishments and they have a significant bearing on institutional performance. Research indicates that a productive organizational culture can facilitate the accomplishment of institutional missions, improve employee morale, and drive employee productivity. It also is known to spark innovation, amplify competitiveness, enhance attentiveness toward customers, and foster financial success [13–18]. Further, it positively influences **organizational climate** [19, 20], the atmosphere or ambiance of an institution derived from the organizational culture operating within, prevailing environmental considerations, and associated influences and impacts of the workforce. A productive organizational culture ultimately affords a key **competitive advantage**, that is, a distinctive capability that gives an organization an edge over its competitors [21, 22]. As healthcare establishments exist in what many view to be the most competitive of industries, the notion that a thoughtfully designed organizational culture can amplify performance makes understanding the concept all the more important.

8.3   The Influences of Organizational Culture

Sometimes referred to as **corporate culture** [10], an organization's culture essentially is a way of thinking which guides employees as they go about addressing their duties and responsibilities within an establishment [23]. This philosophy of operation, in turn, influences all parties circulating in the establishment, revealing a sort of presence or identity that can be felt or sensed within the given organization. When a nurse, reflecting on her employment experience at a particular medical clinic, glowingly describes the camaraderie within the establishment; when a patient, following a successful surgery at a hospital, praises the staff for demonstrating compassion and concern; and when a pharmaceutical sales representative, while making a sales presentation to a physician group, compliments them for creating an environment that exudes innovation, each could be said to be expressing thoughts and feelings arising from the influences of organizational culture.

The influences evoked by an organization's culture emerge from an amalgam of seen and unseen things [8, 24]. Something led the individuals referenced above to arrive at their opinions regarding the given establishments. The nurse perhaps acquired her perspective courtesy of the clinic's hiring of kind and caring employees, its sponsorship of social events that bring employees together and foster bonding, and its support of her when she was injured in an automobile accident on her way to work. The patient noted earlier might have developed his view because of the hospital's patient concierge department which addressed critical needs during his admission, its kind and courteous staff members, and its exceptional care management program. The pharmaceutical sales representative perhaps noted the physician group's incorporation of advanced admissions technologies, its state-of-the-art surgical suites, and its use of the latest robotic surgery technologies.

The observable elements of an organizational culture exist due to unobservable, intangible things, namely, operational values and beliefs, typically portrayed tangibly in mission, vision, and values statements. **Mission statements** are brief documents which succinctly state the purpose of organizations, conveying strategic priorities and other institutional characteristics in a positive, inspiring manner to help guide employees and inform others of institutional aims. **Vision statements** complement mission statements by shifting the focus from present day to tomorrow by expressing what given institutions aspire to become in the future. **Values statements** are documents which succinctly present the core standards, ideals, and principles that guide and direct pursuit of designated missions and visions [25, 26]. These core tenets—essentially **foundations of culture**—drive that which is seen and experienced by those circulating in a given organization, resulting in the communication and transference of the underlying organizational culture [10, 15].

8.4 Positive and Negative Organizational Cultures

The examples expressed earlier in this chapter each portray positive organizational cultures, but it is important to note that negative ones also exist. Depending on the nature of the organizational culture in operation within an establishment, the performance derived from such may be desirable or undesirable, yielding a benefit or detriment to the given enterprise. As such, organizational cultures are often referred to as being strong or weak, positive or negative, healthy or unhealthy, or described in similar fashion. Further, once a particular organizational culture takes root in an institution, it can be very difficult to change [10, 27–29]. Seen in this light, it is not hard to understand why organizational culture is often characterized as being the personality of an organization [30]. Just as the personality of an individual can be good or bad, helping or harming the person, so too can an organization's culture, serving to advance or hinder the institution. Given this, prudent steps must be taken to foster productive organizational cultures within establishments or, if encountered, correct negative ones that have emerged.

8.5   Schein's Model of Culture

To better understand organizational culture, it is helpful to dissect the concept, breaking down its components. This is necessary as organizational culture seems to be a relatively simple concept at face value, but that is not the case. The more one learns about organizational culture, the easier it is to realize that it is actually quite complex, warranting an examination of its various parts to aid in bolstering associated understanding. Arguably the most popular depiction of the components of culture was provided by renowned organizational culture researcher Edgar Schein who developed a framework containing three levels: artifacts, espoused values and beliefs, and basic underlying assumptions. The three levels of Schein's model of culture are explained in the following sections.

8.5.1   Artifacts

Artifacts are visible phenomena, essentially any tangible manifestation that would be said to represent a given institution [8]. Examples of artifacts include an organization's physical environment, such as its architectural style, buildings, and grounds; the appearance and professionalism of its employees, including their grooming and attire; the technologies and other innovations offered by the institution; published mission statements, organizational charts, and related portrayals; and rituals, ceremonies, and protocols which demonstrate institutional priorities, traditions, and practices. Artifacts often are highly diverse, taking many forms, especially in complex medical centers. As observable elements, many times, the meaning of artifacts is very clear to institutional insiders and outsiders alike, as in the case of a hospital's annual employee awards ceremony, an event which obviously is held to honor staff members for performing well. But sometimes the meaning of artifacts cannot be ascertained by those lacking knowledge about the organization and its practices [8]. Take, for example, the bell ringing ceremony often conducted by patients to celebrate the completion of chemotherapy treatment. A hospital visitor with no prior exposure to the ceremony likely would not understand its meaning and would need to inquire to gain an associated understanding. In such cases, deeper knowledge is required to make sense of given observations. All in all, artifacts bring an organizational culture to life by presenting visible elements which represent the underlying philosophy of operation in given institutions.

8.5.2 Espoused Values and Beliefs

Espoused values and beliefs are ideologies which reflect the goals, ideals, viewpoints, and aspirations of given institutions [8]. These are intangible elements, generally informing and motivating the selection of artifacts which visibly represent particular organizations. For example, a medical center's values and beliefs are not directly observable as they are intangibles formulated by and existing within the hearts and minds of the establishment's founders and top executives. They, however, enter the realm of visibility when artifacts are selected to communicate these notions to others circulating in the medical center. Assume, for example, that the medical center embraced a value centered on the delivery of exceptional customer service. This intangible aspiration could be operationalized tangibly by requiring all employees to complete a customer service training program, instituting technologies that reduce wait times and expedite routine care delivery processes, offering amenities such as convenient parking and concierge services which engender goodwill, and incorporating similar features that demonstrate customer service excellence. Each of these artifacts helps to convey to others that customer service is a priority at the medical center, permitting espoused values and beliefs to essentially be seen, albeit via their tangible representations.

8.5.3 Basic Underlying Assumptions

Basic underlying assumptions are magnifications of espoused values and beliefs. They emerge when espoused values and beliefs become so entrenched over time that they become unconscious, automatically governing and guiding the actions of personnel as they go about attending to their assigned duties and responsibilities [8]. In the medical center example above, over time, protocols for handling routine matters in a manner exemplifying exceptional customer service will emerge, but even the nonroutine will be able to be addressed using discretion based on understood operational approaches. The medical center's patient representatives, for example, might regularly offer taxi vouchers when they encounter patients who are experiencing transportation difficulties, with this practice emerging as a result of the governing customer service culture. If, however, they encountered an atypical situation where an out-of-town patient's loved ones could not afford overnight lodging during the admission, they might arrange a hotel voucher, guided simply by basic underlying assumptions emerging from the established culture which dictates acceptable and expected actions. When healthcare organizations observe that basic underlying assumptions are driving thought and action within their halls, the organizational culture is considered to be fully manifested within the establishment.

8.6   Cultural Congruence

Schein's three-level depiction helpfully unveils the innerworkings of organizational culture, permitting associated enlightenment. The levels effectively reveal the components of the concept, affording a greater understanding of its whole. Schein's model also provides a helpful reminder that artifacts must accurately portray the espoused values and beliefs and basic underlying assumptions held by an organization. Such consistency between and among the components of culture is sometimes referred to as **cultural fit** or **cultural congruence** [31]. Organizational cultures, in fact, can witness a mismatch between tangible and intangible components. Consider, once again, the customer service-oriented medical center discussed earlier. Even with excellent intentions, focus can be lost. Perhaps the medical center encountered rapid growth causing short staffing which diminished customer attentiveness. Perhaps new employees were being hired so quickly that customer service training opportunities could not be provided, reducing associated skill sets. Perhaps budget cuts introduced by the medical center reduced the number of amenities available to patients and their loved ones, harming satisfaction levels. Perhaps the erosion of customer service occurred simply due to workplace distractions leading to inattention. In such cases, even though the underlying value of providing exceptional customer service remains, circumstances have diminished its portrayal via tangible artifacts, leading to incongruence between and among the components of culture. Care must be taken to ensure consistency and this requires keen attentiveness and action.

WK Reflections: Branding and Organizational Culture

One of the most exciting aspects associated with developing the organizational culture of a healthcare establishment pertains to the selection of representative cultural artifacts. Here, healthcare providers are tasked with determining how the intangible values and beliefs embraced by a given institution will be expressed tangibly to aid employees, patients, and others in understanding the underlying culture. This step, of course, occurs after values and beliefs have been formulated, something which normally takes place early in the lives of healthcare organizations during strategic planning exercises. In many respects, however, formulation of values and beliefs is a simpler task than that of selecting representative artifacts. A healthcare establishment might, for example, embrace the value of innovation leadership, but how exactly should that be presented tangibly? Ironically, the practice of branding, a concept from the discipline of marketing, offers some helpful insights for approaching this important culture development activity.

Branding is defined as the assignment of elements of identity (e.g., brand names, logos, slogans) to organizations and their product offerings for the purpose of aiding consumers in identifying and understanding associated goods and services. Modern branding practices in health services organizations seek to develop comprehensive brand experiences, often selecting expressions across the full array of senses—sight (e.g., logos, unique color schemes), sound (e.g., branded music-on-hold services), taste (e.g., mints at patient concierge stations, premium meals for patients), touch (e.g., comfortable hospital bedding, signature linens), and smell (e.g., aromatherapy in patient rooms, signature scents within institutions)—as occasions permit [32–35].

Essentially, branding brings tangibility to an otherwise intangible offering by selecting elements to portray and characterize a given healthcare establishment and its services. The practice of choosing cultural artifacts is conducted in similar fashion, requiring the selection of elements to portray and characterize the culture in operation within the establishment. The key difference is that, unlike branding which primarily seeks to address current and prospective patients, artifacts seek to address all stakeholders of given healthcare establishments, notably including employees. Artifacts also delve into deeper aspects of the organization and its operation as they serve both as conveyors and reflections of underlying institutional values and beliefs.

As with branding, the selection of cultural artifacts requires creative thinking. Consider the example of the WK Heart and Vascular Institute, Willis Knighton Health's center of excellence for cardiology. Courtesy of being a component of Willis Knighton Health, the institute embraces innovation leadership as one of its core values and beliefs [1, 36]. Naturally, this requires offering leading technologies for treating heart problems, making for an obvious cultural artifact. Some might think that this would be sufficient, but for optimal results, more is needed. Innovation leadership can be expressed in ways beyond superior technology, further reinforcing underlying values.

The WK Heart and Vascular Institute features, for example, a contemporary architectural design, with its modern appearance suggesting keen innovation. Its servicescapes are equally modern, combining the latest insights on form and function to yield excellent patient experiences. Additionally, continual learning is emphasized with workshops, conferences, and other educational opportunities being provided to staff members to ensure that they stay abreast of the latest developments in the industry. Best practices are embedded into virtually every aspect of operation, further positioning the institute as a citadel of innovation. These and related artifacts were intentionally put into place to support the WK Heart and Vascular Institute's underlying commitment to innovation leadership, and they combine to create an atmosphere that exudes innovation. It can be sensed or felt when walking through the facility, with this indicating that the artifacts are doing their job as intended, tangibly expressing a fundamental element of the establishment's organizational culture.

8   Organizational Culture in Health and Medicine

This brief example nicely illustrates the general approach for selecting cultural artifacts. Similar to a successful branding process yielding elements of identity that accurately represent products, a successful cultural artifact selection process yields an array of tangible elements that accurately represents the underlying values and beliefs of the institution's organizational culture. Viewing this important task through the lens of branding can be very helpful for adding clarity, assisting healthcare organizations in making excellent selections which successfully convey their associated organizational cultures.

8.7   Dominant Cultures and Subcultures

In an ideal institutional environment, the organizational culture of a given healthcare establishment will be uniform across its entirety. In such scenarios, all staff members (e.g., physicians, nurses, administrators, technicians, laborers, etc.) collectively embrace a shared mindset, compliant with institutional values and beliefs, which guides them as they pursue their assigned duties and responsibilities. A united front, of course, enhances a healthcare organization's ability to efficiently and effectively achieve goals and objectives, being freed of the debilitating effects of divisiveness, fractured loyalties, and related factors that diminish productivity. Such a single, uniform, consistent organizational culture, however, is unrealistic in most health and medical enterprises, especially those which are highly complex. More typically, healthcare institutions will see some form of deviation from this ideal, often with a dominant culture and one or more subcultures being present in given establishments. A **dominant culture** is an organizational culture that is embraced by the majority of the members of an institution. This particular variant typically is the one developed and sanctioned by top management [37]. When an institution refers to its organizational culture, it usually is speaking of its dominant culture [38].

A **subculture** is an organizational culture, embraced by a particular subset of the greater workforce, which emerges based on some commonality shared by members (e.g., occupation, department, work location), unifying them in some manner which differs from that of the dominant culture of the institution. The contribution of subcultures is dependent on their nature, with three forms—enhancing, orthogonal, and countercultural—being possibilities. An **enhancing subculture** is one which sees members vigorously champion the dominant culture of the organization, magnifying its impact. An **orthogonal subculture** is one which sees members simultaneously embrace the dominant culture of an organization, as well as a nonconflicting set of perspectives particular to these members. A **countercultural subculture** or **counterculture** is one which is in conflict with the dominant culture, directly challenging the prevailing mindset [37].

The diversity within health and medical organizations, as described earlier in this chapter, creates an almost certainty that subcultures will emerge and exist within given institutions. Opportunities, in fact, abound for subcultures to develop on a range of fronts. When individuals perform the same occupation in a healthcare establishment, bonding on that front can occur, creating the potential for a subculture to develop. Physicians, for example, possess shared experiences with their fellow practitioners dating back to their specialized training programs and extending into the workplace, fostering solidarity that can prompt an associated subculture. The same could be said for most any occupation. Somewhat similarly, particular departments, such as laboratory, imaging, and dietary, can develop unique subcultures based on the experiences of staff members as they go about interacting with other departments within healthcare organizations. Subcultures can also develop by location. A multicampus hospital system, for example, can see the development of subcultures tied to geography. Assume that a particular hospital in the system is located more remotely than the others, resulting in feelings of isolation among its staff members. Such mindsets could easily foster the development of a subculture at that location. Virtually any difference between and among various work groups offers opportunities for the establishment of subcultures.

The emergence of subcultures should not be surprising, as commonalities, especially in highly varied work settings, tend to draw people together. And as long as the subcultures are either the enhancing or orthogonal varieties, their presence is not problematic in given health and medical institutions. However, if a countercultural subculture appears, the healthcare establishment must take action to investigate its emergence and associated causes, rectifying incongruence and restoring unity of purpose across the organization.

Ultimately, regardless of the presence or absence of subcultures, health and medical enterprises must ensure consistent embracement of the institutionally sanctioned organizational culture throughout given establishments, ensuring its dominance, permitting efforts to be directed in unison toward fulfilling associated missions. Indeed, any noted **culture gap**—the difference between the organizational culture desired by the establishment and the actual organizational culture exhibited within the institution—should be narrowed and, ideally, eliminated to foster mission attainment and resulting institutional success. By directing ongoing attention toward organizational culture development and management, healthcare providers set the stage for achieving productive organizational cultures which deliver numerous mutual benefits.

8.8 Developing an Organizational Culture

Many approaches for developing a desired organizational culture have been forwarded over the years. Of these methods, perhaps the simplest, most straightforward approach involves populating its various components, following a logical rationale for assembly. Earlier, Schein's three-level model of organizational culture was presented, depicting a popular rendition of the components of culture, namely, artifacts, espoused values and beliefs, and basic underlying assumptions. This particular model provides an excellent framework for the establishment of a desired organizational culture. Operationalizing this framework via a prudent developmental rationale, such as the four-step method described below, can help healthcare institutions realize a desired organizational culture.

8.8.1 Step 1: Formulate the Espoused Values and Beliefs Which Characterize the Desired Culture

Organizational culture development begins by focusing first on its intangible aspects. The intangible components of Schein's model of culture entail espoused values and beliefs and basic underlying assumptions. As basic underlying assumptions essentially are amplifications of espoused values and beliefs which develop over time, the operative focus during the initial stage of culture development is to concentrate on determining and stipulating an institution's espoused values and beliefs. If well designed and structured, these will eventually become deeply ingrained and evolve into basic underlying assumptions, guiding thought and action.

Espoused values and beliefs very often are expressed in institutional mission, vision, and values statements which emerge through the strategic planning process. Healthcare organizations which have engaged in proper strategic planning activities will find that this step requires little more than conducting a statement review and listing the values and beliefs (e.g., compassionate delivery of care, commitment to technological innovation, timely treatment of patients) which they reference. Those healthcare establishments which have neglected proper strategic planning activities or have decided that former guiding tenets need to be revised, however, must engage in appropriate exercises to yield mission, vision, and values details prior to attempting this cultural development step.

The quantity of espoused values and beliefs selected is dependent on the wishes of the given healthcare organization, as reflected in its mission, vision, and values statements. It is very common for health and medical establishments to embrace multiple, complementary values and beliefs. It also is common for particular subsets of designated values and beliefs to be emphasized. An urgent care clinic, for example, might first and foremost desire being known for its commitment to rapid "no waiting" service and choose to emphasize this above all other values. As such, it is often helpful to rank the values and beliefs selected to aid in determining priorities to emphasize in the organizational culture.

8.8.2 Step 2: Select Artifacts to Communicate and Reinforce the Designated Espoused Values and Beliefs of the Desired Culture

After stipulating espoused values and beliefs, healthcare providers next direct attention toward selecting artifacts, physical manifestations which express the underlying intangibles of the desired culture. With espoused values and beliefs at the forefront of thought, healthcare providers should ask themselves how these aspirations can be expressed tangibly through (1) personnel; (2) buildings, workspaces, and grounds; and (3) items that are placed in and around their facilities. As noted earlier, this process is very similar to that of branding, where marketers select tangible items to portray healthcare services in a desirable manner to patients. And, as with branding, creative thinking is imperative for success in selecting meaningful and relevant artifacts to represent the underlying values and beliefs of the desired culture.

Brainstorming sessions and field trips to other healthcare facilities and even to entities outside of the healthcare industry can be helpful for stimulating creative thinking, yielding potential cultural expressions. Evaluation of artifacts can be aided by role-playing exercises where healthcare providers place themselves in the position of a newly-hired employee, asking themselves if immersion among potential elements will project the espoused values and beliefs of the institution effectively. After assembling a range of options, healthcare providers should select a series of artifacts viewed to effectively convey the espoused values and beliefs of the institution to employees and others circulating about the facility.

8.8.3 Step 3: Determine the Socialization Methods Which Will Be Used to Communicate and Reinforce the Desired Culture

With espoused values and beliefs formulated and artifacts decided, healthcare providers next must determine the socialization methods which will be used to communicate and reinforce the desired organizational culture. In order for the organizational culture to take root, employees must be especially knowledgeable of the espoused values and beliefs of the establishment, along with the meaning of associated artifacts. Given the many demands for time and attention in healthcare settings, sustained efforts are essential. Without such, interest will dwindle and knowledge will fade, diminishing any hopes for cultural assimilation.

Common socialization tools and techniques used regularly within healthcare organizations offer excellent culture conveyance opportunities. Onboarding and orientation sessions are particularly capable avenues for informing new employees of espoused values and beliefs and explaining the meaning of artifacts. Special training sessions, group and individual mentoring, and related educational opportunities offer additional avenues to equip employees with knowledge regarding the desired organizational culture. Periodic reinforcement of the message and meaning of culture during department meetings and other gatherings also aids in fostering desired mindsets.

The particular socialization methods selected for deployment are dependent on the preferences of given health and medical organizations. Healthcare establishments should simply select an array of socialization pathways that they view to be capable of properly introducing and reinforcing the desired organizational culture. As the culture begins to take root in the establishment, communication and transference to others in the institution will occur naturally. Planned socialization activities simply hasten this result, guiding the development of the associated culture.

8.8.4 Step 4: Monitor the Development of the Organizational Culture, Being Especially Alert for Indications That It Is Being Reflected in Basic Underlying Assumptions, Making Adjustments as Needed to Stay on Course

A watchful eye is needed to carefully assess the progress of culture development. With the passage of time, assuming dedicated efforts, the desired culture will become increasingly ingrained. Espoused values and beliefs, expressed via meaningful and relevant artifacts, will become so deeply entrenched that they gravitate into basic underlying assumptions which guide and direct behaviors, with this representing the ultimate proof of assimilation. Anecdotal evidence can be helpful in making this determination, but for best results, formal culture audits, described in the next section, should be conducted at regular intervals as a means of reliably monitoring and evaluating progress.

If experience indicates successful assimilation, the developmental plan can continue unchanged. But if indications suggest that the desired culture is not being embraced, efforts must be taken to determine underlying causes, seek remedies, and reformulate the plan to realize the desired outcome. The causes of unsuccessful assimilation can only be revealed through prudent inquiry and investigation. Perhaps the cultural artifacts are not resonating with employees; perhaps there is incongruence between the artifacts selected and the espoused values and beliefs embraced; perhaps environmental changes have occurred rendering a previously formulated, desired culture invalid, such as in cases involving mergers or acquisitions; or perhaps there is inconsistency in adherence to the desired culture, such as in situations where managers demand cultural compliance from their subordinates, but personally violate associated tenets. Research will shed light on potential impediments.

Healthcare establishments must be particularly vigilant if unproductive subcultures start to emerge, as these can be especially detrimental to efforts to cultivate a desired organizational culture. Depending on the severity of the situation, redirection might be possible with minor modifications or it might require more intensive remedies which call for initiating the culture change process, discussed in a later section. Even once established, organizational cultures must be continually shaped and honed as a matter of practice, so modifications during developmental stages should be expected. By devoting concerted attention to culture development initiatives, realization of a desired organizational culture is entirely possible.

8.9   Culture Audits

A **culture audit** is an evaluation conducted to assess the characteristics and qualities of an establishment's organizational culture, permitting an understanding of its current state, affording opportunities for refinement to ensure desired performance. Such audits are most helpful for purposes of maintaining the integrity of established and desired organizational cultures. They also are beneficial in cases where given organizational cultures are not performing as desired, as audits supply helpful diagnostic information which can inform corrective actions. Further, they can expose subtle flaws that might not yet be detectable via casual observation, permitting them to be proactively addressed. Culture audits essentially entail the collection of information which provides insights regarding the nature of the organizational culture in operation within an establishment [38–40]. At least some of the information required for a culture audit likely will already be in the possession of most healthcare organizations, but additional details will need to be collected in order to gain a comprehensive understanding of the current culture. The three-step culture audit process is explained as follows.

8.9.1   Step 1: Collect Stakeholder Accounts on the State of the Organization's Culture

The first step in conducting a culture audit involves the collection of stakeholder accounts on the state of the organization's culture. Employee and patient satisfaction survey results represent excellent starting points for acquiring this information. Employee satisfaction surveys query staff members about their employer, work settings, job satisfaction, morale, and so on, typically also offering opportunities for them to provide additional comments regarding employment experiences. This information usually offers clear indications of the nature of organizational cultures in operation. Similarly, patient satisfaction surveys, which query customers on their patient experiences, also can provide indications of the status of organizational culture. Additionally, organizational culture surveys and related inquiries can be conducted, querying employees about the state of the establishment's culture, associated strengths and weaknesses, the presence or absence of subcultures, and so on, aiding in assembling a comprehensive profile of the culture in operation.

8.9.2   Step 2: Conduct One or More Culture Walks

Following the collection of stakeholder accounts, culture walks should be conducted. A **culture walk** is a method for observing an organizational culture by literally walking through a given institution, department, or related unit, observing cultural artifacts, interactions between and among employees, dialogues between employees and customers, and the like to provide enlightenment regarding the organizational culture in operation. Culture walks essentially constitute a form of field research completed onsite in active institutional environments, making them very capable knowledge builders [18, 41]. The direct observations afforded by culture walks provide some of the best intelligence possible regarding the state of cultures in organizations.

Culture walks can be conducted by internal members of the organization or by outside parties contracted to engage in such observations. The chief benefit of the latter approach is that when consultants or other outsiders are tasked with conducting culture audits, they have no preconceived notions tied to their observations, permitting fresh perspectives. Further, as they are unknown to staff members, during associated culture walks, employees will be more likely to be carrying out their duties and responsibilities in normal fashion than if, say, a manager or other institutional official is conducting such walks. If done proficiently, culture walks can yield a treasure trove of information about the organizational cultures operating in healthcare establishments, permitting helpful assessments of their associated characteristics and qualities.

8.9.3   Step 3: Prepare a Report Which Comprehensively Presents the Findings of the Culture Audit

The culture audit concludes with the assembly of details collected from stakeholder accounts and culture walks into a comprehensive report of findings. This report is then used to ascertain the state of the establishment's organizational culture. If desired, healthcare establishments can arrange **focus groups**—small assemblies of 8–10 participants, led by a moderator who is charged with engaging them over the course of a brief session, typically lasting an hour or so, for purposes of eliciting perspectives on a given topic—to aid in making sense of findings. Unlike relying on anecdotal evidence, which may or may not provide accurate portrayals, the findings from culture audits are derived from formal analyses which, if conducted properly, supply insights that reflect the true nature of the organizational culture in operation within given establishments. Routine deployments will yield knowledge which can maximize the impact of organizational culture development initiatives.

WK Reflections: The Value of Walking (or Wandering) Around Healthcare Organizations

Intensive immersion in organizational environments is essential for those who are responsible for overseeing healthcare establishments. One could hardly be expected to perform optimally without possessing firsthand familiarity with the organization, its personnel, and its patients. As profiled in Chap. 1, Willis Knighton Health even supports such immersion structurally by placing the offices of its managers, including its top corporate officers, in immediate proximity to care delivery environments. This stands in stark contrast to the approach of some healthcare institutions which opt to erect barriers by officing their leadership teams offsite, far removed from service environments and the insights that they afford. It is the view of Willis Knighton Health that managers with intensive institutional exposure are better at their given jobs because they never lose touch with the ultimate mission of the enterprise.

Culture walks, described in the prior section, serve as a reminder of the importance of immersion within organizational environments. Especially in cases where discretion is needed during these walks, many healthcare establishments have great success using **mystery shoppers** or **secret shoppers**, individuals external to a given organization who are paid to pose as customers for the purpose of evaluating a given customer experience, reporting their findings back to the institution at a later time. But while culture walks can be—and sometimes should be—outsourced to external parties, healthcare managers certainly should not shy away from performing these walks themselves, even if only for purposes of supplementing the findings supplied by contracted parties. Better yet, they should develop a mentality of being in a constant state of evaluation. When combined with environmental immersion, such a mindset dramatically enhances information acquisition potential. Critically, doing so will permit healthcare managers to remain in tune with their given work environments.

The value of immersion in institutional environments is widely acknowledged in the literature of organizational behavior and management. There is even an approach for ensuring routine exposure, referred to as **Management by Walking Around** or **Management by Wandering Around**, abbreviated as MBWA. **MBWA** essentially denotes an approach which sees a manager engage in direct, face-to-face interactions with those under his or her supervision in their actual work settings, permitting an enlightened dialogue and enhanced understanding that can only come through direct observation and engagement. MBWA further permits managers to interact with customers, vendors, and other parties visiting given institutions, providing additional opportunities to gain knowledge. Servicescape assessments, affording evaluations of the form and function of service environments, are also possible through MBWA [18, 41].

Quite obviously, MBWA can support culture walks and much more. It also serves as a unique method for ensuring that healthcare managers do not inadvertently become bound to their given offices, detached from the greater environments of their health and medical organizations. As the MBWA approach is continuous, managers who keep organizational culture at the top of their minds will essentially be privileged to an ongoing assessment that can help to ensure that dominant cultures prevail within their establishments. These results can be compared with the results of periodic, outsourced assessments, supplying another evaluative metric that can help ensure a strong organizational culture. What's more, healthcare managers engaged in such will see their intuition and abilities increase as these exposure opportunities enhance their intellectual and social development as authorities within their respective establishments.

8.10   Changing an Organizational Culture

Health and medical institutions will occasionally find the need to change an established organizational culture. The reasons for such vary. Healthcare providers might find that an organizational culture has deviated from its desired course, perhaps through inattention, infighting, or some other factor. An institution might change its mission, which, in turn, could create incompatibilities with its existing culture. A particular department could be discovered to have developed a counterculture or a related mindset in opposition to the dominant culture. A merger or acquisition might generate culture conflicts which must be resolved for proper and productive assimilation. In these and related cases, changing an organizational culture is a necessary task. Although such alterations are challenging, they are not impossible to realize. The following four-step process provides a helpful framework for transitioning from one organizational culture to another.

8.10.1   Step 1: Conduct a Culture Audit

The process for changing an organizational culture begins by conducting a culture audit, described in detail earlier in the chapter. This particular action is essential, as changing an organizational culture quite obviously requires possessing an accurate understanding of the current mindset in operation. As the magnitude of decisions and actions required for changing an organizational culture is intense, reliance merely on anecdotal evidence characterizing the current culture is insufficient. Instead, formal inquiry and investigation efforts are necessary, with culture audits being capable of providing the required sophistication and accuracy needed for a proper assessment of the current organizational culture.

8.10.2 Step 2: Compare the Current Culture with the Desired Culture, Identify Culture Gaps, and Make Modifications to Close Associated Gaps

Armed with a thorough knowledge of the current culture, provided courtesy of the culture audit, healthcare organizations must then compare the current organizational culture with the desired organizational culture. Specifically, they must identify any culture gaps observed and modify espoused values and beliefs and cultural artifacts to close associated gaps. In some cases, gaps might not be terribly significant, requiring only minor adjustments to achieve aspirations. Other scenarios, however, might require extremely intensive efforts to successfully transition to a new culture. While the magnitude of gaps faced will vary from situation to situation, the activities required are the same: The manifestations of the current culture (i.e., espoused values and beliefs, artifacts) must be modified to reflect the new, desired culture.

8.10.3 Step 3: Inform Employees of the Revised Culture, Outlining Its Features and Benefits, Encouraging Embracement of the New Mindset

Changing mission statements, core values, logos, uniforms, servicescapes, and other intangible and tangible features alone is insufficient to successfully alter a culture. Health and medical establishments must also direct intensive efforts toward informing employees of the revised culture, conveying through orientation sessions and other events the reasons for making the change, the benefits afforded by the alteration, and the necessity for everyone to embrace the new mindset. Patience is required, especially in cases where the desired culture represents a significant departure from the existing culture. In ideal situations, employees will voluntarily embrace the aspirational culture and work to realize its proliferation and potential. Some reluctance and resistance should be expected and, at least up to a reasonable point, tolerated, permitting employees time to acclimate to the change. However, if enduring resistance emerges, harming prospects for successfully achieving the desired culture, healthcare providers will need to take prudent steps to resolve associated roadblocks through additional education, reassignment of personnel, incentivizing compliance, penalizing noncompliance, and related actions.

8.10.4 *Step 4: Engage in Ongoing Monitoring and Evaluation, Making Adjustments as Needed to Realize the Desired Culture*

The process of changing an organizational culture concludes with ongoing monitoring and evaluation. Periodic culture audits, in particular, should be conducted to ensure that progress indeed is being made toward the realization of the desired organizational culture. It should be noted that while the steps associated with changing an organizational culture are fairly straightforward, realizing the desired change in actuality is a highly complex endeavor. As noted earlier, once organizational cultures become established, they are very difficult to change. That said, it is imperative to keep expectations, including timelines for achievement, realistic. Though challenging, healthcare organizations should expect devoted effort and attention directed toward culture change initiatives to pay dividends, permitting the desired culture to replace its predecessor, fulfilling associated aspirations.

8.11 Summary and Conclusions

An organization's culture, if well devised and properly managed, affords health and medical establishments with a strategic asset and key competitive advantage. It plays a pivotal role in determining what the establishment can and cannot achieve. Further, organizational culture educates and enlightens personnel regarding perspectives and practices deemed to be appropriate and acceptable, providing direction as duties and responsibilities are being completed. This is especially important in health and medical settings, as direct oversight is often not possible. Not unlike guidance systems used by rockets journeying into space, ensuring that they stay on course, a productive organizational culture helps healthcare establishments stay on course by creating an institutional mindset that guides employees and their associated decisions and actions. Further, it positively influences patients and their loved ones, setting the stage for mission fulfillment and the realization of institutional success and prosperity. As an organizational culture will develop within an organization, whether guided or not, it is imperative for healthcare providers to proactively endeavor to foster productive mindsets, leaving nothing to chance. A productive healthcare institution results largely from a productive organizational culture, yielding an establishment more capable of serving patients well and reaping the mutual benefits associated with doing so.

Key Terms

- Artifacts
- Basic Underlying Assumptions
- Branding
- Competitive Advantage
- Corporate Culture
- Countercultural Subculture
- Counterculture
- Cultural Congruence
- Cultural Fit
- Culture Audit
- Culture Gap
- Culture Walk
- Dominant Culture
- Enhancing Subculture
- Espoused Values and Beliefs
- Focus Group
- Foundations of Culture
- Management by Walking Around
- Management by Wandering Around
- MBWA
- Mission Statement
- Mystery Shopper
- Organizational Climate
- Organizational Culture
- Orthogonal Subculture
- Schein's Model of Culture
- Secret Shopper
- Socialization
- Subculture
- Values Statement
- Vision Statement

Exercises

1. In your own words, define the concept of organizational culture, identify its components, and discuss its importance in health and medicine.
2. Reflect on your past experiences as either an employee or customer of an organization, whether healthcare related or not. Of these experiences, identify one establishment which you viewed to possess a productive organizational culture and identify another establishment which you viewed to possess an unproductive

organizational culture. Describe your experiences in detail and indicate how they have influenced your perspectives regarding the impact of organizational culture.

3. Reflect on the implications of allowing organizational cultures to develop without any form of guidance in healthcare establishments. What risks are being taken by such an approach and what outcomes would you expect of the resulting organizational cultures?

4. Think deeply about a recent employment experience and describe the culture in operation within the establishment. In your description, speak on each of the components of culture, as identified in Schein's three-level framework, noting artifacts, espoused values and beliefs, and basic underlying assumptions. When you began your employment experience, how did you learn about the culture in operation? How was the culture reinforced over time?

5. Exercise your culture development skills by selecting a particular value or belief which could be embraced by a hypothetical healthcare organization. Then, identify at least five artifacts which could be used to tangibly express this value or belief to others, describing each and supplying justifications for their selection.

6. Suppose that you are the chief executive officer of a hospital which historically has enjoyed a dominant organizational culture that has positively impacted operations. In a recent culture audit, however, you notice signs that an orthogonal subculture has emerged in the laboratory department. What steps would you take, if any, to address this subculture? Why or why not?

7. Suppose that you are the chief executive officer of a hospital which historically has enjoyed a dominant organizational culture that has positively impacted operations. In a recent culture audit, however, you notice signs that a countercultural subculture has emerged in the nursing department. What steps would you take, if any, to address this subculture? Why or why not?

8. Take the opportunity to develop your culture audit skills by visiting a healthcare establishment with which you have little or no familiarity. Conduct a culture walk through its public spaces, observing its architecture, design, symbols, workforce interactions, and more. From your observations, prepare a list of cultural artifacts observed. Then, reflect and report on the espoused values and beliefs which might have motivated selection of the artifacts as expressions of the underlying culture. Based on your observations and analysis, how would you describe the culture in operation?

References

1. Elrod, J. K. (2013). *Breadcrumbs to cheesecake*. R&R Publishers.
2. U. S. Bureau of Labor Statistics. (2022). *Occupational outlook handbook*. Retrieved April 3, 2023, from https://www.bls.gov/ooh/
3. O*NET OnLine. (2023). *Health care and social assistance*. Retrieved April 3, 2023, from https://www.onetonline.org/find/industry?i=62
4. McConnell, C. R. (2020). *Hospitals and health systems: What they are and how they work*. Jones and Bartlett.

5. Shi, L., & Singh, D. A. (2023). *Essentials of the US health care system* (6th ed.). Jones and Bartlett.
6. Kotler, P., Keller, K. L., & Chernev, A. (2022). *Marketing management* (16th ed.). Pearson.
7. Schein, E. H. (1984). Coming to a new awareness of organizational culture. *Sloan Management Review, 25*(2), 3–16.
8. Schein, E. H. (2017). *Organizational culture and leadership* (5th ed.). Wiley.
9. Elrod, J. K., & Fortenberry, J. L., Jr. (2018). Am I seeing things through the eyes of patients? An exercise in bolstering patient attentiveness and empathy. *BMC Health Services Research, 18*(Suppl 3), 41–44.
10. Schein, E. H., & Schein, P. A. (2019). *The corporate culture survival guide* (3rd ed.). Wiley.
11. Groysberg, B., Lee, J., Price, J., & Yo-Jud Cheng, J. (2018). The leader's guide to corporate culture: How to manage the eight critical elements of organizational life. *Harvard Business Review, 96*(1), 44–52.
12. Konopaske, R., Ivancevich, J. M., & Matteson, M. T. (2018). *Organizational behavior and management* (11th ed.). McGraw-Hill.
13. Denison, D. R. (1984). Bringing corporate culture to the bottom line. *Organizational Dynamics, 13*(2), 5–22.
14. Deal, T. E., & Kennedy, A. A. (2000). *Corporate cultures: The rites and rituals of corporate life.* Basic Books.
15. Robbins, S. P., & Judge, T. A. (2019). *Organizational behavior* (18th ed.). Pearson.
16. Kotter, J. P., & Heskett, J. L. (2011). *Corporate culture and performance* (Reprint ed.). The Free Press.
17. Flamholtz, E. G., & Randle, Y. (2011). *Corporate culture: The ultimate strategic asset.* Stanford University Press.
18. Peters, T. J., & Waterman, R. H., Jr. (2004). *In search of excellence: Lessons from America's best-run companies.* HarperBusiness.
19. Ehrhart, M. G., Schneider, B., & Macey, W. H. (2014). *Organizational climate and culture: An introduction to theory, research, and practice.* Routledge.
20. Ashforth, B. E. (1985). Climate formation: Issues and extensions. *Academy of Management Review, 10*(4), 837–847.
21. Fortenberry, J. L., Jr. (2010). *Health care marketing: Tools and techniques* (3rd ed.). Jones and Bartlett.
22. Barney, J. B. (1986). Organizational culture: Can it be a source of sustained competitive advantage? *Academy of Management Review, 11*(3), 656–665.
23. Griffin, R. W., Phillips, J. M., & Gully, S. M. (2020). *Organizational behavior: Managing people and organizations* (13th ed.). Cengage.
24. Trice, H. M., & Beyer, J. M. (1993). *The cultures of work organizations.* Prentice Hall.
25. David, F. R., David, F. R., & David, M. E. (2020). *Strategic management: A competitive advantage approach* (17th ed.). Pearson.
26. Collins, J. C., & Porras, J. I. (1996). Building your company's vision. *Harvard Business Review, 74*(5), 65–77.
27. Neville, L., & Schneider, B. (2021). Why is it so hard to change a culture? It's the people. *Organization Development Review, 53*(1), 41–46.
28. Cameron, K. S., & Quinn, R. E. (2006). *Diagnosing and changing organizational culture: Based on the competing values framework* (Rev ed.). Jossey-Bass.
29. Smircich, L. (1983). Concepts of culture and organizational analysis. *Administrative Science Quarterly, 28*(3), 339–358.
30. Schein, E. H. (2016). The concept of organizational culture: Why bother? In J. M. Shafritz, J. S. Ott, & Y. S. Jang (Eds.), *Classics of organization theory* (8th ed., pp. 301–313). Cengage.
31. Cameron, K. S., & Freeman, S. J. (1991). Cultural congruence, strength, and type: Relationships to effectiveness. In R. W. Woodman & W. A. Pasmore (Eds.), *Research in organizational change and development* (Vol. 5, pp. 23–58). JAI Press.

32. Elrod, J. K., & Fortenberry, J. L., Jr. (2018). Driving brand equity in health services organizations: The need for an expanded view of branding. *BMC Health Services Research, 18*(Suppl 3), 23–28.

33. Lindstrom, M. (2005). *Brand sense: Build powerful brands through touch, taste, smell, sight, and sound.* The Free Press.

34. Hulten, B. (2017). Branding by the five senses: A sensory branding framework. *Journal of Brand Strategy, 6*(3), 281–292.

35. Agarwal, S. (2015). Customer sense: How the five senses influence buying behaviour. *Journal of Consumer Marketing, 32*(4), 307–308.

36. Elrod, J. K., & Fortenberry, J. L., Jr. (2017). Centers of excellence in healthcare institutions: What they are and how to assemble them. *BMC Health Services Research, 17*(Suppl 1), 15–24.

37. Martin, J., & Siehl, C. (1983). Organizational culture and counterculture: An uneasy symbiosis. *Organizational Dynamics, 12*(2), 52–64.

38. McShane, S. L., & Von Glinow, M. A. (2019). *Organizational behavior* (4th ed.). McGraw-Hill.

39. Wilkins, A. L. (1983). The culture audit: A tool for understanding organizations. *Organizational Dynamics, 12*(2), 24–38.

40. Hitt, M. A., Miller, C. C., Colella, A., & Triana, M. D. C. (2018). *Organizational behavior* (5th ed.). Wiley.

41. Peters, T., & Austin, N. (1985). MBWA (Managing by walking around). *California Management Review, 28*(1), 9–34.

Chapter 9
Organizational Structure and Design in Health and Medicine

Learning Objectives

After examining this chapter, readers will have the ability to:

- Define organizational structure and discuss its importance in health and medical establishments.
- Define organization design, understand its key areas of concentration, and discuss its impact in healthcare organizations.
- Identify and discuss the building blocks of organizational structure, including work specialization, chain of command, span of control, centralization, and formalization.
- Understand common methods of departmentalization and their resulting organizational structures, including the simple structure, the functional structure, the divisional structure, and the matrix structure.
- Understand hub-and-spoke networks and discuss their use and application in the healthcare industry.
- Understand centers of excellence and discuss their assembly and application in the healthcare industry.
- Appreciate the value of organizational charts, understand what they portray, and recognize steps for their productive assembly.

J. K. Elrod, J. L. Fortenberry, Jr., *Organizational Behavior and Management in Health and Medicine*, https://doi.org/10.1007/978-3-031-61823-9_9

WK Reflections: Willis Knighton Health's Hub-and-Spoke Network

As an institution with a century of history, Willis Knighton Health has seen its organizational structure and design evolve tremendously over time. Structure and design decisions of practically every type and variety imaginable have been addressed by the establishment through the years, but none has had the lasting impact of a single decision dating back several decades which continues to deliver value today. That particular decision pertained to the manner in which Willis Knighton Health organized its growing multi-campus system.

From its origin in 1924 through to the early 1980s, Willis Knighton Health consisted of a single site, Willis Knighton North (formerly known as Willis-Knighton Medical Center), located in west Shreveport, Louisiana. In the 1970s, however, a vision of growth emerged, with executives committing to its pursuit and realization. The foremost concern of the era involved elevating Willis Knighton North's infrastructure and service array, permitting the establishment to attract and retain more patients. In a relatively brief period of time, success was achieved on this front, and Willis Knighton North began to enjoy a burgeoning patient population and high customer loyalty. With things going very well for the establishment, attention then was directed toward examining expansion options, permitting Willis Knighton North to extend its reach within the community. A comprehensive market assessment was conducted, indicating very high growth in south Shreveport. What's more, no hospital was serving the area at the time. These positive attributes ultimately compelled Willis Knighton North to select this area for establishing its first expansion hospital. This vision was indeed realized in 1983 with the introduction of Willis Knighton South, yielding a multicampus system covering west and south Shreveport [1].

In the months and years leading up to Willis Knighton South's presentation in the market, planning focused on scores of intensive organizational structure and design decisions, but an important foundational decision first had to be made. Specifically, the institution had to determine the manner in which healthcare delivery relationships between Willis Knighton North and Willis Knighton South would operate. Organization designs which duplicated operations at each location were popular expansion models during the era, but this avenue was considered to be inefficient. A more attractive plan was viewed to entail sharing services in some manner to better economize, with this ultimately resulting in adopting the hub-and-spoke organization design [1, 2].

The **hub-and-spoke organization design** arranges service delivery components into a network made up of an anchor establishment (hub) which offers a full array of services, complemented by secondary establishments (spokes) which offer more limited service arrays, routing patients who are in need of more intensive services to the hub for treatment [2–4]. It yields a healthcare network featuring a main campus and one or more satellite campuses. Through strategic centralization of the most advanced medical services at a single site and distribution of basic services via secondary sites, the hub-and-spoke model has the ability to maximize efficiency and effectiveness. A well-designed **hub-and-spoke network** fulfills patient care needs completely, yet it does so in a manner that promotes resource conservation, return on investment, service excellence, and enhanced market coverage [2, 4–7].

Embracing the hub-and-spoke model, the institution designated Willis Knighton North as the hub or home campus and Willis Knighton South as the spoke. Willis Knighton North, as the network's hub, would offer comprehensive clinical services, the most advanced technologies, and associated administrative support services, such as human resource management and marketing, with this site providing the full operational array of services and support within the system. Willis Knighton South, as a satellite, concentrated exclusively on a more limited array of clinical services, looking to Willis Knighton North for complementary services and support, thus eliminating duplication between sites and affording greater economies. When patients at Willis Knighton South needed more intensive technologies, say, in cardiology or cancer treatment, they would be routed to Willis Knighton North for care. Having resolved all issues associated with organizational relationships between the two entities, attention turned toward developing Willis Knighton South's organizational chart, the traditional task associated with organizational structure and design, arranging departments and people in a manner to productively carry out the new institution's mission.

Willis Knighton Health's decision to use the hub-and-spoke model worked superbly in its initial two-facility arrangement, but it continued to yield benefits over time. As hub-and-spoke networks are highly scalable, satellites can be added as needed [2, 4, 7]. This attribute proved very helpful as the institution continued its expansion in following decades. Willis Knighton Health's hub-and-spoke network now includes five hospitals and one retirement community, entailing nearly 1300 beds. Notably, Willis Knighton Health's many general and specialty medical clinics also serve as spokes linked to the main campus hub. These clinics are located across the region and aid in the institution achieving comprehensive market coverage. As with hospital spokes, clinic spokes concentrate on providing a more limited array of services, looking to Willis Knighton North as their resource for the system's most advanced technologies, various support services, and related complementary offerings.

All in all, the hub-and-spoke organization design has benefited Willis Knighton Health significantly. Interestingly, the model was originally developed for use in the transportation industry, best known for its deployment by air carriers which, due to significant financial burdens, sought an efficient system to accomplish more with less [8, 9]. Beyond healthcare, the model of organization has been successfully operationalized in many other industries, including retailing and education [2, 10–13]. While system-level, multisite organizational structure and design tasks might not be among the most commonly encountered in health and medicine, an awareness of such can be helpful in understanding the more commonly encountered tasks associated with arranging people, places, and things within given healthcare establishments. It also nicely illustrates the variety of tasks associated with organizational structure and design.

9.1   Background

Establishing a health services organization represents a profoundly complex challenge, requiring a seemingly unending array of decisions and actions to realize an operational entity. To the casual observer, such a pursuit would call for things such as formulating a viable business plan, securing proper funding, acquiring authorization from policy bodies, procuring a building to house operations, outfitting the building with furnishings and fixtures required to address patients, and hiring personnel to carry out assigned duties and responsibilities. While these steps are necessary, such top-of-mind perspectives represent just the tip of the iceberg. Deeper pursuits remain, with some of the most essential centering on the framework, design, and operational characteristics of the organization [1, 2, 14].

The best of property, plant, and equipment in the hands of the most educated and capable of employees counts for very little if the methods for organizing and accomplishing work are not equally well addressed and initiated. Chief among these operational challenges is that of determining the healthcare organization's structure, including its chain of command, arrangement of departments, and reporting relationships, leading to the development of the establishment's organizational chart. Further, processes and procedures for carrying out work must be determined. Such pursuits are among the most critical in organizational life, as they ultimately outline pathways leading to mission fulfillment. If the institution is part of a larger network, then arrangements between and among sites must also be determined [15, 16].

Effectively, a blueprint of operations must be formulated at the onset of a healthcare establishment's life, addressing the who, how, why, and when questions associated with the provision of health and medicine in a manner to realize designated missions. Going forward, this blueprint must remain viable, changing to accommodate conditions faced to ensure that the institutional structures and work processes permit operations to proceed unfettered [2, 15–17]. Skills associated with assembling and maintaining institutional frameworks and related mechanisms fall under the auspices of organizational structure and design, the focus of this chapter.

9.2 Defining Organizational Structure and Design

The **organizational structure** of an establishment refers to an institution's hierarchy, depicting its chain of command, arrangement of departments, and associated reporting relationships within the organization. It is presented via a diagram known as an **organizational chart**, which typically uses a series of boxes and lines to illustrate structural arrangements within an institution. Organizational structure activities, including organizational chart assembly, represent the most notable pursuits of **organization design**, a component of organizational behavior and management which focuses on the process of formulating, implementing, and evaluating institutional structures, activities, and operations in a manner which facilitates the fulfillment of an organization's mission. An organization's structure serves as the foundational framework governing institutional operations. Organizational structures also communicate power relationships, indicating where authority resides. Further, organizational structures often are presented publicly via organizational charts, making them objects of attention both internally and externally. Beyond organizational chart assembly and modification tasks, organization design activities entail engineering and reengineering interorganizational and intraorganizational relationships, formulating and modifying work protocols and processes, and similar actions, with these ultimately impacting underlying organizational structures [15, 17–20].

Organizational structure and design skills and abilities have been, are, and always will be requirements for any type of establishment; they are timeless essentialities. Every institution exists to achieve some sort of mission, with accomplishment requiring structure, order, processes, procedures, protocols, and the like. Through organizational structure and design pursuits, structural and operational blueprints emerge, detailing organizational arrangements of people and departments, permitting the work of given establishments to be conducted. Ultimately, these efforts are aimed at ensuring that healthcare organizations properly set and maintain a designated course, regardless of circumstances or situations encountered, permitting associated missions to be realized. As such, organizational structure and design efforts are strategic matters, necessitating that those engaged in the practice possess an intimate knowledge of the mission, vision, values, and other strategic directives of given institutions. This requires executive-level attention, informed by multidisciplinary perspectives, given that decisions in even a single area of structure and design often have far reaching implications in other areas [2, 15–17].

Those involved in organizational structure and design activities must possess a particularly deep understanding of the building blocks of organizational structure. They also must have a thorough knowledge of methods of departmentalization and their resulting organizational structures. Additionally, techniques for the proper assembly of organizational charts must be understood. Numerous decisions must be made on each of these fronts, with associated efforts ultimately yielding the operational framework of the organization. These areas and more are profiled in the following sections.

9.3   Building Blocks of Organizational Structure

Complex things naturally are made up of numerous building blocks, assembled together in a manner to create a cohesive whole capable of addressing a particular issue or concern. As complex mechanisms, organizational structures are no different, requiring numerous decisions across a range of areas constituting building blocks. The building blocks of organizational structure include work specialization, chain of command, span of control, centralization, and formalization [21]. These five areas each must be addressed proficiently by healthcare providers as they go about assembling the organizational structures of their given establishments.

9.3.1   Work Specialization

Described in detail in Chap. 1, the concept of **work specialization**, also known as **division of labor**, references the manner in which the tasks of an institution are divided into separate jobs [21]. The ultimate aim of specialization is for work to be divided in a manner to permit employees to specialize in particular areas of responsibility. Employees perform part of an activity, rather than its whole. Doing so allows for more and better work to be produced, courtesy of attention being devoted to specific duties rather than diluted across a range of differentiated obligations [22, 23]. Much of the work specialization occurring within the healthcare industry emerges as a product of licensure and certification mandates, permitting only those possessing certain qualifications to perform particular activities. Other occupations within the healthcare industry are treated similarly to those within broad business and industry, with specialization not being mandated by policy, but voluntarily pursued to capitalize on its benefits. Take, for example, a hospital's marketing department. In such settings, it is very common for a director or manager to coordinate a group of individuals specializing in particular marketing functions, such as strategy, graphic design, photography, web programming, and so on, permitting efficiency and effectiveness to be maximized. Healthcare institutions ultimately must look at tasks required to achieve given missions and break down those tasks into jobs systemwide which can be pursued productively by staff members.

9.3.2   Chain of Command

Also described in Chap. 1, the **chain of command**, also known as the **scalar chain**, refers to the unbroken line of authority extending from the very top officer within an organization to the lowest ranks of the establishment [17, 22]. This chain is very obvious when examining most organizational charts, as one literally can follow the lines of authority through their graphical depictions of hierarchies. Structuring this chain requires the extension of **authority**—the right to give orders and the power to mandate compliance—to managers. But with this authority, managers also must take **responsibility**, accepting accountability for outcomes. The exact form and composition of the chain of command is dependent on the preferences of healthcare establishments, with the ultimate goal being to arrive at a model that ensures order, but is not so restrictive that it creates inefficiencies. This requires a delicate balance. Whatever the resulting design, fine-tuning may be required after enacting initial designs in order to arrive at the best fit for the organization and its needs. And certainly as healthcare organizations evolve, so too must their chains of command. A chain of command that works well today might not work well tomorrow, depending on internal and external environmental factors, requiring ongoing attentiveness.

9.3.3 Span of Control

Another building block of organizational structure which must be addressed when designing organizational charts is that of span of control. **Span of control** refers to the number of employees a manager supervises. This determines the number of managers employed by an organization and the number of levels within the organization's hierarchy, as reflected in the organizational chart. A wider span of control means that a manager supervises a larger number of employees. A narrower span of control means than a manager supervises a smaller number of employees. By placing more employees under the supervision of managers, organizations ultimately can reduce levels within the organizational hierarchy, creating a flatter organization, as opposed to a taller organization. The trend in recent decades has been for organizations to become flatter, as wider spans of control mean that organizations can hire fewer managers. Communications also are more efficient as flatter organizations have fewer layers that communications must travel. This particular characteristic can expedite decision-making, increasing institutional agility. However, there are limits to how far a manager can be stretched before oversight burdens become too great. Having too few employees to supervise can also be problematic. In cases of overly narrow spans of control, managers can be tempted to micromanage employees, diminishing their autonomy, causing dissatisfaction. A balance is required, with this often necessitating trial-and-error, as optimal spans of control will vary between and among institutions and even among types of work in given institutions [15, 21]. Some types of work in healthcare establishments have the benefit of staffing ratio guidance, which can inform span of control decisions, but other types of work have no such luxuries, necessitating use of inference and experience to guide decisions.

9.3.4 Centralization

The concept of **centralization** refers to where in the organizational structure of an institution decisions are formally made [21]. **Centralized organizations** concentrate power and decision-making authority at the top of their given institutional hierarchies. A relatively small number of individuals, typically those occupying executive ranks, retain tight control over the institution and its operations. **Decentralized organizations** distribute power and decision-making authority, at least to some degree, to managers at lower levels in their given institutional hierarchies [15, 21]. Institutions usually are not perfectly centralized or decentralized. As such, it can be helpful to view centralization as a continuum, ranging from high to low, as it very often is a matter of degree [24].

Centralized organizations have the advantage of control, with top oversight ensuring that procedures and practices conform with institutional expectations. As decentralized organizations grant decision-making authority to managers lower in institutional hierarchies, the control afforded by centralized structures cannot be as confidently assured in decentralized scenarios. When authority is decentralized, however, organizations can more quickly address problems when and where they are encountered, as managers possess the autonomy to do so. Decentralization also increases input from multiple parties, potentially improving decisions. Further, decentralized structures can diminish the prospect of managers feeling alienated as a result of decisions being handed down to them from those higher in the organizational hierarchy [17]. The "centralization versus decentralization" question is resolved not by simply stipulating a particular proportion but instead by determining the optimal degree required to successfully accomplish given goals and objectives. Ascertaining a proper balance is necessary for achieving the best outcomes [22].

9.3.5 Formalization

The concept of **formalization** refers to the degree to which an establishment standardizes work by rules, guidelines, formal training, and related parameters [25, 26]. Formalization fosters consistent job performance, as employees are guided by rigid protocols for completion of work assignments. It is a necessary ingredient for producing a standardized product or delivering a standardized service [21]. Autonomy is reduced, as employees cannot decide how they wish to perform given operations, but the resulting consistency is often viewed as an acceptable trade-off. Formalization tends to increase as organizations grow in size, as direct supervision becomes more limited, diminishing managerial oversight and necessitating guidance through written rules and regulations [25].

Degree of formalization sometimes is the prerogative of the institution, based on its preferences for organizing work. At other times, however, formalization is dictated by external influences, such as governmental policy or other regulations [25]. This is very often the case in the healthcare industry. Clearly, clinical occupations fall into this category, but other work also involves prominent practice regulations, such as those associated with accounting and human resource management. Even outside of external mandates, healthcare organizations routinely require employees to follow best practices, derived from either institutional or industry experience, all to ensure standardization in outputs produced in pursuit of patient care excellence.

9.4 Types of Organizational Structures

Organizational structures emerge through a process known as departmentalization. Formally defined, **departmentalization** refers to the manner in which activities are grouped within an establishment [25]. It is through departmentalization that the look and design of the organizational chart takes shape and ultimately is assembled. Departmentalization can occur on many bases, yielding a variety of organizational structures. Some of the more common organizational structures include the simple structure, the functional structure, the divisional structure, and the matrix structure.

9.4.1 The Simple Structure

Simple structures are very basic institutional frameworks that are used to organize operations of minimal complexity. In a simple structure, hierarchies typically are very flat, having only two or three levels. Spans of control are wide and authority is highly centralized, with power usually being held by a single individual. Formalization is low and employees are few [17]. Consider the simple structure of an independent retail pharmacy focused on the dispensing of drugs and over-the-counter medicines, complemented by sales of a limited selection of convenience goods. Here, a single owner-manager provides all oversight and direction, with three pharmacists, a business office manager, four customer service representatives, and two cashiers all reporting to him. Simple structures permit quick decision-making, they are economical in that managerial expenses are minimal, and they clearly indicate who is in charge. They can be effective for as long as operations remain simple, but with growth, these structures break down as they cannot accommodate increased complexity. Despite a number of advantages, the simple structure carries a degree of risk in that operations typically are overseen by a single individual. If this person dies, becomes ill, or encounters any other hardship which hampers oversight, operations can come to a standstill, jeopardizing viability [17]. Still, for organizations of limited complexity, the simple structure is suitable and appropriate.

9.4.2   The Functional Structure

The **functional structure** organizes jobs by type of work performed, placing them into departments by given function or specialty [15]. It is well suited for growing operations and can even accommodate large organizations, including those with multiple hierarchical levels [17]. Power typically is centralized in functional structures [15]. Consider the case of a rural hospital which elected to establish a series of departments covering a range of occupational specialties (e.g., medicine, nursing, respiratory therapy, laboratory, pharmacy, dietary, housekeeping, finance, human resources, marketing, etc.). Each department featured a director who reported to a chief operating officer who, in turn, reported to a chief executive officer, with the directors working collaboratively with each other to deliver services. In these structures, since jobs are arranged by specialty, efficiencies are realized, making functional departmentalization a very productive structural method. Functional structures can prove challenging in that by grouping employees into departments by specialty, **silos** can form where employees focus on the issues and concerns of their assigned departments, losing sight of the wants and needs of the greater organization [27]. Additionally, communication barriers can emerge between and among departments in such an arrangement. This, however, typically can be overcome by employing managers committed to ensuring productive interdepartmental and intradepartmental relations. With intensive formal controls and coordination, functional structures can be highly effective [25].

9.4.3   The Divisional Structure

The **divisional structure** groups jobs by their place or location (i.e., **geographic departmentalization**), the goods or services they produce (i.e., **product departmentalization**), or the customers they serve (i.e., **customer departmentalization**) [17]. To illustrate geographic departmentalization, consider the case of a cosmetic surgery center located in Jackson, Mississippi, which decided to grow its footprint by opening two new centers, one in New Orleans, Louisiana, and the other in Memphis, Tennessee. To do this, it opted to replicate the functional organizational structure established at its original location (Jackson) at each of the new locations (New Orleans and Memphis), essentially forming Mississippi, Louisiana, and Tennessee divisions, each featuring a division administrator reporting to the top corporate officer.

As an illustration of product departmentalization, consider the case of a newly established medical clinic which opted to departmentalize by product line, deciding to create three product divisions—pediatric medicine, adult medicine, and geriatric medicine—with each division housing identical arrays of departments, each focused on delivering tailored care. Structuring operations in this manner affords institutions with opportunities to offer enhanced patient experiences, with employees focusing of designated product lines. The efficiencies of this approach are reduced due to duplication of services across divisions, resulting in the loss of economies of scale. The benefits of customized care, however, could outweigh the benefits of those particular efficiencies. Customer departmentalization works similarly to that of product departmentalization, structuring divisions by customer group served (e.g., pediatric patients, adult patients, geriatric patients).

As these examples illustrate, the divisional structure can easily accommodate growth. New divisions can simply be created when and where warranted. If, for example, the geographically departmentalized cosmetic surgery center noted above observed numerous clients driving in from Birmingham, Alabama, and wanted to capitalize on that market, it could simply establish a Birmingham division, without disrupting other divisions. The product departmentalized medical clinic might perhaps add a product line focusing on a particular health condition afflicting many in the given community, with this addition not intruding on other lines. The divisional structure also is beneficial in reorganization scenarios, as divisions that are no longer of interest to an enterprise can be sold or, if no longer viable, simply shut down. The chief advantage afforded by the divisional structure centers on the ability of divisions to concentrate on their respective areas of focus. Knowledge sharing within divisions is enhanced, but between divisions, it can be diminished, as silos can develop. Generally, divisional structures are more costly to operate than functional structures, as they often replicate services across divisions [25].

9.4.4 The Matrix Structure

The **matrix structure** combines elements of functional departmentalization and product departmentalization in an attempt to capitalize on the benefits of both. Matrix organizations achieve this by essentially superimposing a horizontal structure of authority onto a vertical structure [27]. Assume in the medical clinic example presented earlier that the administrator believed that performance would improve with additional oversight. He, therefore, decided to overlay a functional departmentalization structure containing departments by occupational specialty (e.g., nursing, laboratory, human resources, etc.) over the existing product departmentalization structure (e.g., pediatric medicine, adult medicine, geriatric medicine). This arrangement effectively placed personnel in both a functional department (e.g., nursing, laboratory, human resources, etc.) and a particular product group (e.g., pediatric medicine, adult medicine, geriatric medicine). In such scenarios, employees effectively report to two managers, one from their functional department and the other from their product group. This, of course, violates the principle of unity of command, necessitating that functional and product managers work in an especially collaborative manner to ensure consistency and order in directives forwarded to subordinates. Managerial collaboration is essential to overcome problems which can emerge from violating the principle of unity of command.

The matrix structure works well when pressures exist to focus on multiple areas, in situations of high work complexity or interdependence necessitating intensive coordination, and in situations where resources must be shared in order to achieve the greatest efficiencies [15]. Given dual reporting relationships, however, it can create confusion among staff members and generate power struggles between managers [17]. Further, the additional management layer associated with matrix structures increases the costs associated with this form of departmentalization [24]. Pure matrix structures are relatively rare compared to traditional forms of organization, but its characteristics often are integrated within more traditional forms. Many healthcare establishments, even if they are predominantly structured in traditional form, incorporate at least some cross-collaborative mechanisms reminiscent of matrix organizations.

9.5   Assembling Organizational Charts

Organizational structure activities culminate in the assembly of an organizational chart, arguably the most widely recognized activity of organizational structure and design. Many routes for assembly are possible, with a helpful seven-step framework being presented in the sections that follow.

9.5.1   Step 1: Acquire a Comprehensive Understanding of the Work Produced by the Organization

Arguably the most important step in assembling an organizational chart involves first acquiring a comprehensive understanding of the work produced by the given organization. Chart developers specifically must possess knowledge of the organization's mission, the tasks and processes required for accomplishing work, the categories of personnel needed to complete the work, the names of all departments housing personnel, the titling schemes selected for different managerial levels, and related insights. Such acumen regarding the work carried out by the organization is especially important because possessing this knowledge frees up parties engaged in organizational chart development to focus specifically on the core activity at hand, namely, the development of a viable organizational structure that arranges departments and people in such a way to foster the accomplishment of the given institution's mission. Backtracking to gather details on how work is completed would not be necessary for the informed. Of course, given the complexities of the healthcare industry, it is understood that even highly knowledgeable, dedicated individuals engaged in organizational chart development occasionally will encounter intricacies of work that are not fully understood. The operative point is that knowledge gaps should be closed prior to beginning chart assembly work, with this often necessitating fact-finding and observation activities to fully grasp the nature of the work, bolstering chart development efforts.

9.5.2 Step 2: Acquire a Thorough Understanding of the Fundamentals of Organizational Structure and Design

Having acquired a comprehensive understanding of the work produced by the organization, the next step in organizational chart assembly involves ensuring a thorough understanding of the fundamentals of organizational structure and design. Those involved in organizational chart development must be knowledgeable of the building blocks of organizational structure, as described earlier in the chapter, as they must address matters pertaining to work specialization, chain of command, span of control, centralization, and formalization as they go about formulating the associated framework. Organizational chart developers also must possess an understanding of departmentalization and resulting types of organizational structures, also described earlier in the chapter, as they must make fitting selections in chart assembly. Further, they must keep in mind that structure must follow strategy; that is, organizational charts must be designed in a manner to fulfill designated missions, with this being kept at the forefront of thought throughout assembly [15, 18]. This foundational knowledge of organizational structure and design will afford chart developers with an awareness of points of focus and available options as they work their way through the assembly process.

9.5.3 Step 3: Acquire Tools for Illustrating the Envisioned Organizational Chart

Organizational charts depicting the structures of modern healthcare institutions must be illustrated in a professional manner, necessitating acquisition of associated tools of the trade. This is obvious when one considers several generally accepted guidelines for chart construction. Organizational charts ideally should be presented on a single page, permitting one to easily view operations in their entirety. This also facilitates displaying organizational charts, which very typically are framed and placed throughout institutions. Simplicity of presentation is encouraged, allowing individuals to easily understand the framework. It should be self-explanatory even on cursory examination. Boxes and lines represent the chief devices used to illustrate structural relationships in organizational charts. Within each box, a brief descriptor is placed, with this often being a department name (e.g., Nursing Services) or job title (e.g., Director of Nursing). Some institutions opt to use employee names and, occasionally, their photographs are added. Boxes should be of uniform size across the entire organizational chart. Solid lines are used to connect boxes, with these denoting direct reporting relationships. Indirect reporting relationships typically are expressed using dotted lines. In traditional, hierarchical organizational charts, levels are used to indicate authority, with higher levels denoting greater authority than lower levels. A solid line running from a higher position to a lower position indicates a superior-subordinate relationship and vice versa.

As one easily can surmise from the visual presentation of organizational charts, assembly can be greatly aided by using organizational chart software, such as Microsoft Visio, permitting the professional presentation of these frameworks. Use of such software also facilitates making updates to charts as healthcare institutions and their associated organizational structures evolve. These software offerings provide pathways for creating attractive looking organizational charts, but they also typically supply helpful tools which guide the development process. Such software should be considered mandatory whenever engaging in the activity of developing and refining organizational charts. Armed with foundational insights and now the tools of the trade, those involved in organizational chart assembly are ready to take their first steps as illustrators.

9.5.4 Step 4: Using the Acquired Insights and Tools, Draw an Initial Illustration of the Organizational Chart

With insights gained and tools acquired, organizational chart developers make their first attempt at illustrating the structure of the organization. The operative starting point for assembling an organizational chart begins with the top authority of the establishment (e.g., CEO, President), placing this box at the top of the presentation page. *(Note that in this example, the titles of managerial personnel are incorporated, but if desired, department names could be used instead.)* One layer down, positions reporting directly to this top position (e.g., VP of Operations, VP of Nursing, VP of Marketing) are presented, each in its own separate box, with solid lines directly connecting each position to the superior position. This process continues to the next layer and the next until all managerial positions have been presented, along with associated lines of authority, concluding chart development. If desired, additional organizational charts can be prepared for individual departments within the establishment, complementing the institution-wide organizational chart and offering opportunities to better understand reporting relationships within these given units. Doing so is especially helpful for understanding staffing within departments, as nonmanagerial positions are revealed in such microlevel analyses. If matrix structures, hybrid structures, or other unique forms of organization are desired, resulting depictions must mirror as closely as possible the associated reporting relationships. By the conclusion of this step, an initial illustration of the organizational chart should be in hand.

It is understood that chart assembly can be somewhat intimidating, given the many decisions required and natural concerns regarding potential missteps. Fortunately, such concerns can be allayed quite easily by investigating the manner in which peer healthcare establishments have been designed. Doing so, in fact, can help to jumpstart organizational chart initiatives even for experienced developers.

As noted earlier in the chapter, health and medical organizations often publicly post their organizational charts in annual reports and personnel policy manuals, on corporate websites, and in similar locations, providing an easily accessible source of intelligence. By studying the organizational charts of peer establishments, healthcare providers can acquire an understanding of common structural practices embraced by similar facilities, aiding them in formulating ideas for their own organizational charts. On identifying particularly desirable organizational charts, healthcare providers might even decide to engage these establishments, contacting their executives to request additional insights. Competitive sensitivities might prohibit this on the local level, but out-of-market institutions would likely welcome such a dialogue, potentially even leading to strategic alliances. For good measure, organizational chart developers might wish to explore the structural techniques embraced by institutions outside of those in the healthcare industry, giving another useful pool of intelligence. This simple but highly effective method for jumpstarting organizational chart assembly can dramatically build confidence and ability, expediting the development of an accurate structural illustration.

9.5.5 Step 5: Envision How the Illustration Will Translate into Actual Practice, Refining the Organizational Chart as Needed

Following the development of the initial rendition of the organizational chart, it is critical to thoroughly examine the resulting design, making refinements as needed. Specifically, those involved in development must carefully envision how the illustration will translate into actual practice. Namely, they must think carefully through the placement of departments and the arrangement of reporting relationships and determine if they accurately depict the desired structure of the institution. Of course, it is vital for the organizational chart to reflect the totality of organizational operations. Does the illustration as presented permit the work of the institution to be accomplished? Are any components missing from the diagram (e.g., departments inadvertently overlooked)? Does the resulting organizational chart conform with earlier decisions regarding work specialization, chain of command, span of control, centralization, and formalization? Is the form of departmentalization that was selected at the onset of chart assembly conveyed as intended? Attention also must be directed toward considering how employees and other stakeholders will view the depiction. Is it anticipated that they will be able to easily follow lines of authority and understand the reporting relationships between and among departments? By the conclusion of this step, a refined illustration of the organizational chart should be in hand.

9.5.6 Step 6: Permit Others in the Organization to Examine the Organizational Chart and Offer Feedback, Refining the Organizational Chart as Needed

As a further check on the accuracy of a given depiction, newly developed organizational charts should be circulated to a sample of managers and employees for their review and commentary. This certainly is possible in cases where existing healthcare organizations are being reengineered structurally, given that personnel will already be on staff and accessible. In cases where organizational charts are being created for new healthcare establishments which have not yet been opened, opportunities to acquire feedback will be more limited, but still are possible. In the formative days of a healthcare organization's life, it is not uncommon for establishments to make early hires, affording at least a small pool of employees who can be asked for feedback. Ultimately, when and where possible, organizational structure and design initiatives, including the construction of organizational charts, should be informed by multidisciplinary perspectives [15]. Especially in healthcare establishments, coordination and communication are essential between and among departments, necessitating effective structures. As such, insights from clinical and administrative personnel are most helpful in crafting appropriate and effective frameworks [15, 18].

9.5.7 Step 7: Finalize the Organizational Chart, Publicize It, and Structure Departments and Work Relationships, Accordingly, Evaluating the Illustration Periodically to Ensure Its Accuracy

The final step of organizational chart assembly is an operational stage, involving finalization of the illustration, followed by its publication. For all-new healthcare organizations, the resulting organizational chart is then used to structure departments and reporting relationships in a manner compliant with the decisions noted in the approved depiction. For existing healthcare organizations involved in restructuring operations, the resulting organizational chart is used to guide modifications which will see the current structure being replaced by the revised version. Assuming a successful launch, organizational charts should be monitored periodically to ensure that they accurately reflect the structure of given healthcare establishments. Organizational structures indeed change over time through growth, retrenchment, mission adjustments, and so on. As such, organizational charts should be considered to be "living documents" subject to change when and where warranted.

WK Reflections: Centers of Excellence

Discussions on the topic of organizational structure and design very often concentrate most heavily on elements leading to the development of organizational charts. This is for good reason, given the importance of these documents, but it is imperative to realize the equivalent importance of organization design matters beyond chart assembly. As noted earlier, organization design prominently includes activities such as determining interorganizational and intraorganizational relationships and crafting work protocols and processes. The chapter started off by profiling a unique organizational arrangement concerning Willis Knighton Health's hub-and-spoke network. It will conclude with another unique organizational arrangement, namely, Willis Knighton Health's development of centers of excellence as a means of delivering the highest quality care in given specialty areas to patients.

A **center of excellence** is a specialized program within a healthcare organization which supplies an exceptionally high concentration of expertise and related resources on a particular front of medicine which is delivered in a comprehensive, interdisciplinary manner, often within a single building. It essentially is a place where excellence in a particular area of medicine is housed and made available to patients. In such arrangements, personnel, technologies, and other resources associated with addressing a particular medical condition are compartmentalized in an organizational subunit. This subunit—the center of excellence—is responsible for delivering the full continuum of care and, in many respects, operates as an institution within an institution [28–30].

The WK Cancer Center, for example, offers patients the utility and convenience of visiting a single site on Willis Knighton Health's main campus for receipt of all services related to their care and treatment, ranging from patient education seminars to social services to pharmacy to chemotherapy to one of the most advanced cancer treatment technologies available, proton therapy. This approach starkly contrasts with traditional delivery methods where care components from multiple departments are strung together to carry out medical interventions, often necessitating that patients visit multiple buildings on campuses or even multiple locations within communities to realize the continuum of care [28].

Organizing care via the center of excellence model carries a number of benefits. It maximizes patient convenience via consolidation of care within a single servicescape, fosters specialization and high performance in that personnel are focused exclusively on a particular medical condition, promotes collaboration across disciplinary lines to ensure joint accountability for outcomes, and pools resources which would otherwise be distributed more broadly, making for greater efficiency and effectiveness [28, 31, 32]. These benefits are highly desired in health and medicine, compelling many healthcare institutions to make the investments required to establish and operate centers of excellence. Willis Knighton Health, in fact, considers the center of excellence delivery model to be a vital component of its service mix, crediting the model with fueling growth which led to its current market leadership position.

The center of excellence model of healthcare delivery represents a highly unique organizational arrangement, illustrating the variety of activities falling under the auspices of organization design. Notably, it demonstrates the value of creativity when making associated decisions regarding how to structure not just healthcare organizations but also the work within them. Doing so has the potential to positively impact operations, yield competitive advantages, and facilitate the delivery of outstanding patient care and attention. As such, healthcare providers are encouraged to intensively study organizational structure and design and deeply explore methods of organization used by establishments both within and outside of the healthcare industry to better understand options and opportunities that can be applied in their own institutions for associated gains.

9.6   Summary and Conclusions

The organizational structure of an establishment refers to an institution's hierarchy, depicting its chain of command, arrangement of departments, and associated reporting relationships within the organization. Organizational structure activities, including organizational chart assembly, represent the most notable pursuits of organization design, a component of organizational behavior and management which focuses on the process of formulating, implementing, and evaluating institutional structures, activities, and operations in a manner which facilitates the fulfillment of an organization's mission. When healthcare organizations are established, a full range of decisions and actions concerning institutional structures and work processes are required. As they mature, these operational facets must evolve to accommodate any changes encountered. While options abound for structuring and designing organizations in manners desired, as with anything, prudent decisions must be made in order to realize success. The better designed a healthcare establishment, the better able it will be to perform. By deploying associated knowledge and skills, healthcare providers will be able to aid their given institutions in harnessing the power of organizational structure and design, affording opportunities to execute operations successfully, ultimately leading to mission fulfillment.

Key Terms

- Authority
- Center of Excellence
- Centralization
- Centralized Organization
- Chain of Command
- Customer Departmentalization
- Decentralized Organization
- Departmentalization
- Division of Labor
- Divisional Structure
- Formalization
- Functional Structure
- Geographic Departmentalization
- Hub-and-Spoke Network
- Hub-and-Spoke Organization Design
- Matrix Structure
- Organization Design
- Organizational Chart
- Organizational Structure
- Product Departmentalization
- Responsibility
- Scalar Chain
- Silo
- Simple Structure
- Span of Control
- Work Specialization

Exercises

1. In your own words, define the concept of organizational structure and discuss its importance in health and medical establishments.
2. In your own words, define the concept of organization design, identify its key areas of concentration, and discuss its impact in healthcare organizations.
3. Identify and discuss the five building blocks of organizational structure.
4. In your own words, define the concept of departmentalization and discuss its role in organizational structure and design.
5. Place yourself in the role of a healthcare entrepreneur establishing a new durable medical equipment company. Demonstrate your understanding of the simple structure by preparing a hypothetical organizational chart for this new entity.

6. Define and discuss the matrix structure. How might this particular form of departmentalization be used effectively in health and medical organizations? What are the risks of such a structure?
7. In your own words, define the hub-and-spoke network and discuss how this particular organization design is used in the healthcare industry.
8. Broaden your knowledge of the various types of organizational structures used by healthcare institutions by visiting the physical locations or websites of hospitals, clinics, and other health and medical establishments, seeking their organizational charts. Identify three and study them using your newfound knowledge regarding departmentalization and related organizational structure and design facets. Prepare a summary report, identifying the organizational charts reviewed and the observations gleaned from your investigation and analysis.

References

1. Elrod, J. K. (2013). *Breadcrumbs to cheesecake*. R&R Publishers.
2. Elrod, J. K., & Fortenberry, J. L., Jr. (2017). The hub-and-spoke organization design: An avenue for serving patients well. *BMC Health Services Research, 17*(Suppl 1), 25–33.
3. Porter, M., & Lee, T. (2013). The strategy that will fix health care. *Harvard Business Review, 91*(10), 50–70.
4. Ahlquist, G., Saxena, S. B., Belokrinitsky, I., & Kapur, A. (2012). *Charting a clear course in rough seas: A new view on hospital and health systems strategy*. Strategy&.
5. Govindarajan, V., & Ramamurti, R. (2013). Delivering world-class health care, affordably. *Harvard Business Review, 91*(11), 117–122.
6. Devarakonda, S. (2016). Hub and spoke model: Making rural healthcare in India affordable, available and accessible. *Rural and Remote Health, 16*(1), 1–8.
7. Roney, K. (2012, November 28). Four emerging models provide strategy roadmap for future transactions. *Becker's Hospital Review*. Retrieved April 6, 2023, from http://www.beckershospitalreview.com/hospital-transactions-and-valuation/4-emerging-models-provide-strategy-roadmap-for-future-transactions.html
8. Lin, M., & Kawasaki, A. (2012). Where to enter in hub-spoke airline networks. *Papers in Regional Science, 91*(2), 419–436.
9. Skipper, J., Cunningham, W., Boone, C., & Hill, R. (2016). Managing hub and spoke networks: A military case comparing time and cost. *Journal of Global Business and Technology, 12*(1), 33–47.
10. Banjo, S. (2013, June 18). Wal-mart: A pro in physical-store retail logistics. *Wall Street Journal, 19*, B2. Retrieved April 6, 2023, from https://www.wsj.com/articles/SB10001424127887323566804578553300075547368
11. Millar, L. (2014). Use of hub and spoke model in nursing students' practice learning. *Nursing Standard, 28*(49), 37–42.
12. Scalise, A., Pierangeli, M., Calamita, R., Tartaglione, C., Bolletta, E., Grassetti, L., & Di Benedetto, G. (2015). An example of a hub and spoke network system in plastic surgery: The regional reference center for non-healing wounds in Ancona (Italy). *Igiene e Sanità Pubblica, 71*(1), 51–72.
13. Elrod, J. K., & Fortenberry, J. L., Jr. (2017). The hub-and-spoke organization design revisited: A lifeline for rural hospitals. *BMC Health Services Research, 17*(Suppl 4), 29–35.
14. McConnell, C. R. (2020). *Hospitals and health systems: What they are and how they work*. Jones and Bartlett.

15. Anderson, D. L. (2019). *Organization design: Creating strategic and agile organizations*. Sage.
16. Burton, R. M., Obel, B., & Hakonsson, D. D. (2020). *Organizational design: A step-by-step approach* (4th ed.). Cambridge University Press.
17. Robbins, S. P., & Judge, T. A. (2019). *Organizational behavior* (18th ed.). Pearson.
18. Galbraith, J. R. (2014). *Designing organizations: Strategy, structure, and process at the business unit and enterprise levels* (3rd ed.). Jossey-Bass.
19. Hitt, M. A., Miller, C. C., Colella, A., & Triana, M. D. C. (2018). *Organizational behavior* (5th ed.). Wiley.
20. Stanford, N. (2018). *Organization design: The practitioner's guide* (3rd ed.). Routledge.
21. Colquitt, J. A., Lepine, J. A., & Wesson, M. J. (2019). *Organizational behavior: Improving performance and commitment in the workplace* (6th ed.). McGraw-Hill.
22. Fayol, H. (2016). General principles of management. In J. M. Shafritz, J. S. Ott, & Y. S. Jang (Eds.), *Classics of organization theory* (8th ed., pp. 53–65). Cengage.
23. Shafritz, J. M., Ott, J. S., & Jang, Y. S. (Eds.). (2016). *Classics of organization theory* (8th ed.). Cengage.
24. Griffin, R. W., Phillips, J. M., & Gully, S. M. (2020). *Organizational behavior: Managing people and organizations* (13th ed.). Cengage.
25. McShane, S. L., & Von Glinow, M. A. (2019). *Organizational behavior* (4th ed.). McGraw-Hill.
26. Burns, T. R., & Stalker, G. M. (1961). *The management of innovation*. Tavistock.
27. Konopaske, R., Ivancevich, J. M., & Matteson, M. T. (2018). *Organizational behavior and management* (11th ed.). McGraw-Hill.
28. Elrod, J. K., & Fortenberry, J. L., Jr. (2017). Centers of excellence in healthcare institutions: What they are and how to assemble them. *BMC Health Services Research, 17*(Suppl 1), 15–24.
29. Rodak, S. (2013, March 4). Is center of excellence investment the silver bullet healthcare has been looking for? *Becker's Hospital Review*. Retrieved April 6, 2023, from http://www.beckershospitalreview.com/hospital-key-specialties/is-center-of-excellence-investment-the-silver-bullet-healthcare-has-been-looking-for.html
30. Molden, M., Brown, C., III, & Griffith, B. (2013). At the heart of integration: Aligning physicians and administrators to create new value. *Frontiers of Health Services Management, 29*(4), 3–16.
31. Kuo, L., Simmons, K., & Kelz, R. (2015). Bariatric centers of excellence: Effect of centralization on access to care. *Journal of the American College of Surgeons, 221*(5), 914–922.
32. Bonow, R. O., & Adams, D. H. (2016). The time has come to define centers of excellence in mitral valve repair. *Journal of the American College of Cardiology, 67*(5), 499–501.

Chapter 10
Organizational Change in Health and Medicine

Learning Objectives

After examining this chapter, readers will have the ability to:

- Define organizational change and change management and discuss their role and importance in the healthcare industry.
- Compare and contrast planned and unplanned change, as well as evolutionary and revolutionary change, supplying examples of each.
- Understand the role played by the environment in initiating change in health and medicine.
- Define environmental scanning and discuss its importance in the change management initiatives of healthcare establishments.
- Outline the process of change by describing models of change and their illustrative steps leading to organizational transformations.
- Identify and discuss common sources of resistance to change and methods used to deal with that resistance, noting approaches that can be deployed to ensure that change initiatives are successful.

WK Reflections: Change in Practice

In 1990, Willis Knighton Health introduced the Willis Knighton Physicians Network, a new form of organization designed to benefit its medical staff and the greater institution. Historically, Willis Knighton Health's medical staff members operated independent practices exclusively, with physicians being responsible for all aspects of their given establishments, ranging from the clinical elements to the administrative ones. With the emergence of the Willis Knighton Physicians Network, this traditional practice management mindset was profoundly changed, with physicians no longer being independent prac-

J. K. Elrod, J. L. Fortenberry, Jr., *Organizational Behavior and Management in Health and Medicine*, https://doi.org/10.1007/978-3-031-61823-9_10

titioners, but instead, becoming employees of the institution. Participation in the network was voluntary; it was an option for physicians to consider which carried several unique and highly desirable benefits [1].

By joining the Willis Knighton Physicians Network, physicians were afforded with the benefits typically expected of employment (e.g., salaried compensation, retirement benefits, paid vacations, health insurance, malpractice insurance), providing significant, worry-free stability to members. Perhaps even more compelling, however, was that through network membership, Willis Knighton Health would assume responsibilities for the administrative aspects of associated medical practices (e.g., billing, collections, staffing, marketing), permitting physicians to concentrate exclusively on the delivery of medicine. In fact, this very attribute—freedom from the administrative bureaucracy of operating medical practices—served as the primary impetus for pursing this new direction, courtesy of earlier requests for such being forwarded by a few solo practitioners. These physicians welcomed the prospects of exclusively focusing on clinical matters. They also believed that higher performance would be possible by turning over the administrative side of practice management to experts at Willis Knighton Health [1].

While the benefits available to medical practitioners via the Willis Knighton Physicians Network happened to be sizeable, they also extended to Willis Knighton Health. While acquisition of practices carried associated costs, including ongoing employment and practice infrastructure expenditures, the institution benefited by garnering the productivity and revenue generated by these operations. Such models bolster both inpatient and outpatient admissions, courtesy of the employed cadre of physicians on staff. Referrals to specialists, too, are boosted, as are referrals to rehabilitation, long-term care, hospice, and other services provided internally, enhancing associated revenues. By combining multiple practices under a universal management framework, economies of scale, too, are realized, hastening performance. Further, the combined power of a large group of physicians enhances an institution's ability to negotiate with third-party payers, further justifying this model of operation [1].

As implementation of the network ensued, great care had to be taken, given the monumental change which was introduced. Notably, significant developmental work was necessary to roll out a model that would be effective, with this requiring major investments on the part of Willis Knighton Health. Proper vetting of the pathway was essential, increasing the likelihood that the target audience—physicians—would welcome the change and join the network. Further, the physicians themselves had much to consider, especially regarding concerns that their autonomy might be compromised by joining the network. In anticipation of this, Willis Knighton Health took preemptive steps, ensuring open and robust communications in describing the network and its operation, coupled with a complete commitment to transparency, with this greatly allaying physician concerns. Additionally, Willis Knighton

Health's employees impacted by the looming acquisitions and increased management responsibilities needed to be informed about the change, necessitating presentation of comprehensive details and the provision of assurances of support, further bolstering implementation success.

On the network's introduction, interest was piqued among physicians and membership growth ensued immediately. Now over 30 years old, the Willis Knighton Physicians Network has been and continues to be a resounding success, affording a major competitive advantage for Willis Knighton Health. Today, network members number over 500. Had Willis Knighton Health not respected the change initiated by instituting the Willis Knighton Physicians Network, along with the impacts of the change on the institution, its personnel, and its stakeholders, the positive outcomes derived from the network's introduction and development would not have been possible. As change is pervasive in the healthcare industry, knowledge of change and proficiencies in change management are vital for anyone serving in managerial capacities within health and medicine.

10.1 Background

Of all descriptors used to characterize the healthcare industry and its operation, change is arguably the most frequently one mentioned. Change indeed is pervasive in health and medicine; it is unyielding and, by many accounts, actually increasing in prevalence. Beliefs that practicing in accordance with the status quo will lead to enduring success are futile, as operations will invariably change, usually sooner rather than later [2–6]. Such persistent change as witnessed in the halls of medicine comes from many sources. Some changes frequently experienced by health and medical establishments are similar to those witnessed by most any institution: a new CEO is hired, an establishment is acquired by another, two organizations decide to merge, new technologies are purchased, customer groups demand new offerings, a key supplier raises prices, and a new competitor enters the market. Such changes and scores of those similar are common experiences in organizational life across business and industry, including those focused on the delivery of medical services [3, 6–8].

Other changes, however, are the result of the unique nature of health and medicine, distinctively impacting its particular establishments. The extensive health policy framework governing the healthcare industry, for example, is frequently modified, impacting operations. When life and limb are at stake, intensive oversight and scrutiny from policy bodies should be expected, resulting in myriad regulations that are subject to change over time [1, 3, 9]. Financing mechanisms, too, are unique in the healthcare industry and are subject to frequent adjustments by public and private third-party payers, making it essential for healthcare providers to be change agile [1, 3, 10]. Additionally, clinical and administrative technologies are constantly evolving, requiring regular updates and enhancements. Even the state of community health is unpredictable, as evidenced by periodic public health crises, with this necessitating alterations in practice patterns and attention [1, 7]. In many respects, change could be said to be more prevalent in the healthcare industry than in any other industry [6].

Such a change-rich environment naturally plays havoc with operations, necessitating keen attentiveness, accurate assessments of impact, and swift action to address any and all influences encountered. As changes often directly impact those serving in health and medical establishments, a premium also is placed on getting the support and commitment of staff members to embrace whatever change is encountered, permitting operations to continue unfettered. Healthcare providers must have the ability to adapt institutional operations efficiently and effectively, ensuring that healthcare organizations stay on course [1, 5, 6, 8]. This chapter directs comprehensive attention toward organizational change, permitting healthcare providers to understand associated fundamentals and put them into practice for the benefit of their organizations and patients.

10.2 Defining Organizational Change

Organizational change concerns the alteration of operations within an institution. It typically is prompted by circumstances and situations encountered in external and internal environments, with organizations maneuvering themselves in a manner to accommodate or adjust to these influences [11]. For example, a medical clinic which receives demands from its patients to expand hours of operation might possibly decide to grant the request, adding evening and weekend coverage. Likewise, a forthcoming reimbursement change which bolsters payments for rehabilitative services would constitute an environmental change potentially compelling a hospital to expand its rehabilitation offerings to capitalize on this positive development. Instances such as these would constitute **planned change** in that the organizations are taking deliberate steps to address pressing developments in pursuit of some desired state. It is also possible for change to occur without the deliberate extension of efforts, with this constituting **unplanned change** [12]. A hospital that witnessed a competitor's unexpected closure, dramatically increasing its patient volume and rocketing it to market leadership, would be an example of such a change. It did not actively seek the patient volume and resulting market leadership, but circumstances led to its occurrence, necessitating associated attention.

Great skill is required to proficiently address change in healthcare organizations. At face value, change-related activities in institutions might seem to be somewhat problem-free endeavors, but that is not the case. In fact, change is almost universally described as being difficult [13]. Success requires intensive knowledge of change processes, keen surveillance abilities, problem-solving prowess, and implementation acumen, among many other things. Some change is easier to effect than others, with magnitude of change being a key determinant. **Evolutionary change** refers to change that involves incremental adjustments, with these sometimes being termed "baby steps." This type of change contrasts sharply with **revolutionary change**, defined as comprehensive, sweeping change that profoundly alters the status quo. Evolutionary change is easier to implement than revolutionary change, as modest adjustments are more easily tolerated than are more robust modifications [14]. Both variants occur regularly within healthcare establishments, so health and medical providers must be capable of managing both types.

Since change is a pervasive and enduring feature of organizational life, healthcare managers cannot evade responsibilities for handling change. Its level of prominence is so pronounced that many institutions seek to proactively guide and direct change initiatives by engaging in a formal process known as **change management**. Managers ideally must become so proficient in overseeing change initiatives that they become recognized as **change agents**, individuals who have mastered change management, proving themselves capable of building bridges within their establishments which lead people, places, and things from a current state to one that is desired. They are catalysts for change within their organizations. Arriving at such a lofty position requires one to thoroughly develop acumen associated with change and its many facets [15].

10.3   Change and the Environment

Change within healthcare institutions typically is prompted by change in the environment. As environments are in the state of constant change, any institution situated within given environments will regularly face the need to adapt to applicable changes in order to remain relevant and viable. Successfully adapting to change will permit healthcare establishments to actively pursue their given missions, productively serving patients, even in the context of ever-evolving and often highly tumultuous settings. Change, of course, can be positive (e.g., burgeoning patient volume) or negative (e.g., reimbursement reductions), but regardless of variety, current practices are impacted, forcing operational adjustments and accommodations. Due to the potential for change to impact operations, notably including critical workflow processes and procedures, health and medical providers must be vigilant in monitoring developments, permitting quick attention whenever change is encountered [5, 6, 16, 17].

In order to stay abreast of changes, healthcare institutions must engage in **environmental scanning**, an activity which also is referred to as **environmental surveillance** or **environmental analysis**. Described comprehensively in Chap. 6, environmental scanning refers to the activity of surveilling the environment for purposes of identifying opportunities and threats, permitting them to be proactively addressed by an organization. It is an essential skill of change management. Surveillance efforts must be directed both internally and externally, as disruptive influences can arise from both within and outside of given healthcare establishments [6, 18, 19].

Common tools for environmental scanning include the PEST analysis and the SWOT analysis. The **PEST analysis** focuses on the **external environment** or **macroenvironment** and specifically seeks to identify political, economic, social, and technological forces that have the potential to impact given organizations. The **SWOT analysis** adds **internal environment** or **microenvironment** attention. Also known as a **situation analysis** because it depicts the state of affairs of an organization, the SWOT analysis identifies institutional strengths, weaknesses, opportunities, and threats. Strengths and weaknesses pertain to internal environmental factors, while opportunities and threats relate to external ones, affording the SWOT analysis with the capability of portraying an organization's microenvironment in the context of its macroenvironment. Both of these analyses afford opportunities for healthcare establishments to remain apprised of the state of their given environments, permitting them to detect associated changes [6, 18, 19].

Proactive attention through active environmental scanning efforts represents one of the best methods for productively managing change, permitting healthcare organizations to capitalize on opportunities and diminish or eliminate threats. Addressing change in a proactive, rather than reactive, fashion should be the goal of any healthcare provider, as doing so affords institutions with time to study associated change and plan how best to address its impacts.

10.4   Lewin's Model of Change

Whenever a change looms, it is useful to consult models of change, as these can be most helpful in gaining an understanding of what lies ahead as efforts to transform healthcare organizations ensue. Models of change essentially map the process of change, providing step-by-step guidance for how transformations from a current state to a desired state are achieved. These models often are aggregated under a particular area of organizational behavior and management known as organizational development. **Organizational development** focuses on guiding and directing efforts that build and enhance organizational effectiveness, with a special emphasis being placed on change management [20]. Organizational development draws on many disciplines, including **action research** which seeks to effect change by diagnosing current problems, applying interventions to resolve those problems, and studying the outcomes to evaluate the effectiveness of the interventions [21]. Many models of change exist, with researchers offering their perspectives on the process of realizing transformation based on their beliefs and experiences. Some view change negatively, as a problem in need of resolution, while others view change positively, as an opportunity for advancement [22]. Social psychologist Kurt Lewin introduced a landmark model of change which specifically focused on preparing for change, implementing change, and reinforcing change. The model consists of three stages: unfreezing, changing, and refreezing.

10.4.1   Stage 1: Unfreezing

Unfreezing, the first stage of Lewin's model of change, seeks to break status quo approaches, opening the door for change to occur. The goal of this stage is to prepare for change by instilling a motivation to change in all parties involved in the desired transformation. In doing so, organizations often will make a case for change by supplying evidence that it is needed [23–25]. For example, a medical clinic desirous of introducing evening and weekend hours of operation to complement its weekday hours of operation might point to patient requests for options to visit outside of normal business hours. The clinic also might point to competing clinics which are either planning to offer increased hours of operation or are already doing so. Additionally, the clinic might demonstrate that patient volume has dwindled, suggesting that increased hours of operation will help stem loss of share, noting also that layoffs could be forthcoming if losses do not cease. These are very compelling motivations for change which should encourage clinic employees to embrace desired alterations positively, certainly as the consequences of not doing so arguably would place each of them in a far worse situation.

10.4.2   Stage 2: Changing

Changing, the second stage in Lewin's model of change, focuses on implementation. During this stage, staff members are directed to learn different processes and do different things. The implements of change—new equipment and technology, new policies and procedures, new evaluation systems, and so on—are also put into place during this stage. Training is essential and patience, at least up to a point, must be extended, allowing employees time to acclimate to given changes. It must be remembered that personnel are being called to relinquish prior approaches, familiar processes, and established routines, with this proving to be very difficult for many. In the medical clinic example noted earlier, extension of hours certainly can hardship staff members. New work schedules must be arranged, with this potentially being favorable to some, but not to others, depending on their personal preferences and obligations. Goals must be clear, assurances must be high, and support must be thorough. During the changing stage, a clear pathway toward a desired end must be mapped out and shared with those expected to change [23–25].

10.4.3   Stage 3: Refreezing

Refreezing, the third and final stage of Lewin's model of change, involves reinforcing the change that took place in the prior stage. This stage calls for organizations to support the efforts of staff members as they go about accommodating the required change. Efforts particularly must be directed toward reinforcing initiated modifications, helping employees become accustomed to new changes. Rewards and recognitions are very useful during the refreezing stage, with these acknowledgments providing further reinforcements which support changes that have been made. Extending the earlier clinic example, employees assigned to work evening and weekend hours perhaps could be offered extra pay or other incentives for agreeing to work these new schedules. **Role modeling** also can be helpful, with managers leading by example. The clinic's managers should at least periodically be present during the extended hours, conveying the importance of the new schedule to others and indicating that they, too, are sharing the burden of the change. Successful completion of the refreezing stage draws Lewin's model of change to a close. By the conclusion of this stage, the desired change should now be established, becoming the new routine until another need for change appears, starting the process once again [23–25].

10.5 Kotter's Eight-Stage Process of Creating Major Change

John Kotter, a noted leadership and change expert, offered a typology of change management consisting of eight stages, namely, establishing a sense of urgency, creating a guiding coalition, developing a vision and strategy, communicating the change vision, empowering broad-based action, generating short-term wins, consolidating gains and producing more change, and anchoring new approaches in the culture. The first four stages effectively defrost the status quo. New practices are introduced in stages five to seven. The final stage grounds the change in the organizational culture. The process is sequential; stages cannot be skipped without likely consequences that can diminish or derail change efforts [13, 26, 27]. The process supplied by Kotter, in many respects, is a more detailed version of the one offered by Lewin. Stages 1–4 equate with Lewin's unfreezing stage, stages 5–7 equate with Lewin's changing stage, and Stage 8 equates with Lewin's refreezing stage. Kotter's model of change heavily emphasizes the importance of implementation in the change process, as he viewed associated faults to be the major shortcoming which derails change management initiatives [28].

10.5.1 Stage 1: Establishing a Sense of Urgency

Stage 1 of Kotter's change model—establishing a sense of urgency—is a most crucial step for gaining cooperation necessary for change to occur. As change is inherently difficult, those involved in the process must shed complacency and view the need for change to be an urgent matter. This will elevate attentiveness to and acceptability of forthcoming changes. Frank discussions are helpful during this stage. Revelations that failure to change can lead to circumstances far worse than the inconveniences associated with the change can prove very motivating [13, 26, 27]. Salary reductions, layoffs, and facility closures resulting from declining patient volume, for example, can go a long way toward waking up those who are not taking the change mandate seriously, bolstering vital attentiveness to looming crises.

10.5.2   Stage 2: Creating a Guiding Coalition

The second stage of Kotter's change model—creating a guiding coalition—essentially entails selecting a group of individuals to lead the transformation effort. Importantly, change initiatives should not be solo concerns. While a single individual, such as a highly regarded CEO, certainly is capable of making headway, the complexity of change initiatives necessitates a broader group to ensure that transformation efforts take root. Guiding coalitions must be composed of individuals holding position power, keen expertise, and high credibility. They also should be viewed by others to be leaders, holding personal power and related positive attributes. These qualities provide the foundational skills required for effecting change. They also imbue individuals with the formal and informal authority necessary to upend dissatisfaction and remove any roadblocks encountered. Management and leadership skills both are essential for effecting change; management skills control the change process and leadership skills drive the change [13, 26, 27].

10.5.3   Stage 3: Developing a Vision and Strategy

Stage 3 of Kotter's change model—developing a vision and strategy—effectively presents the direction of the change and the means for its achievement. **Vision** essentially refers to a picture of the future tied to a narrative that expresses the reasons people should strive to create that future. A good vision serves three purposes: it clarifies the direction for the change, it motivates individuals to take proper action, and it coordinates the actions of many. Care must be taken to strategically map out this vision as this points to the ultimate destination resulting from the forthcoming change initiatives. It should be compelling and convincing, sufficiently vetted to ensure that the desired state represents an improvement over the current state, pointing to a better future for the organization and its employees [13, 26, 27].

10.5.4   Stage 4: Communicating the Change Vision

Communicating the change vision—the fourth stage of Kotter's change model—is essential as change will not be possible unless everyone involved in the process possesses a clear understanding of its goals and direction. When such an understanding is achieved, transformation becomes possible, as a shared sense of a desirable future is revealed. Communications used to broadcast the planned change should be simple, eliminating jargon and other confusing terms, and highly illustrative, using helpful analogies and examples. Conveyances should be delivered via multiple channels, such as large and small group meetings, memos, and individual interactions; they should be repetitive, facilitating awareness through multiple exposures; and they should be bidirectional, with two-way communication being essential for proper dialogues to occur. Further, communications should be open and forthcoming, with change agents explaining any seeming inconsistencies to build confidence in all [13, 26, 27].

10.5.5   Stage 5: Empowering Broad-Based Action

The fifth stage of Kotter's change model—empowering broad-based action—calls for organizations to enlist many in the change process, as internal transformation rarely happens with few involved. Employees must be empowered to assist. As such, organizations seeking change must remove as many barriers to transformation as possible, facilitating actions which will see the desired change realized. Empowerment for change is facilitated by reinforcing awareness of the vision through robust communications with personnel, revising organizational structures to be compatible with this vision, providing training to foster knowledge associated with the change, aligning all institutional systems (e.g., human resources, accounting and finance, quality control) with the vision, and confronting managers who are unsupportive of the change, seeking to either gain their commitment or block their resistance [13, 26, 27].

10.5.6   Stage 6: Generating Short-Term Wins

Generating short-term wins—the sixth stage of Kotter's change model—is critical because change often takes significant time. If progress is not observed along the way, it can be demoralizing and potentially destroy the change initiative. As such, efforts must be directed toward generating and publicizing short-term gains to illustrate that the vision is being realized. Short-term wins should be visible, permitting everyone to see the given results for themselves; unambiguous, with clarity defusing any arguments that gains are not as presented; and clearly associated with the change effort, with the result convincingly tied to the broader change that is being sought. Short-term wins prove that sacrifices are paying off, they reward change agents and initiators marshalling the cause, and they help direct vision and strategies. They also frustrate cynics and other resisters, they strengthen the support of leaders, and they foster momentum [13, 26, 27].

10.5.7   Stage 7: Consolidating Gains and Producing More Change

Consolidating gains and producing more change—the seventh stage of Kotter's change model—is critical as momentum can quickly be lost. Celebrating short-term wins must be followed up by assertions that more work is needed, generating continued momentum to realize the transformation. At this stage, the broad change initiative must advance, using short-term wins as motivation. Leaders should reemphasize urgency and ensure that responsible managers in the organizational hierarchy continue their change management endeavors. Efforts also should be directed toward reducing any unnecessary interdependencies in the organization, eliminating needless bureaucracy to hasten the transformation [13, 26, 27].

10.5.8   Stage 8: Anchoring New Approaches in the Culture

The eighth and final stage of Kotter's change model—anchoring new approaches in the culture—ultimately solidifies the initiated change, making it a stable feature of the organization. Here, it is vitally important to remember that if the change achieved proves to be incompatible with the organization's underlying culture, it will be doomed to fail. This necessitates that the transformation be anchored in the associated culture, an activity occurring in the final stage of the change process as the majority of alterations in norms and values occurs at this point. Anchoring is advanced when the results of the change become evident, clearly revealing that the new approach works better than the old one. It is facilitated by robustly communicating the validity of practices, evidenced by the gains achieved via the change. Notably, conveyances should emphasize how the positive impacts of the change are benefiting all institutional stakeholders. Signs of disenchantment, if observed, should be stifled, as they can undermine the anchoring process. For example, if employees refuse to accept and support the new way of operating, disciplinary measures, up to and including termination, must be initiated. Such steps are critical for facilitating anchoring, institutionalizing the transformation and rounding out the change process [13, 26, 27].

10.6   Sources of Resistance to Change

Any form of change has the potential to be challenging and, as such, resistance should be expected whenever a change is announced. Given the frequency of change experienced in health and medicine, healthcare providers must strive to fully understand sources of resistance to change and methods for dealing with that resistance in order to ensure that their institutions remain change agile. Resistance to change can come from a variety of sources, with four of the most common ones being narrow-minded self-interest, misunderstanding and lack of trust, different assessments of the value of change, and low tolerance for change [29], as explained below.

10.6.1   Narrow-Minded Self-Interest

Narrow-minded self-interest is one of the most frequently experienced sources of resistance to change, stemming simply from an individual's belief that a particular change will not benefit him or her personally; that something of value will be lost as a result of the alteration. Because people in such contexts are operating in their own interest, rather than in the interest of their given organizations, resulting resistance is often expressed by acting out politically, placing pressure on those initiating the change in an effort to thwart the planned transformation. This sort of behavior also incites power struggles [29]. A good example of this form of resistance would be that of a hospital announcing a new method for scheduling nurses, permitting better, more consistent coverage for patients, yet the staff nurses, who will be forced by the change to abandon their comfort zones, protest it vigorously. Their mindset is self-serving, rather than focused on serving patients, which is what they were hired to do.

10.6.2   Misunderstanding and Lack of Trust

Misunderstanding and lack of trust are certainly instigators of resistance to change. When change and its implications are not fully understood, resistance to change can be expected to be high, especially in cases where individuals view the looming change to cost them more than they will gain. This is all the more the case when distrust between supervisors and subordinates is high. Complete cohesion between supervisory personnel and their subordinates is somewhat of a rarity in organizational life. This distrust fosters the potential for misunderstandings to occur. Therefore, when a change is communicated, those impacted by the change are naturally skeptical which automatically generates resistance [29]. In the healthcare industry, the relationship between administrators and physicians, for example, is often stressed, with parties sometimes viewing each other with skepticism and distrust. At least some of this stems from enculturation in their respective programs of study, with mindsets acquired through socialization in academia often being transferred into practice. Regardless of its origin or presence, the mindsets of parties involved in change initiatives must be taken into consideration when planning transformations in an effort to build bridges and establish collegial interactions which will foster change.

10.6.3   Different Assessments of the Value of Change

Change resistance can stem from different assessments of the value of change. In such cases, those impacted by the change do not see its impact in the same light as those who are initiating the change. They, in essence, view the change to carry more costs than benefits on at least an individual level and, very often, on an institutional level. Those initiating the change sometimes assume that they possess the same facts as those impacted by the change, but very often this is not the case, setting the stage for different assessments of the value of change [29]. Consider the case of a hospital deciding to outsource its laboratory operations, resulting in the department's current employees continuing to work onsite, but under the employ of a privately contracted laboratory management company. While hospital executives would clearly understand the change, likely motivated by desires for maximizing efficiency and effectiveness, the laboratory department's employees would not possess such information without associated disclosures. The absence of such detail would lead them to focus mostly on the employer shift and its potential consequences to their livelihoods. To diminish resistance to change in such scenarios, change agents and initiators would need to ensure that all parties impacted by the change possess equivalent details, permitting each side to be fully informed, reducing the potential for resistance.

10.6.4   Low Tolerance for Change

Low tolerance for change stems from insecurities associated with one's ability to adjust to change and acquire new skills and behaviors that can accommodate the transformation. The potential to adjust and adapt to change differs between and among individuals, with some being more capable than others. Limited tolerance for change, courtesy of personal limitations, leads to natural resistance to change. As the reasons for limited tolerance are numerous, change agents and initiators must develop proficient diagnostic abilities in order to bridge associated gaps and reduce dissent [29]. Consider, for example, older employees possessing many years of experience in given healthcare establishments. Compared to their younger, less tenured counterparts, the routines and associated comfort zones of senior employees have been established for lengthy periods of time, creating increased burdens for breaking away from such patterns. Care indeed must be taken whenever change mandates are issued. Seeing the change from the perspective of those impacted and anticipating their stumbling blocks to acceptance can be helpful in devising methods to allay their concerns and foster desired transformations.

10.7   Methods for Addressing Resistance to Change

Since resistance to change is commonplace in health and medical institutions, healthcare providers must be able to address it successfully. Several methods for dealing with resistance to change are available, including education and communication, participation and involvement, facilitation and support, negotiation and agreement, manipulation and cooptation, and explicit and implicit coercion. Skillful change management endeavors typically call for a combination approach, with the exact formulation being dependent on the environmental context of the scenario [29]. Each of the noted strategies for addressing resistance is explained in following sections.

10.7.1   Education and Communication

Education and communication are excellent pathways for addressing resistance to change. By fully informing employees of forthcoming changes and the reasons they are necessary, concerns regarding associated transformations can be reduced or eliminated. This particular strategy option is very helpful in situations where resistance stems from inadequate or inaccurate information [29]. Consider the case where two hospitals in a particular city decide to merge. Such a pursuit naturally will spur serious questions from impacted parties. Aside from the complex analyses and investigations required to properly vet such a comprehensive initiative, the respective institutions would need to meaningfully engage their employees, educating and enlightening them, addressing any associated concerns, and conveying full support throughout the change process. Taking such steps will help to calm employees and break change resistance, with the time and money spent ensuring understanding, paying dividends as given transformations roll out.

10.7.2   Participation and Involvement

Participation and involvement can allay resistance by essentially granting a voice to those involved in the forthcoming change. By listening to suggestions and making use of advice from impacted parties, resistance can be diminished significantly. This approach is particularly helpful when change agents believe that they need additional details to help them implement the transformation, warranting insights from others. This is especially the case when full commitment will be required to effect the change [29]. In the merger initiative noted earlier, opportunities abound for organizing the two healthcare establishments. As leaders go about crafting an associated organizational structure for the merged entity, they could be benefited by the perspectives of employees, calling on employee interviews, focus groups, or similar means to present ideas and acquire feedback. Permitting such participation can not only improve outcomes but also diminish change resistance, given that impacted parties have been given a voice in devising the transformation.

10.7.3   Facilitation and Support

Facilitation and support services are invaluable for reducing or eliminating resistance to change, with this essentially seeing the managers behind the change be supportive of those facing the change. This is particularly helpful in situations where fear and anxiety are driving resistance. Here, organizations offer employees assistance to help them adjust to the transformation at hand [29]. Continuing the merger initiative noted earlier, assume that it is determined that one of the two facilities will close after completion of a construction project at the other campus which will expand its capacity. The employees who are based at the campus targeted for closure likely will feel concerned and threatened by the plans, with fears that their jobs will be lost dominating their thoughts. Such fears can be diminished or reduced entirely by providing meaningful assistance and support to those impacted. In this case, the leadership team could provide assurances to employees that the closure will not result in significant layoffs, pledging to offer new work opportunities in other areas of operation to anyone who is released from their current job as a result of the change. For those employees facing increased commute times as a result of the closure, the institution could temporarily offer shuttle services, reducing associated financial challenges and permitting staff members time to relocate closer to their work. Such measures, aimed squarely at facilitating and supporting personnel throughout the change process, will increase employee confidence, helping to break associated resistance.

10.7.4   Negotiation and Agreement

Reduction or elimination of resistance to change can be achieved through the strategy of negotiation and agreement. This entails considering what resisters view to be valuable and offering it in return for their agreement and support. A bonus or some other type of incentive might perhaps be granted for those shouldering significant change burdens. Other possibilities include paid time off or even work from home opportunities, depending on the nature of the job and whether such perks can be accommodated. This strategy is particularly helpful in situations where change will hardship specific parties who have bargaining power due to their importance in work processes [29]. Continuing the merger example, assume that strife appeared to be building across both campuses, with employees increasingly becoming disenchanted with the new direction. Leaders could perhaps develop a new and improved employee benefits package to be offered on completion of the transformation. Such an incentive, particularly if well devised, could dramatically soften any resistance experienced, fostering broad acceptance and support for the change initiative.

10.7.5   Manipulation and Cooptation

Manipulation and cooptation constitute covert attempts to influence others. This often involves selective conveyance of information associated with the change in an attempt to garner acceptance. **Cooptation** is a form of manipulation where resisters are given key roles in the change process, effectively bringing them into the fold for purposes of gaining their support. This does not constitute participation, however, as change agents are not interested in acquiring or using the opinions of coopted individuals. They simply want their support for the change initiative. This can be called for when other strategies are viewed be incapable of reducing resistance [29]. Assume, for example, that the merger initiative noted earlier required the support of several key departments which were notoriously resistant to change, regardless of its merit. By granting the managers of those departments a seat at the decision-making roundtable, resistance can be diminished and change potentially could even be bolstered by this cooptation effort. Such strategies, however, must be used with caution, as they can backfire if those targeted read the given approaches for what they are—manipulation—with the discovery of this almost certainly magnifying resistance [29].

10.7.6   Explicit and Implicit Coercion

Managers occasionally force change through explicit and implicit coercion. Threats of demotion, pay reductions, and even terminations are examples of mechanisms used to coerce others into accepting new initiatives. This particular strategy, however, is risky, as individuals inherently dislike change being forced upon them. Organizations, though, will often assume such risk in cases where speed is essential and when the given change will not be popular or accepted, regardless of how it is introduced. Situations encountered dictate strategies used [29]. This particular strategy, along with manipulation and cooptation, should only be used as last resorts. Certainly, pressing demands might warrant their use in health and medical organizations, but with proper attentiveness and proactivity, such pathways can be minimized and perhaps avoided entirely. Achieving such should be an aspiration of everyone serving in healthcare management roles.

WK Reflections: Change as a Reminder of Interconnectivity

Change is an interesting component of organizational behavior and management in that it so very clearly draws upon and necessitates use of virtually all components of the discipline. This makes change a nexus point of sorts, given that its appearance prompts one to tap into knowledge from across organizational behavior and management. While interconnectivity is common to all of the discipline's components, its obvious presentation in change provides the perfect opportunity to emphasize the intricate linkages between and among the components of organizational behavior and management. Indeed, an understanding and appreciation of this facet is essential as it illustrates that mastery of organizational behavior and management cannot be achieved without fully understanding its various components.

Addressing a single component in isolation from other components is a rarity at best. Consider the earlier discussion profiling the Willis Knighton Physicians Network. A single change—the establishment of the network—prompted Willis Knighton Health's executives to call on virtually every aspect of organizational behavior and management. They, for example, had to strategize to develop the concept of the network, envision its operation, and craft an appropriate organizational structure and design. Communication with impacted parties had to be robust to accurately convey the nature of the change and what it meant for all. In order to foster acceptance of the change, motivational techniques had to be devised. Further, executives had to demonstrate excellent management and leadership to shepherd the project through to its operationalization. Be sure to remember the interconnected nature of the components of organizational behavior and management, and let this serve as motivation to build skills across each area, permitting enhanced abilities to manage and lead healthcare establishments.

10.8 Summary and Conclusions

Given the perpetual change associated with the healthcare industry and its many organizations, health and medical providers must endeavor to develop skill sets that help them navigate tumultuous environments. For operations to be conducted consistently and productively, change must be addressed and managed properly. In order to make this a reality, healthcare providers must maintain situational awareness at all times by engaging in active and ongoing environmental surveillance. Additionally, the process of change must be clearly understood, affording skills associated with plotting each and every step necessary for successful transformations. Further, skills associated with understanding and overcoming resistance to change are necessary for facilitating acceptance of change, successfully advancing healthcare entities from current to desired states. With such acumen, healthcare providers can encourage personnel and acquire their support to embrace whatever change is warranted, permitting operations to continue without fail.

Key Terms

- Action Research
- Change Agent
- Change Management
- Changing
- Cooptation
- Environmental Analysis
- Environmental Scanning
- Environmental Surveillance
- Evolutionary Change
- External Environment
- Internal Environment
- Kotter's Eight-Stage Process of Creating Major Change
- Lewin's Model of Change
- Macroenvironment
- Microenvironment
- Organizational Change
- Organizational Development
- PEST Analysis
- Planned Change
- Refreezing
- Revolutionary Change
- Role Modeling
- Situation Analysis
- SWOT Analysis
- Unfreezing
- Unplanned Change
- Vision

Exercises

1. In your own words, define organizational change and change management and discuss their role and importance in the healthcare industry.
2. Compare and contrast planned and unplanned change, as well as evolutionary and revolutionary change. Reflect on your recent work experiences and provide examples illustrating each of these types of change.

3. Define change agent and discuss your personal strengths and weaknesses in such a capacity. As all managers should strive to become change agents on behalf of their organizations, what steps are you taking to develop associated skills?
4. Define environmental scanning and discuss its importance in the change management processes of healthcare establishments. How might you go about establishing an environmental scanning program in a healthcare organization? What methods would you use to operationalize the practice and ensure situational awareness?
5. Compare and contrast Lewin's model of change and Kotter's eight-stage process of creating major change. Which do you prefer and why?
6. Identify and discuss common sources of resistance to change. Based on your personal and professional experiences, which of the common sources of resistance presented in the chapter have you most often encountered? Provide associated details.
7. Outline and briefly summarize common methods used to address resistance to change. Following this, describe a situation where you encountered resistance to change, indicate how it was addressed, and communicate the resulting outcome. Based on the information supplied in the chapter, could any improvements have been made in your attempts to break resistance? Share associated insights.
8. Define cooptation and describe its use in overcoming resistance to change. Reflect on your work experiences and answer the following questions: Have you ever been coopted? Have you ever coopted another party? Have you ever observed cooptation? What are your overall thoughts on cooptation? Share associated experiences and insights.

References

1. Elrod, J. K. (2013). *Breadcrumbs to cheesecake*. R&R Publishers.
2. Walston, S. L., & Johnson, K. L. (2021). *Healthcare in the United States: Clinical, financial, and operational dimensions*. Health Administration Press.
3. McConnell, C. R. (2020). *Hospitals and health systems: What they are and how they work*. Jones and Bartlett.
4. Ginter, P. M., Duncan, W. J., & Swayne, L. E. (2013). *Strategic management of health care organizations* (7th ed.). Jossey-Bass.
5. Kotler, P., Stevens, R. J., & Shalowitz, J. (2021). *Strategic marketing for health care organizations: Building a customer-driven health system* (2nd ed.). Wiley.
6. Fortenberry, J. L., Jr. (2010). *Health care marketing: Tools and techniques* (3rd ed.). Jones and Bartlett.
7. Shi, L., & Singh, D. A. (2023). *Essentials of the US health care system* (6th ed.). Jones and Bartlett.
8. Hillestad, S. G., & Berkowitz, E. N. (2020). *Health care market strategy: From planning to action* (5th ed.). Jones and Bartlett.
9. Wilensky, S. E., & Teitelbaum, J. B. (2023). *Essentials of health policy and law* (5th ed.). Jones and Bartlett.

10. Reiter, K. L., & Song, P. H. (2021). *Gapenski's healthcare finance: An introduction to accounting and financial management* (7th ed.). Health Administration Press.
11. Konopaske, R., Ivancevich, J. M., & Matteson, M. T. (2018). *Organizational behavior and management* (11th ed.). McGraw-Hill.
12. Hitt, M. A., Miller, C. C., Colella, A., & Triana, M. D. C. (2018). *Organizational behavior* (5th ed.). Wiley.
13. Kotter, J. P. (2007). Leading change: Why transformation efforts fail. *Harvard Business Review, 85*(1), 96–103.
14. Burke, W. W. (2018). *Organization change: Theory and practice* (5th ed.). Sage.
15. Griffin, R. W., Phillips, J. M., & Gully, S. M. (2020). *Organizational behavior: Managing people and organizations* (13th ed.). Cengage.
16. Killpack, K. (2017). *Change Rx for healthcare: Your prescription for leading change.* CRC Press.
17. Toussaint, J., & Barnas, K. (2021). *Becoming the change: Leadership behavior strategies for continuous improvement in healthcare.* McGraw-Hill.
18. Elrod, J. K., & Fortenberry, J. L., Jr. (2017). Peering beyond the walls of healthcare institutions: A catalyst for innovation. *BMC Health Services Research, 17*(Suppl 1), 35–38.
19. Elrod, J. K., & Fortenberry, J. L., Jr. (2018). Catalyzing marketing innovation and competitive advantage in the healthcare industry: The value of thinking like an outsider. *BMC Health Services Research, 18*(Suppl 3), 45–48.
20. Cheung-Judge, M., & Holbeche, L. (2015). *Organization development: A practitioner's guide for OD and HR* (2nd ed.). Kogan Page.
21. McShane, S. L., & Von Glinow, M. A. (2019). *Organizational behavior* (4th ed.). McGraw-Hill.
22. Cooperrider, D. L., & Whitney, D. (2016). Appreciative inquiry. In J. M. Shafritz, J. S. Ott, & Y. S. Jang (Eds.), *Classics of organization theory* (8th ed., pp. 334–339). Cengage.
23. Gold, M. (Ed.). (1999). *The complete social scientist: A Kurt Lewin reader.* American Psychological Association.
24. Crosby, G. (2021). *Planned change: Why Kurt Lewin's social science is still best practice for business results, change management, and human progress.* Routledge.
25. Kinicki, A., & Fugate, M. (2018). *Organizational behavior: A practical, problem-solving approach* (2nd ed.). McGraw-Hill.
26. Kotter, J. P. (2012). *Leading change.* Harvard Business Review Press.
27. Kotter, J. P., Akhtar, V., & Gupta, G. (2021). *Change: How organizations achieve hard-to-imagine results in uncertain and volatile times.* Wiley.
28. Robbins, S. P., & Judge, T. A. (2019). *Organizational behavior* (18th ed.). Pearson.
29. Kotter, J. P., & Schlesinger, L. A. (2008). Choosing strategies for change. *Harvard Business Review, 86*(7/8), 130–139.

Chapter 11
Organizational Learning in Health and Medicine

Learning Objectives

After examining this chapter, readers will have the ability to:

- Define organizational learning, discuss its importance in health and medicine, and identify characteristics and qualities typifying learning organizations.
- Define exploitative learning and exploratory learning, provide examples of each in health and medicine, and convey why healthcare establishments must engage in both types of learning.
- Identify and describe the three levels of learning in healthcare organizations and discuss the imperative for knowledge to be shared broadly across institutions, rather than confined to individuals, departments, or other subsets.
- Demonstrate an understanding of the organizational learning process by identifying and defining its three stages.
- Identify and discuss the action steps for becoming a learning organization and reflect on their application in health and medicine.
- Discuss the role played by organizational culture in the development of healthcare establishments as learning organizations.

WK Reflections: Enhancing Organizational Learning Through Strategic Partnerships

When one ponders the topic of organizational learning, there is a tendency to focus on educational initiatives occurring within healthcare institutions. Examples of such endeavors include employee onboarding and orientation, skill-building workshops, coaching and mentoring, and the like. These pursuits and much more are discussed in this chapter, but while reflecting on concepts presented herein, it will be helpful to maintain an open mind regarding the sources available for developing intellectual capital, ensuring

J. K. Elrod, J. L. Fortenberry, Jr., *Organizational Behavior and Management in Health and Medicine*, https://doi.org/10.1007/978-3-031-61823-9_11

particularly that external relationships are not neglected in efforts to build and maintain a capable workforce. The highly technical, multidisciplinary nature of the healthcare industry creates significant educational challenges for healthcare providers, as it demands attention across so many areas. The educational needs of healthcare organizations typically are so robust that they simply cannot be sufficiently provided by internal means alone, necessitating that at least some learning opportunities be outsourced to external education providers, notably institutions of higher learning.

Partnerships between healthcare organizations and institutions of higher learning offer clear pathways for bolstering the intellectual prowess of employees, hastening organizational learning. Such arrangements permit healthcare providers to delegate responsibilities for employee development to the very institutions which specialize in delivering educational experiences, usefully complementing internal initiatives. Some of the opportunities which dedicated educational providers offer cannot be replicated by healthcare institutions, notably including the issuance of college credits to demonstrate accomplishments and the conveyance of college degrees evidencing achievements. Additionally, some learning requirements might necessitate external delivery simply because command of the associated subject matter might not be in the possession of anyone inside given healthcare organizations. Especially complex educational initiatives very often are best suited for delivery by external specialists possessing the resources to convey the latest insights which then can be transferred into given healthcare establishments by the employees receiving the associated training and development.

Today, it is quite common for healthcare institutions to offer tuition reimbursement programs, permitting employees opportunities to pursue, at reduced or no cost, programs of study deemed to be beneficial to their respective employers. Such arrangements may be all that healthcare organizations require from external parties to support employee development, but if deeper needs remain, more intensive arrangements can be structured. For example, healthcare institutions with numerous employees in need of a particular educational experience might consider entering into partnerships with colleges and universities to deliver coursework for critical programs onsite at given healthcare establishments. Aside from being a great convenience for employees, healthcare providers might also be able to negotiate better tuition rates for the classes offered.

Creative thinking is especially helpful when pondering healthcare provider/education provider partnerships. Over the years, Willis Knighton Health has established many highly creative partnerships with institutions of higher learning in a bid to bolster health and medical education in northwest Louisiana. The institution has invested in numerous educational endeavors, with several notable examples including programs in medicine, health administration, and nursing at LSU Medical School, LSU Shreveport, and Northwestern State University of Louisiana, respectively. By supplying funds to establish or strengthen healthcare-related academic and technical programs through professorships, salary support for faculty recruitment and retention, student scholarships, and the like, the supply of individuals capable of serving proficiently in health and medical roles is increased, aiding Willis Knighton Health in staffing its various facilities. This also bolsters learning opportunities for the institution's current employees, permitting them to pursue coursework and develop new skills, enhancing their potential to take on greater responsibilities in the workplace. Many of the educational programs receiving support from Willis Knighton Health would be scaled back or eliminated entirely without the associated resources, diminishing the labor force and negatively impacting healthcare providers and patients alike. The investments have paid significant dividends, amplifying knowledge acquisition opportunities and accelerating organizational learning, benefiting Willis Knighton Health and the greater community [1, 2].

The contributions forwarded by Willis Knighton Health to develop the health and medical educational infrastructure of northwest Louisiana quite obviously are of extreme magnitude. While such investments might be difficult or impossible for some healthcare providers to make, opportunities abound for scaled back versions of such partnerships or the development of all-new creative arrangements that see the educational needs of healthcare establishments being addressed in unique and helpful fashions. Whenever educational needs present themselves and they cannot be addressed by internal means, be certain to look externally for opportunities to ally with educational providers to close gaps and shore up organizational learning. Partnerships, ranging from the simple to the highly complex and creative, likely can be arranged, aiding healthcare providers in the vital duty of ensuring a capable workforce.

11.1 Background

Health and medical establishments are citadels of knowledge, with keen expertise constituting perhaps the most critical resource necessary for successfully delivering patient care. Knowledge is the foundation of most any pursuit, and it is especially vital in complex environments such as those commonly observed in health and medicine where there is little to no leeway for error. Organizational prowess results from many things, with the most notable source arguably being highly trained staff members who bring diverse, specialized skill sets into their respective healthcare organizations. Over time, through enculturation and other methods which foster high-intelligence environments, the knowledge brought into healthcare organizations by individuals becomes institutionalized, producing competencies typifying given establishments. Especially in comprehensive medical centers and other very complex settings, these competencies are extensive and highly varied, ranging from clinical prowess to administrative expertise to technical know-how, with each bit of knowledge contributing to the comprehensive pool of acumen possessed by and available to given healthcare institutions [2–6].

Knowledge, however, is a precarious resource, requiring great care and attention in its management. Knowledge, for example, can be incomplete, impeding institutional operations and reducing competitiveness. Knowledge also can become stagnant if efforts are not taken to ensure that it remains current, drawing on the latest tools, techniques, and trends to positively impact operations. Even in cases where knowledge is current, its circulation within given institutions can be limited, diminishing its potential to benefit healthcare establishments. While wide circulation is helpful, it does not guarantee that knowledge possessed will actually be used, representing a further challenge associated with knowledge management. As knowledge is closely held by and tied to individuals, it also can be fleeting, departing quickly through employee turnover unless care is taken to institutionalize this resource [7–10]. These and related nuances of knowledge, learning, and development are addressed in a component of organizational behavior and management known as organizational learning, the focus of this chapter.

11.2   Defining Organizational Learning

Organizational learning refers to the practice of actively acquiring, circulating, using, and retaining knowledge within an institution as a means of informing current and future pursuits, permitting enhanced performance across given establishments. It serves as the foundation of **knowledge management**, concerted efforts taken by organizations to build and maintain institutional intelligence and acumen. Institutions which successfully incorporate organizational learning into their operations are known as **learning organizations**. A basic understanding of organizational learning and the learning organization is possible merely by reflecting on one's own personal learning experiences, as the associated benefits are similar to those of individual learning. A learned individual is one who has acquired knowledge and demonstrates that knowledge in daily life, with this acumen benefiting the person as he or she goes about navigating the world. A learned organization operates in similar fashion and experiences similar benefits which, at the level of the institution, translates into greater innovation, increased competitive advantages, enhanced performance, and so on as the establishment conducts operations over time. Parallels between organizational and individual learning should come as no surprise as organizations are collections of people. Just as learning develops people, it also develops organizations [7, 8, 11–13].

The characteristics and qualities typifying learning organizations are quite extensive and highly comprehensive. Learning organizations specifically have become proficient in seeking and capturing information of benefit to their establishments (i.e., **knowledge acquisition**), assessing its impact and discovering methods for its application in the workplace. Additionally, they are skilled at circulating knowledge (i.e., **knowledge transference**), ensuring that it reaches all parties who might potentially benefit from associated insights within their given establishments. Further, learning organizations have operationalized knowledge gained by integrating it into activities within their institutions (i.e., **knowledge deployment** or **knowledge integration**), permitting their establishments to benefit from the derived acumen. This is critical, as knowledge acquired but unused provides no meaningful impact on operations. Learning organizations also are proficient in institutionalizing knowledge in a manner that ensures its availability on demand and prevents its departure when employee turnover inevitably occurs (i.e., **knowledge storage** or **knowledge retention**), affording what is known as **organizational memory**. As such, organizational learning helps to stave off **organizational forgetting**, the seepage and eventual loss of institutional knowledge occurring over time as a result of employee turnover, inattentiveness, and related disruptions which ultimately break down knowledge management systems and erode organizational memory. Ultimately, organizational learning affords healthcare institutions with what is referred to as **intellectual capital**, knowledge held by an organization which is so well developed and comprehensive that it is considered to be an asset, positively influencing operations, supplying competitive advantages, and amplifying performance [9, 10, 14–17].

11.3 Types of Learning

Learning can be characterized as being exploitative or exploratory. Both types of learning are vitally needed in healthcare establishments, and both are mandatory in order for institutions to be considered to be learning organizations. **Exploitative learning** seeks to make better use of existing knowledge within an organization, effectively exploiting currently held resources to derive maximum benefits. Assume, for example, that a medical clinic developed a dashboard capable of monitoring the external environment, permitting the establishment to better capitalize on opportunities and avoid or eliminate threats. Assume also that this valuable resource has only been used on a limited basis because the individual responsible for its implementation has been overburdened with other duties hampering full deployment of the dashboard and complete realization of its potential. Exploitative learning would see the medical clinic take active steps to make full use of the dashboard, seeking to identify and remove any impediments to full deployment which, in this case, likely would involve restructuring job duties or hiring additional personnel to facilitate its implementation. Knowledge held often is not used to its fullest, representing lost opportunities. Exploitative learning strives to generate the maximum return on investment from existing knowledge, permitting advancements that otherwise would not be possible [17].

By contrast, **exploratory learning** seeks to identify and secure new knowledge for use within an organization, permitting innovation and advancement, courtesy of these novel insights. Assume that the medical clinic noted above witnessed significant expansion, adding several satellite clinics across the region, complementing its home campus. Assume also that the establishment decided to centralize new employee orientation, bringing new hires from across the system to the home campus for a day of training, but quickly noticed associated hardships, as time and travel increased expenses and contributed to numerous absences. These hardships prompted exploratory learning, with executives seeking methods for better administering orientation programs, eventually compelling the medical clinic to purchase an online learning platform, permitting new employees quick and convenient access to the orientation program regardless of their location. Exploratory learning typically requires establishments to look outside of their organizations and, very often, outside of their industries for knowledge which can be transferred either directly or with modification into their respective institutions [17–19]. It is an essential form of learning, complementing exploitative learning, permitting healthcare organizations to derive knowledge from both internal and external sources.

11.4   Levels of Learning

Learning in establishments exists on individual, group, and organizational levels [20, 21]. Healthcare providers naturally are desirous of facilitating learning at the organizational level. The broader the distribution of knowledge across organizations, the greater the opportunity for that intelligence to generate a meaningful impact on operations. Knowledge beneficial to an establishment which resides exclusively in the hands of individuals or groups is problematic as its benefits extend only to those limited parties rather than the greater organization [13, 20]. Consider a hospital executive who discovers an excellent resource for grants but decides to keep this resource to himself, refraining from sharing this knowledge with others. As the knowledge was acquired via **individual learning**, it resides at the individual level, and since it is unshared, it benefits only the holder of the information. Suppose, however, that the executive decides to share details about this grant resource with the managers of the departments under his authority. Here, the benefits are extended to the group level, constituting a form of **group learning**. Forwarding this information to the hospital at large would see the benefits extend to the organizational level, constituting **organizational learning**. If, however, knowledge of this resource is withheld from the greater hospital, its potential to benefit the establishment is not fully reached and organizational learning is prohibited.

The reasons behind the limited circulation of knowledge within healthcare institutions are highly varied. In some cases, restrictions are motivated by selfishness at the individual or group level. Competition within organizations might be so pronounced that it pits parties against each other, prompting them to seek advantages whenever and wherever possible, even at the expense of greater institutional good. Situations such as this are all too common in health and medicine, often emerging when incentives designed to promote healthy competition inadvertently result in unhealthy competition. Failures to share knowledge also can be the result of **political gamesmanship**, where individuals or groups seek to elevate themselves for purposes of acquiring or maximizing power, typically at the expense of the organization. Additionally, it can result from the development of **silos** within establishments where departments or other units focus on themselves while neglecting the greater organization, compelling self-centered behaviors. Withholding knowledge can also occur innocently and unintentionally. Perhaps healthcare organizations have not established proper mechanisms for sharing knowledge, creating barriers in doing so which strand acquired knowledge at individual or group levels. Or perhaps institutions have not adequately encouraged all to actively share knowledge across given organizations. Regardless of cause, healthcare organizations are shortchanged whenever knowledge does not flow freely throughout establishments, something which impedes their ability to emerge as learning organizations. By building a culture which emphasizes sharing knowledge, complete with mechanisms to foster its distribution, healthcare institutions can make great strides in circulating knowledge broadly [2, 7, 18].

11.5 The Organizational Learning Process

Organizational learning is typically measured by **learning curves**—also known as **experience curves**—which essentially are depictions of the knowledge building process, generally communicating that as learning or experience increases, performance does, as well. Assuming that healthcare institutions are dealing with willing, motivated personnel, the quicker individuals acquire knowledge and put it to use, the quicker organizations can realize associated performance improvements. Realizing enhanced performance represents the ultimate goal of organizational learning, but this lofty accomplishment does not occur instantaneously. It instead results from a process, consisting of cognitive, behavioral, and performance improvement stages [22]. These stages are applicable to any learning endeavor in healthcare establishments, whether strategic or tactical. Speed of movement through these stages defines the learning curves associated with a particular new idea or insight. As productivity and performance ultimately result from successful learning experiences, healthcare providers quite obviously are desirous of hastening the organizational learning process.

The **cognitive stage** initiates the process of organizational learning. Here, employees are introduced to new ideas and they begin to build an associated awareness. Consider, for example, the introduction of a new electronic medical records system in a hospital. As employees attend seminars and other training opportunities designed to acclimate them to the new system, their knowledge increases. This expansion of knowledge then starts to impact and influence their thinking. At this point, the changes resulting from learning are intangible, occurring within the hearts and minds of employees. Soon, however, their knowledge enters the realm of tangibility, being observable through actions, signifying advancement to the **behavioral**

stage. At this point, the new ideas have been internalized by employees and they begin to alter their work habits and patterns in observable manners. Continuing the electronic medical records example, once the new system is rolled out, knowledge gained during the cognitive stage is applied in practice, with staff members making use of the system in competent fashion. The **performance improvement stage** concludes the process, as enhanced behaviors, informed by new knowledge, result in heightened performance [22]. Here, if learning has been successful, the hospital at last reaps the benefits it envisioned when it purchased the new electronic medical records system.

Given the importance of organizational learning, healthcare institutions must not leave its development to chance. Active assessments are required, evaluating progress across the stages of the organizational learning process to ensure advancements along learning curves. During the cognitive stage, surveys, questionnaires, and interviews are particularly helpful assessment devices. Quizzes and other forms of examination which test knowledge retention also can be useful. Each of these pathways gives insights into the depth of understanding possessed by employees. During the behavioral stage, the assessment devices used during the cognitive stage continue to have value, but direct observation is also quite helpful where supervisors monitor the actions of employees to ensure that acquired knowledge is used as intended. Once new knowledge is fully operationalized, an overall assessment of the performance improvements is in order. This calls for a comprehensive **learning audit**, an evaluation of learning endeavors designed to compare desired outcomes with observed results. This is a vital activity as it provides critical information regarding the success of organizational learning pursuits, providing guidance for initiating any needed improvements. It also enhances intelligence which can aid in designing future organizational learning efforts [22].

11.6 Action Steps for Becoming a Learning Organization

Becoming a learning organization is possible for any healthcare establishment committed to incorporating into operations a range of action steps known to foster the proliferation and management of institutional knowledge. Profiles of these action steps are presented in the following sections.

11.6.1 Adopt the Practice of Solving Problems in an Orderly, Systematic Fashion

The process through which healthcare organizations solve problems very often is conducted in an unsystematic, haphazard fashion, dominated by subjectivity. Given that much needed order is missing from this approach, outcomes achieved are inconsistent at best. Further, the spotty methods deployed to resolve matters in such cases yield almost no knowledge, with this proving to be an extreme disservice to both current and future problem-solving initiatives. Better outcomes are possible by addressing problem-solving in a systematic, orderly manner, reliant on objective measures and rooted in the scientific method. Learning organizations are well aware of the benefits of such an approach and work to embed systematic problem-solving skills into institutional operations. The key pathway for this rests with enhancing the problem-solving skill sets of employees, especially those who hold managerial duties and responsibilities [22].

Training programs designed to enhance problem-solving skills often do so via practical exercises and case studies. These educational activities importantly must train staff members to look beyond the superficial, ensuring that they identify underlying causes of problems, as only when root causes are identified and addressed is resolution possible. This training equips employees with equivalent, capable skill sets, permitting a common language and approach for systemically resolving issues encountered. As problems are addressed in a scientific manner, outcomes are improved. Further, opportunities for knowledge acquisition are enhanced, as the defined approach and the results derived from such can be analyzed, permitting opportunities for refinement which can improve future problem-solving initiatives [22]. As such, healthcare institutions desirous of becoming learning organizations must make prudent investments in workforce development initiatives which bolster the ability of employees to resolve any problems encountered in systematic fashion.

11.6.2   Embrace the Practice of Experimentation as a Means of Expanding Horizons

Knowledge very often is derived from **experimentation**. This essentially involves the testing of new knowledge as a means of expanding one's horizons. Experimentation can occur on very narrow fronts, such as a trial conducted within a single clinic of a medical center to assess the potential of a new admissions protocol, or very wide fronts, such as a systemwide test to evaluate a new onboarding technique within the medical center. Such trials provide treasure troves of information, building knowledge and guiding operations, informed by direct experience rather than untested assumptions. Prominent requirements which foster experimentation include the establishment of an infrastructure supportive of experiments, including leadership support, incentives which encourage innovation, and resources sufficient to conduct trials; the hiring and development of employees capable of conducting and evaluating experiments in their respective areas of operation; and the development of an organizational culture which encourages the free flow of ideas and information, fostering the compilation of options which can be considered for experimentation. Routine experimentation serves as an excellent defense against status quo operations and their debilitating effects, encouraging innovation and advancement, courtesy of trials, tests, demonstration projects, and more [22].

11.6.3   Examine Past Institutional Successes and Failures as a Means of Informing Current and Future Pursuits

Learning from past experience represents one of the most essential knowledge resources in healthcare organizations. As such, it is a critical activity required of learning organizations. Whether prior endeavors proved to be successes or failures, rich information can be gleaned from these experiences, permitting health and medical institutions to shape and hone their approaches going forward. Past successes obviously can reveal avenues which experience suggests are capable of generating desired outcomes. Failures can show pathways which history suggests should be avoided, given results which fell short of expectations [22]. This critical information is available to most any healthcare organization merely by directing time and attention toward evaluating past experiences. Optimal approaches for ensuring that past experiences are analyzed and associated knowledge captured typically require some sort of formalized process designed to assess efforts on a routine basis. This arrangement deeply ingrains the evaluative process within healthcare organizations, helping to ensure that proper reflection is never neglected. Formalization also aids in ensuring that evaluative efforts continue even when work obligations become especially intense. As reflection is important within each and every unit of operation in healthcare establishments, managers at all levels must be assigned responsibilities for conducting evaluations of efforts in their respective departments, sharing insights both within and outside of these units, fostering organizational learning systemwide.

11.6.4   Seek Out Opportunities to Learn from External Parties to Gain New Insights and Understanding

Opportunities to learn are not limited to internal experiences. They also are available externally, both within and outside of the healthcare industry. As for opportunities within the healthcare industry, case studies and other accounts in trade and scholarly journals focused on health policy, health administration, and related areas offer obvious pathways for acquiring insights. The same is true of tours of healthcare establishments which sometimes are possible through grand openings, open houses, and related events. Few pathways, however, offer better learning opportunities than firsthand accounts shared directly between parties [22]. Gaining these perspectives, however, can be difficult, given competitive sensitivities, especially within one's own market, but possibilities for this increase when looking to external markets for insights. A good starting point involves identifying comparable institutions in external markets and inquiring about the possibilities of establishing an information-exchange type of relationship. Even a single relationship with a peer establishment will offer great potential for knowledge acquisition, making these pursuits worthwhile. And as addressed earlier in the chapter, the value of learning via relevant programs of study offered through educational institutions certainly should not be overlooked as such pathways offer immense potential for enhancing knowledge.

Another fruitful avenue for learning from others entails gleaning insights from organizations outside of the healthcare industry. Innovations, problem-solving techniques, and other types of knowledge emerge from a variety of industries. If attention is only directed toward one's own industry, key opportunities will be missed [22]. **Insular mindsets**—perspectives which are so intensively focused inwardly that they crowd out attention directed toward the greater environment—are quite common in health and medicine. As such, peering beyond the walls of the healthcare industry can yield insights that not only inform but also afford competitive advantages. Many times, tools and techniques from outside of the healthcare industry can be transferred directly into healthcare organizations without any form of modification. At other times, they can be altered for use within health and medical establishments without too much difficulty. As learning organizations seek knowledge at every possible opportunity regardless of source, healthcare organizations desirous of becoming citadels of knowledge must be open to pursuing both traditional and nontraditional avenues for acquiring insights as a means of building intelligence and acumen [18, 19]. This pathway is explored more deeply later in the chapter.

11.6.5 Develop Proficiencies in Circulating Knowledge Intraorganizationally

Successfully transferring knowledge requires that healthcare organizations efficiently and effectively forward insights to all parties within their given institutions who might potentially benefit from the associated knowledge. Doing so is a hallmark of learning organizations. Knowledge, however, is always at risk of being stranded in particular corners of healthcare establishments, hampering its impact potential. Consider the case of a compliance officer who attends a seminar concerning upcoming accreditation changes impacting her hospital, but fails to circulate the information to others on her return. Here, the hospital, through its agent, successfully acquired critical knowledge, but failed to adequately share these details broadly between and among parties who could have benefited from the associated insights, representing a missed learning opportunity. The same would be true for a particular hospital within a greater health system which devised admission system improvements, but neglected to share these innovations with its sister hospitals, permitting all to benefit.

To avoid losses associated with knowledge circulation failures, learning organizations incorporate mechanisms which encourage and facilitate the successful transfer of ideas and insights within their establishments. Mechanisms vary, but they usually involve establishing an organizational culture which emphasizes systemwide teamwork and places a premium on sharing knowledge. Complementing this culture are specific methods which foster knowledge transfer, such as workforce development programs aimed at conveying cutting edge insights, personnel rotation programs which permit employees to observe knowledge discoveries outside of their areas of operation for potential transference into their own, and similar information-sharing applications. These techniques facilitate the comprehensive circulation of knowledge within establishments, fostering learning environments [22]. Associated investments have the potential to deliver outstanding returns, courtesy of their ability to distribute knowledge broadly across healthcare organizations.

11.6.6 Ensure That Knowledge Is Being Used to Its Fullest Intraorganizationally

Knowledge which is successfully acquired and circulated represents a key strategic asset for any healthcare establishment, but a crucial additional element is required to fully benefit from this resource. Specifically, knowledge must be deployed competently; that is, it must be used properly by its holders to address organizational matters for which the knowledge applies [14, 15]. It is not uncommon for individuals to possess a full understanding of what is required to properly address a given matter but do the opposite of what they have learned. Consider the case of a laboratory manager who has been trained in properly handling departmental human resource management issues, but fails to follow institutional protocols when addressing an employee infraction. In this case, the laboratory manager is not properly using his knowledge, making it count for nothing, representing a significant loss both for the manager and his healthcare institution. Learning organizations ensure that knowledge is not only possessed by employees but also used properly, permitting its full benefits to be derived. Knowledge deployment excellence occurs partially through training, ensuring that throughout the learning process, proper applications of knowledge are emphasized, and partially through supervision, ensuring that in actual practice, employees properly make use of acquired knowledge to effect desired outcomes. Infractions can be addressed constructively through the provision of additional guidance or, if necessary, via the disciplinary process.

11.6.7 Safeguard Organizational Knowledge and Insights by Developing Proper Retention Systems

Of particular importance in fostering organizational learning is the safeguarding of institutional knowledge, ensuring that it does not disappear, even in the face of employee turnover, lapsed concentration, or any other influence with the potential to erode organizational memory. Learning organizations institutionalize knowledge, permitting its retention within organizations and accessibility by employees [14, 15]. This often is achieved by a combination of centralized and decentralized measures. Centralized measures typically involve establishing a learning center within healthcare organizations and appointing a manager, such as a chief learning officer, director of education, or similar executive, possessing oversight duties and responsibilities. Often housed in human resource departments, given their traditional focus on workforce development, such centers typically work to aggregate knowledge across given establishments, compiling insights and other discoveries, placing them into an institutional database for retrieval as needed. This archival activity nicely complements other activities commonly assigned to learning centers, including conducting and coordinating workforce development initiatives and linking employees with external learning opportunities, such as college degree or certificate programs. Decentralized measures complement centralized ones, with these generally occurring at the department level across organizations, enlisting managers within their respective units to take steps to ensure that expertise, know-how, and other intelligence are preserved. Aside from efforts to archive knowledge departmentally, managers within learning organizations also take steps to ensure that knowledge does not reside solely in the hands of single individuals. Defenses against such risks notably involve **cross-training** employees, permitting the replication of skill sets to ensure that knowledge is possessed by more than one person, increasing its endurance potential over time. As knowledge is an institutional asset, it should be treated as such, which, among other things, requires its preservation and protection.

WK Reflections: Peering Beyond the Walls of Healthcare Institutions

Of all of the action steps required to become a learning organization, the one that perhaps is most elusive is that of acquiring knowledge from external parties, especially when it hails from institutions which are not involved in the delivery of health and medicine. Earlier discussion on this topic referenced the tendency for healthcare providers to possess insular mindsets. These highly compartmentalized perspectives have the capacity to lead those serving in healthcare organizations to focus on developments within their given industry of operation, often with such voracity that the greater environment of business and industry is neglected. The reasons for this are understandable when one reflects on the occupational lives of those working in healthcare organizations. Healthcare employees typically work hand-in-hand with others involved in like pursuits, hold memberships in healthcare-focused professional societies, read newsletters and other publications which concentrate on health and medical care, and participate in conferences and other professional development opportunities centered on health matters. These and similar activities and engagements foster a tremendous degree of industry solidarity. This is highly beneficial for building acumen regarding the operation of healthcare facilities, but such concentrated focus can prove to be quite limiting in other important contexts [18, 19, 23–28].

Focusing exclusively on the healthcare industry diminishes one's exposure to industries outside of health and medicine, limiting awareness of associated advancements, insights, and know-how. Such externally derived tools and techniques might be disregarded by those in health and medical organizations, with these developments being declared to be nontransferable due to the unique nature of the healthcare industry. This, however, is not always the case. As noted earlier in the chapter, many innovations indeed emerge from outside of the healthcare industry and these often are transferrable, either directly or with slight modifications. If one is not looking for them, however, they will be missed, along with their associated benefits. Those healthcare organizations desirous of being the best must ensure that they keep a watchful eye not only on developments within the healthcare industry but also on developments outside of the healthcare industry [18, 19, 24, 28, 29].

Had Willis Knighton Health been solely focused on monitoring developments within the healthcare industry, some of its most enduring accomplishments and advancements would never have been achieved. Its broad environmental surveillance permitted the system to adopt numerous innovations well in advance of its peers, generating numerous benefits, many of which continue to deliver value to this day. Its hub-and-spoke network—the organization design embraced by Willis Knighton Health and profiled in Chap. 9—was derived from the transportation industry. While many healthcare organizations use this framework today, Willis Knighton Health was among the first to deploy it successfully and reap associated benefits, all due to efforts to look beyond the healthcare industry for transferrable practices of value [18, 19, 30]. Willis Knighton Health also was one of the first hospitals to model patient experiences after hotel guest experiences, incorporating value-added offerings, such as concierge services, complimentary lodging for the loved ones of out-of-town patients, and free transportation, sparked by insights gained from the hospitality industry [18, 19, 31]. The institution, too, was a pioneer in using advertising, especially that which makes use of billboards, to promote healthcare services, mirroring the marketing communication techniques that were being deployed by general business and industry. Advertising now is a staple of the healthcare industry, but when Willis Knighton Health initiated its use, it was a rarity in health and medicine [18, 19, 32, 33].

These noted instances are complemented by many more examples illustrating Willis Knighton Health's early adoption of insights and approaches emerging from outside industries, affording significant recognition, experience, and lasting benefits for the institution. Healthcare establishments desirous of leading in their respective markets will want to ensure that they do not neglect to peer beyond the walls of healthcare institutions for potentially transferable tools and techniques [18, 19]. Organizational learning efforts will be notably enhanced, increasing the potential to generate competitive advantages and, most importantly, elevating opportunities to enhance patient care and attention.

11.7   Organizational Learning and Organizational Culture

When healthcare establishments incorporate the action steps for becoming a learning organization, the stage is set for them to engage in productive knowledge management endeavors. They are well on their way to emerging as learning organizations. Healthcare providers, however, must proceed with caution. For there to be any hope of achieving long-term success, organizational learning efforts during this formative period must be shepherded very carefully, ensuring devoted focus and attention. The best defense against lost momentum rests with developing an organizational culture that places a value on knowledge management [34, 35]. For this to occur, organizational learning must be elevated from being a mere program within a healthcare establishment to a valued, mission-critical initiative firmly embedded in its organizational culture [36, 37]. When this is accomplished, organizational learning will be shared (i.e., embraced by broad groups of employees), pervasive (i.e., prevalent across the institution), enduring (i.e., lasting over time in the organization), and implicit (i.e., understood by those operating in the organization) [38]. It also will be perpetuated over time, handed down from employee to employee, courtesy of **socialization**, a process through which individuals come to realize and understand the expectations of a group, permitting them to adjust their behaviors in a manner to foster acclimation and approval [39, 40]. Healthcare establishments which successfully incorporate organizational learning into their respective organizational cultures can expect lasting organizational learning successes. They indeed will emerge as learning organizations and reap all of the benefits associated with such.

11.8   Summary and Conclusions

Knowledge arguably is the chief foundational asset required for successful pursuits within health and medicine. Knowledge drives virtually every process and operation within healthcare organizations, and especially when possessed broadly by staff members across given establishments, its impact potential is unparalleled. As such, knowledge acquisition, retention, and related educational endeavors must be prioritized by healthcare providers. This calls for intensive attention to be directed toward organizational learning, given its focus on knowledge management and all that it entails. Ideally, healthcare establishments should seek to become so proficient in knowledge management that they become known as learning organizations. This requires healthcare organizations to incorporate into operations a range of action steps known to foster institutional knowledge, elevating also organizational learning as a component of the given institution's organizational culture. If this is done, the power of knowledge can be harnessed by healthcare establishments, with expectations of its continuation as an institutional asset for as long as organizations remain dedicated to ensuring that the tenets of organizational learning remain intact.

Key Terms

- Behavioral Stage
- Cognitive Stage
- Cross-Training
- Experience Curve
- Experimentation
- Exploitative Learning
- Exploratory Learning
- Group Learning
- Individual Learning
- Insular Mindsets
- Intellectual Capital
- Knowledge Acquisition
- Knowledge Deployment
- Knowledge Integration
- Knowledge Management
- Knowledge Retention
- Knowledge Storage
- Knowledge Transference
- Learning Audit
- Learning Curve
- Learning Organization
- Organizational Forgetting
- Organizational Learning
- Organizational Memory
- Performance Improvement Stage
- Political Gamesmanship
- Silo
- Socialization

Exercises

1. In your own words, define organizational learning, discuss its importance in health and medicine, and identify characteristics and qualities typifying learning organizations.
2. Discuss the concept of knowledge management, detailing its impact and influence in healthcare establishments. Reflect on your current employer's knowledge management practices and assess its associated performance. What are its knowledge management strengths? What are its weaknesses? What improvements would you recommend and why?

3. Define exploitative learning and exploratory learning and discuss the necessity for healthcare institutions to be proficient in both types of learning. Further demonstrate your understanding by describing from your recent work experiences a situation that called for exploitative learning and a situation that called for exploratory learning.

4. Identify and describe the three levels of learning in healthcare organizations and discuss the imperative for knowledge to be shared broadly across institutions, rather than confined to individuals or groups. Reflect on a recent employment experience and describe your employer's knowledge sharing proficiencies. What improvements would you suggest and why?

5. Define learning curves and discuss their use in health and medicine as indicators of organizational learning. What techniques does your employer use to expedite organizational learning, hastening advancement along learning curves?

6. Demonstrate your understanding of the organizational learning process by identifying and defining its three stages. Does your current employer address organizational learning in a manner consistent with this formal process? If so, indicate how it aligns with the process. If not, indicate how it deviates from the process. What suggestions would you offer your employer for improving its organizational learning efforts?

7. Identify and discuss the action steps required for becoming a learning organization. For each action step, assess your current employer's associated proficiencies, noting strengths and weaknesses and indicating any recommended improvements.

8. Discuss the role played by organizational culture in the development of healthcare establishments as learning organizations. Is organizational learning a component of your current employer's organizational culture? What evidence do you have to support your assertion? What enhancements would you recommend and why?

References

1. Elrod, J. K., & Fortenberry, J. L., Jr. (2017). Tithing programs: Pathways for enhancing and improving the health status of the underprivileged. *BMC Health Services Research, 17*(Suppl 4), 15–22.
2. Elrod, J. K. (2013). *Breadcrumbs to cheesecake*. R&R Publishers.
3. Shi, L., & Singh, D. A. (2023). *Essentials of the US health care system* (6th ed.). Jones and Bartlett.
4. Walston, S. L., & Johnson, K. L. (2021). *Healthcare in the United States: Clinical, financial, and operational dimensions*. Health Administration Press.
5. McConnell, C. R. (2020). *Hospitals and health systems: What they are and how they work*. Jones and Bartlett.
6. Flynn, W. J., Valentine, S. R., & Meglich, P. A. (2022). *Healthcare human resource management* (4th ed.). Cengage.
7. Senge, P. M. (2006). *The fifth discipline: The art and practice of the learning organization*. Doubleday.

8. Marquardt, M. J. (2011). *Building the learning organization: Achieving strategic advantage through a commitment to learning* (3rd ed.). Nicholas Brealey Publishing.
9. Argyris, C. (1999). *On organizational learning* (2nd ed.). Blackwell.
10. Argote, L., & Levine, J. M. (Eds.). (2020). *The Oxford handbook of group and organizational learning*. Oxford University Press.
11. Griffin, R. W., Phillips, J. M., & Gully, S. M. (2020). *Organizational behavior: Managing people and organizations* (13th ed.). Cengage.
12. Robbins, S. P., & Judge, T. A. (2019). *Organizational behavior* (18th ed.). Pearson.
13. Massingham, P. (2020). *Knowledge management: Theory in practice*. Sage.
14. McShane, S. L., & Von Glinow, M. A. (2019). *Organizational behavior* (4th ed.). McGraw-Hill.
15. Kinicki, A., & Fugate, M. (2018). *Organizational behavior: A practical, problem-solving approach* (2nd ed.). McGraw-Hill.
16. Flores, L. G., Zheng, W., Rau, D., & Thomas, C. H. (2012). Organizational learning: Subprocess identification, construct validation, and an empirical test of cultural antecedents. *Journal of Management, 38*(2), 640–667.
17. Hitt, M. A., Miller, C. C., Colella, A., & Triana, M. D. C. (2018). *Organizational behavior* (5th ed.). Wiley.
18. Elrod, J. K., & Fortenberry, J. L., Jr. (2017). Peering beyond the walls of healthcare institutions: A catalyst for innovation. *BMC Health Services Research, 17*(Suppl 1), 35–38.
19. Elrod, J. K., & Fortenberry, J. L., Jr. (2018). Catalyzing marketing innovation and competitive advantage in the healthcare industry: The value of thinking like an outsider. *BMC Health Services Research, 18*(Suppl 3), 45–48.
20. Gill, S. J. (2019). *The manager's pocket guide to organizational learning*. HRD Press.
21. Ford, J. K. (2021). *Learning in organizations: An evidence-based approach*. Routledge.
22. Garvin, D. A. (1993). Building a learning organization. *Harvard Business Review, 71*(4), 78–91.
23. Gamble, M. (2013). How much should we expect healthcare to mimic other industries? *Becker's Hospital Review*. Retrieved May 13, 2023, from http://www.beckershospitalreview.com/hospital-management-administration/how-much-should-we-expect-healthcare-to-mimic-other-industries.html
24. Samet, K., & Smith, M. (2016). Thinking differently: Catalyzing innovation in healthcare and beyond. *Frontiers of Health Services Management, 33*(2), 3–15.
25. Quinn, J. B., Anderson, P., & Finkelstein, S. (1996). Managing professional intellect: Making the most of the best. *Harvard Business Review, 74*(2), 71–80.
26. Natarajan, R. N. (2006). Transferring best practices to healthcare: Opportunities and challenges. *TQM Magazine, 18*(6), 572–582.
27. Fortenberry, J. L., Jr. (2011). *Cases in health care marketing*. Jones and Bartlett.
28. Armada, A., & Martin, A. (2016). Business model disruption: Innovation as a catalyst. *Frontiers of Health Services Management, 33*(2), 39–44.
29. Kaissi, A. (2012). "Learning" from other industries: Lessons and challenges for health care organizations. *The Health Care Manager, 31*(1), 65–74.
30. Elrod, J. K., & Fortenberry, J. L., Jr. (2017). The hub-and-spoke organization design revisited: A lifeline for rural hospitals. *BMC Health Services Research, 17*(Suppl 4), 29–35.
31. Elrod, J. K., & Fortenberry, J. L., Jr. (2018). Establishing Good Samaritan programs in healthcare institutions: A method for enhancing patient experiences and increasing loyalty. *BMC Health Services Research, 18*(Suppl 3), 9–16.
32. Elrod, J. K., & Fortenberry, J. L., Jr. (2020). Advertising in health and medicine: Using mass media to communicate with patients. *BMC Health Services Research, 20*(Suppl 1), 1–8.
33. Elrod, J. K., & Fortenberry, J. L., Jr. (2018). Healthcare establishments as owner-operators of digital billboards: Making the most of excellent roadside visibility and high traffic counts to better connect with patients. *BMC Health Services Research, 18*(Suppl 3), 29–40.
34. Cook, S. D. N., & Yanow, D. (1993). Culture and organizational learning. *Journal of Management Inquiry, 2*(4), 373–390.

35. Schein, E. H. (1996). Three cultures of management: The key to organizational learning. *Sloan Management Review, 38*, 9–20.
36. Schein, E. H. (2017). *Organizational culture and leadership* (5th ed.). Wiley.
37. Schein, E. H., & Schein, P. A. (2019). *The corporate culture survival guide* (3rd ed.). Wiley.
38. Groysberg, B., Lee, J., Price, J., & Cheng, J. Y.-J. (2018). The leader's guide to corporate culture: How to manage the eight critical elements of organizational life. *Harvard Business Review, 96*(1), 44–52.
39. Konopaske, R., Ivancevich, J. M., & Matteson, M. T. (2018). *Organizational behavior and management* (11th ed.). McGraw-Hill.
40. Schein, E. H. (1984). Coming to a new awareness of organizational culture. *Sloan Management Review, 25*(2), 3–16.

Chapter 12
Groups and Teams in Health and Medicine

Learning Objectives

After examining this chapter, readers will have the ability to:

- Define groups, discuss their prevalence in health and medicine, and detail their importance in delivering patient care.
- Compare and contrast groups and teams and provide examples of each in health-care organizations.
- Demonstrate an understanding of formal groups and informal groups by defining both types, identifying and describing associated subcategories, and supplying examples of each in health and medicine.
- Discuss the concept of diversity and its role, influence, and impact on groups in health and medicine.
- Identify and describe the group development process and discuss its application in healthcare organizations.
- Identify and discuss qualities which enhance group performance and describe methods for ensuring their presence in groups within health and medical establishments.

12.1 Background

Healthcare establishments are no place for **lone wolves**, individuals who prefer working independently and in isolation, unconnected to and unconcerned for others. This is because the services provided by health and medical institutions are amalgams requiring input from multiple parties who must work together in order to produce desired results. A person responsible for a piece of the puzzle obviously must be concerned for his or her own production, but also for the production of those responsible for other pieces, permitting completion. Such collective efforts

J. K. Elrod, J. L. Fortenberry, Jr., *Organizational Behavior and Management in Health and Medicine*, https://doi.org/10.1007/978-3-031-61823-9_12

also produce all-important **synergies** which allow far more to be accomplished than that possible by the combined efforts of individuals working alone [1–3]. Indeed, the multidisciplinary, highly specialized nature of health and medicine necessitates that those working within healthcare establishments shed natural tendencies for independence in favor of mindsets where they see themselves as components of a greater, comprehensive whole. This, however, does not diminish the importance of the individual and individuality. While tasks are often collaborative, at other times, they are highly independent. But even so, much like the cogs making up a wheel, eventually one's production must be passed on to another, culminating in the delivery of a given healthcare service to a particular patient. Collaboration is a necessary and expected ingredient of health and medicine [1, 4–8].

While it is with near certainty that the vast majority of those serving in the healthcare industry clearly realize that they must be capable of working productively with others, the reality is that circumstances and situations occurring both within and outside of workplaces often lead to less than desirable on-the-job behaviors, clouding better judgment. Personality differences are ever present, work schedules typically are long and difficult, and physical and emotional fatigue on both personal and professional fronts is pervasive, leading some to lose sight of the bigger picture and focus on themselves and their particular concerns as ends unto themselves. Much of this is accidental, resulting from the rigors of life's complexities unfolding in highly challenging environments. Nevertheless, resulting attitudes and behaviors can and often do lead to barriers which damage collegiality and diminish institutional productivity [1, 9–11]. One of the best defenses against this entails acquiring an understanding of groups and their associated characteristics. Healthcare organizations, after all, are collections of people, necessitating an understanding of the fundamental operation of groups in work settings.

12.2   Defining Groups

Broadly defined, a **group** is a collection of two or more individuals who share one or more characteristics, goals, or purposes. Over the course of one's life, individuals are members of numerous groups. Some are joined by choice, others by circumstance. Membership may last a lifetime or it may be fleeting. One's race, education, religion, occupation, hobbies, tastes, preferences, or any other attribute or quality characterizing an individual can serve as the basis of group membership [12, 13]. In organizational behavior and management, attention quite obviously focuses on groups in work contexts. Knowledge of groups is particularly important in organizational life as establishments effectively are mass assemblies of people. As such, understanding organizations, in essence, necessitates that one understands groups. Chief concerns center on things such as methods for productively organizing people to work together effectively, understanding **group dynamics** (i.e., interactions and exchanges between and among individuals when they are organized into groups), techniques for directing diverse arrays of people to collaboratively pursue an institution's mission, and the like. Knowledge of groups and their operation effectively constitutes a foundation of organizational behavior and management as associated details inform many other aspects of the discipline, including leadership, motivation, communication, and much more [12–15].

Both within organizations and across broad society, the term group is often used interchangeably with the term team. Doing so generally is harmless, but technically, the two terms are quite distinct. A **team** is a small group of individuals whose members work in an especially close and collaborative fashion in pursuit of a particular goal or objective for which they hold themselves collectively accountable [16]. Teams have been described as being mature groups, an advanced arrangement of individuals connected more intensively than their broader counterpart [17]. Consider, for example, the senior management of a hospital. These particular individuals would be said to belong to a broader group, namely, hospital personnel, which is composed of all who are employed by the given organization. They also would fall into a smaller group, namely, hospital executives, which includes those holding managerial duties in both senior and junior capacities across the institution. But due to their interconnectivity, intensive working relationships, common mission, and mutual accountability, the members of senior management also would constitute a team, consisting solely of those occupying the top ranks within the hospital.

Similarly, the surgery department of a medical center would feature a broad array of employees who each work toward delivering a particular service within the institution. This broad collection of employees would constitute a group. Within that group, however, there invariably will be teams organized to deliver specific components of the broader mission, necessitating more intensive interactions, with surgical teams offering perhaps the best example of such. It is helpful to remember that all teams are groups, but not all groups are teams. Still, much of the theory and practice of groups applies equally to teams [15]. Despite the technical difference between groups and teams, for purposes of simplicity, this chapter is structured to support using the two terms interchangeably.

12.3 Types of Groups

Groups in healthcare organizations can broadly be divided into two types: formal groups and informal groups. As implied by their associated descriptors, these two types of groups are distinguished by their formality or lack thereof. **Formal groups** are assemblies of people which are purposely created by an organization to perform the work required by the establishment. Membership in formal groups is assigned by supervisory authorities who place personnel in designated groups as a means of populating the workplace to permit mission fulfillment. Organizational goals are the preeminent focus of formal groups; something understandable as the very reason for their existence is to accomplish institutional duties and responsibilities [17]. When viewing the organizational charts of healthcare establishments, one effectively is observing mass collections of formal groups which inhabit given organizations.

Formal groups can be further divided into command groups and task groups. **Command groups** are formal groups consisting of supervisors and their designated subordinates. These particular groups are determined and defined by the organizational structure of the establishment which stipulates its chain of command, arrangement of departments, positions of employment, and reporting relationships. Most any department within a healthcare establishment, such as nursing services, housekeeping, information technology, and the like, would constitute a command group. **Task groups** are formal groups consisting of employees, often from different organizational units, who interact with one another for the purpose of accomplishing a particular goal or objective [17]. Such groups may or may not be identified in a given healthcare establishment's organizational chart, with this being dependent on the level of detail expressed in particular depictions. A hospital's quality assurance task force, drawing on personnel from across the establishment, represents an excellent example of a task group. Campus beautification committees, often featured in healthcare organizations and populated by a range of employees dedicated to ensuring that campuses look their best, also would constitute a task group. Whether of the task or command variety, each operates in an official, organization-sanctioned capacity, making them formal groups.

Informal groups are the second broad assembly of people found in healthcare organizations, with these groups emerging through social interactions between and among employees in an establishment. Informal groups are not formally authorized or assembled by the organization in which they exist. As such, organizational goals are not the focus of informal groups. Very often, however, matters associated with the organization and its operation are the subject of discussion by the members of these groups. Visiting a medical center's cafeteria during lunchtime reveals many informal groups. Employees who regularly eat together effectively constitute informal groups. These groups are not limited to lunches, though, nor are they required to meet on campus. Several physicians who practice medicine at a particular hospital and meet regularly to play golf at a local country club would constitute one such example of this. These types of informal groups are known as **friendship groups**, as friendship is the basis of their formation [17].

Interest groups are another type of informal group that exists within healthcare establishments, with these groups forming as a result of mutual interests shared by their members. A group of medical clinic employees who discover a mutual interest in reading might, for example, start a book club, inviting other members of their organization to join them as they explore selected works. A grassroots effort to collect food for the homeless, spurred by like-minded employees of a particular hospital, would also constitute an interest group. Be they friendship or interest-based, the formation of informal groups is largely motivated by the need that employees have for social contact. Although they exist solely on an unsanctioned basis, informal groups have the potential to influence cohesion between and among employees and foster performance, accordingly. Work matters, even in social contexts, will invariably come up, making informal groups influential and impactful in given organizations [17].

12.4 Diversity and Groups

A particular composition that contains a variety of different elements, characteristics, or qualities is said to possess **diversity**. Diversity, in fact, is an attribute that handily and accurately describes the healthcare industry, with virtually every aspect of operation involving at least some level of differentiation. The delivery of healthcare services, even in establishments focusing on concentrated areas of medicine, requires extensive occupational diversity. This, in turn, calls for healthcare establishments to hire individuals possessing vastly different backgrounds, skills, and abilities, with each carrying varying levels of authority, prestige, and market value. This notable occupational diversity, unique to the healthcare industry, combines with the personal diversity characterizing the staffs of most any industry to create a true institutional melting pot. Healthcare personnel typically exhibit a vast range of demographic variables (e.g., age, gender, race, nationality), psychographic qualities (e.g., social class, personality), and behavioral attributes (e.g., attitudes, loyalties, outlooks). With such diversity inhabiting the halls of medicine, it stands to reason that most any group within healthcare institutions will feature a profound level of diversity [1, 4, 5, 18–21].

As diversity across myriad fronts characterizes the healthcare industry and its establishments, healthcare providers can benefit from knowing about its impact, especially on groups within their given organizations. Perhaps the most prominent benefit of diversity stems from its gathering of multiple differentiated perspectives, with this having the potential to improve decision-making, innovation, and more, helping healthcare establishments to advance. This is because the multiple perspectives of those possessing different backgrounds and experiences permit a wider range of knowledge than that possessed by individuals possessing like backgrounds and experiences. Another benefit of diversity is that it expands the technical capacity of groups, permitting them to accomplish far more than that possible without a differentiated pool of talent [22]. Indeed, health and medical organizations could not perform at all without healthy diversity, given the extensive division of labor required to deliver patient care.

Diversity, however, can pose challenges in groups. Notably, the greater the diversity exhibited in groups, the longer it will take for its members to assimilate into a unified entity. This is because individuals must first familiarize themselves with those who are dissimilar before bonding can occur. This, of course, takes time. In homogenous groups, the learning curve leading to assimilation is not as lengthy because members possess an inherent understanding of those who are similar, hastening the bonding process. Not surprisingly, **fault lines**—divisions based on some characteristic or quality which result in the emergence of subgroups within a larger group—also are more likely to emerge when diversity is extensive in given assemblies, as there are more opportunities for these lines to be drawn [2, 12]. Fortunately, the employees of the healthcare industry are well known for their professionalism and compassion, fitting qualities for those pursuing patient care, one of the noblest of missions [1, 9]. These qualities aid employees in bonding with one another, even in highly diverse group settings.

12.5 Tuckman's Model of Group Development

The process through which groups develop in health and medical organizations is of keen interest to healthcare providers, as this knowledge can aid them in facilitating cohesion between and among group members, yielding productive, mission-dedicated cadres of employees. Many models have been devised to depict group development, but arguably the most popular and highly publicized of these is known as Tuckman's model of group development. This model, originating in the 1960s, views group formation to occur via a process consisting of five sequential stages, namely, forming, storming, norming, performing, and adjourning [23–25]. Some groups move through the stages rather quickly; others proceed more slowly. Regardless of speed, patience is required, as group assimilation ultimately is a learning process which takes time. Success is not guaranteed and some efforts to assemble productive groups are never realized, with assimilation stalling somewhere across the stages of group development. An awareness of the process, however, fosters an associated understanding that can position healthcare organizations to achieve desirable outcomes. The five stages of Tuckman's model are explained in the following sections.

12.5.1 Stage 1: Forming

The **forming** stage constitutes the very beginning of Tuckman's group development process. This essentially is an ice-breaking stage where individuals are first introduced to the group. Here, they get to know their new peers, the group's leadership, its mission, and its purpose. Forming happens to be one of the most recognized stages of group development, as many can vividly recall their initial days acclimating to a new work group. High levels of uncertainty typically distinguish the forming stage, as members strive to understand the characteristics and fundamentals associated with their new environment and its operation. Understandably, mutual trust is very low during this stage, as cautious attitudes prevail in settings unfamiliar to individuals. Particular attention is centered on understanding one's role and responsibilities within the group. The qualifications of peers, their respective roles in the group, and their personalities also are examined, giving members a better sense of the overall assembly of the group [25, 26]. Quite a bit of trial and error occurs during the forming stage, as various approaches and interactions are forwarded by members in an effort to gauge methods that will resonate with the greater group, fostering collegiality and collaboration. Members tend to be polite to each other in this early stage, putting their best foot forward to get along with peers. As indicated earlier, the more diverse the group, the longer the duration of the forming stage, as more effort is required to understand those who are dissimilar. The forming stage concludes when people begin to see themselves as being members of the group [17, 22].

12.5.2 Stage 2: Storming

The second stage of Tuckman's group development process is known as **storming**. During this stage, the honeymoon-like period characterizing the forming stage disappears, with cordiality giving way to conflict, confrontation, and competition between and among the members of the group [17, 25]. Here, individuality asserts itself within the group, with this understandably leading to friction, as ideas and actions begin to clash. Internal strife can occur on myriad fronts. Group members might be upset over the perceived fairness of their given assignments. They might disagree over courses of action about to be taken by the group. They might encounter incompatible personalities which stifle interactivity. Group members also might waiver in their commitment and dedication to the mission of the group. Subgroups or other factions might form during this stage, further contributing to the contentious environment characterizing storming [25, 26].

In many respects, the storming stage represents a "shaking out" period, requiring members to forgo individual tastes and preferences in favor of mindsets which are compatible with the group, effectively conceding a "my way" perspective for one that reflects "our way." Very often, group members are able to survive this tumultuous period, with some groups weathering storms better than others. However, there certainly are those situations where compatibility simply cannot be achieved, creating a collective of individuals incapable of bonding, threatening the prospects of successful group assembly. Outright rebellion is not unheard of during this stage [26]. Fortunately, cooler heads tend to prevail, with dedicated employees productively working through their personality differences and any other points of contention. When this is achieved, the storming stage ends and the norming stage begins.

12.5.3 Stage 3: Norming

Norming is the third stage of Tuckman's group development process. During this stage, individual members overcome their personal and professional differences and bond as a group. The conflict, confrontation, and competition characterizing the prior stage cease, being replaced by cooperation and collaboration. Information is freely exchanged between and among members, members work to find common ground in all pursuits, and differences of opinion are accepted. As collegiality reigns, groups begin to bond, permitting the membership to operate as one, realizing the synergies possible through the establishment of an effective group. This atmosphere permits the establishment of **norms**, standards of practice which essentially stipulate what attitudes and behaviors are and are not acceptable to the group, effectively constituting somewhat of a group culture that governs its operation. This stage effectively concludes when all of the individuals composing the group consider themselves to be fully on board and ready to work collaboratively to fulfill designated missions and other directives assigned to the given unit [17, 25, 26].

12.5.4   Stage 4: Performing

Performing, the fourth stage of Tuckman's group development process, sees a group realize its full potential, functioning as a cohesive unit, directing its complete attention toward fulfilling the mission assigned to the given unit [17, 25, 26]. Established, productive departments in healthcare organizations essentially are operating at the performing stage of group development, delivering the value expected of them, courtesy of the positive group dynamics that permit goals and objectives to be accomplished. Despite this achievement, groups which successfully reach the performing stage continue to have upside potential. As experience builds, opportunities for enhanced performance are possible, and the very best of groups within health and medical establishments will continue to evolve for the better with the passage of time. Of course, performance can also dwindle if care is not taken to secure gains achieved. Something as seemingly harmless as a personnel change, for example, can alter group dynamics and send performance spiraling downward into oblivion. Vigilance indeed is required when the performing stage has been reached by groups, protecting what ultimately should be considered to be a strategic asset of healthcare establishments.

12.5.5   Stage 5: Adjourning

The final stage of Tuckman's group development process is known as **adjourning**. During this stage, the group effectively disbands, drawing the group development process to a conclusion. Many groups never reach this stage, however, as they are permanent fixtures in their respective organizations [17, 25]. Long-established, productive departments in viable healthcare institutions clearly fit this profile. Once arranged, they simply continue operation in perpetuity. Other groups, however, are temporary, being established for a specific purpose which, once resolved, cease operation. Task forces arranged to manage particular matters, such as a public health crisis or a pending merger, offer excellent examples of fleeting groups which eventually will adjourn. And there, of course, are those situations where groups once thought to be permanent suddenly and unexpectedly find themselves adjourning, as in cases when medical centers close or when mergers call for reorganization. Adjourning, especially when associated with groups possessing lengthy histories, often is met with mixed feelings on the part of group members. On one hand, members might experience feelings of pride and accomplishment, courtesy of the successes achieved by the group. On the other hand, feelings of sadness and remorse might be experienced, given that the relationships developed between and among members are drawing to a conclusion [17]. Regardless of the reasons for adjournment, healthcare providers should reflect on group accomplishments and express associated appreciation, permitting impacted parties closure as given groups conclude operations.

12.6   Qualities which Enhance Group Performance

Groups, regardless of their type, size, focus, or mission, must perform well in order for them to make desired contributions within their given healthcare establishments. The array of characteristics which enhance group performance is quite extensive. Of these, several qualities are particularly vital. These include excellent leadership, clarity of mission, proper organizational structure and design, open and robust communication, strong group cohesion, intensive organizational learning, and strong accountability. These qualities are described below.

12.6.1   Excellent Leadership

Guidance for any group is critical, having a direct bearing on its associated performance. This guidance, first and foremost, is derived from managers charged with oversight duties and responsibilities. In modern healthcare establishments, these individuals are expected to possess leadership skills and abilities, using this acumen to advance designated managerial initiatives. Group performance also is enhanced by those members who do not hold formal managerial roles but nevertheless are viewed to be leaders due to their knowledge, charisma, or other personal factors. Performance can be fueled further by giving group members a voice in how the work of the group is to be conducted, with this effectively constituting a form of **shared leadership** [26]. The criticality of excellent leadership within groups applies equally to both permanent and temporary groups. While it is important to focus mostly on departments, divisions, locations, and other core groups, healthcare providers certainly should not neglect applying equal attention toward fleeting groups, such as temporary task forces, committees, and other briefly convened versions, given that these units also are impactful on greater operations within health and medicine. When excellent leadership permeates groups, they are positioned to deliver their very best [1, 27].

12.6.2   Clarity of Mission

In order for groups to thrive, the mission to be fulfilled by them must be crystal clear and well understood by each and every group member, from the highest rank to the lowest. Ultimately, group members must possess an intimate knowledge of the purpose of the work of the group and how it fits into the bigger picture of organizational operations. Timelines for providing the operational components supplied by given groups also must be carefully devised, accurately conveyed, and clearly understood by all members. While clarity of mission is important in any industry, it arguably is all the more vital in health and medicine, given the intensive specialization and epic degree of interdependency required in patient care. Pressure to perform is justifiably high. By ensuring that groups are fully aware of their assigned missions, members will possess knowledge of what is at stake should oversights, omissions, or other failures occur. Such an understanding can compel group members to amplify their performance, even in highly challenging circumstances and situations, elevating both group and organizational outcomes [1, 14, 26].

12.6.3   Proper Organizational Structure and Design

The need for proper organizational structure and design is vital not only at the macro-organizational level; it also is vital at the micro-organizational level [28, 29]. Quite obviously, as components of greater organizations, the groups making up healthcare establishments must be organized effectively in order to flesh out their highest levels of performance. This naturally requires determining the group's hierarchy, chain of command, and associated reporting relationships. The importance of this is obvious in formal groups, but it also is critical for informal groups, as proper attention directed toward structure and design permits order and order is a prerequisite for performance. Attention must also be directed toward ensuring that the size of the group permits it to function effectively, a task that requires trial and error, as no pat formulas exist for making such determinations [1, 12, 14]. All in all, the structure and design characteristics of groups must be addressed properly in order to realize optimal results.

12.6.4   Open and Robust Communication

Communication which freely and robustly flows between and among the members of a group bolsters its potential for performance. This makes sense even at face value, as productive dialogues must be realized in order for work assignments to be carried out effectively. Group members must, for example, be able to issue and receive instructions, provide and receive feedback, encourage and motivate each other, and accomplish scores of additional tasks which are dependent on successful communication. However, vigorous communication offers impacts far beyond its most obvious applications. Notably, it facilitates trust between and among group members. When accurate and sufficient communication flows freely, the informational needs of group members are fully met, removing information gaps that can hamper progress, diminish confidence, and divide. Rich communication naturally diminishes the opportunities for conflict to develop, and even when disagreements within groups occur, open dialogues supply the primary avenue for resolving encountered difficulties. Open and robust communication serves as a pathway for amplifying group performance, justifying investments of time and money to ensure that groups feature ongoing and productive dialogues as they go about accomplishing their designated missions [26, 30, 31].

12.6.5   Strong Group Cohesion

Group cohesion refers to a notable and highly desirable attribute of a group, characterized by the formation of bonds between and among its members, permitting them to pursue goals and objectives in a unified manner. Recall that group cohesion appears during the performing stage of Tuckman's model of group development, as profiled earlier, with its presence indicating the pinnacle of group development. Groups achieving this lofty quality feature high levels of collaboration, with members operating in a friendly, collegial manner. Members are extremely dedicated to each other, their assigned duties and responsibilities, and their group's mission, with accomplishment being a top concern and priority [12, 26]. Once cohesion is realized by groups, however, continued vigilance is required to ensure that performance is maintained and even advanced. Healthcare providers also must make certain that traps which effectively see groups operate as individuals are avoided. **Groupthink**—a phenomenon where group members opt to go along with particular courses of action in an effort to maintain consensus rather than engage in open and meaningful discussions to vet pathways under consideration—is an ever-present threat to group performance. Care must be taken to ensure that cohesion does not veer into blind conformity [2, 32].

12.6.6   Intensive Organizational Learning

Group performance is bolstered by the state of the group's knowledge, including lessons learned by its members over time, making organizational learning of vital importance for the achievement of optimal results. **Organizational learning** refers to the practice of actively sharing knowledge, insights, and experiences between and among institutional members as a means of informing current and future pursuits, permitting enhanced performance. In the same way that organizational learning is used broadly across establishments to enhance institutional performance, it can be used departmentally or in other group contexts to enhance group performance. As knowledge within groups develops, associated performance capabilities naturally flourish, affording increased potential to realize success [33, 34]. An essential component of organizational learning, robust circulation of knowledge, for example, is vitally needed within groups, permitting everyone to possess equivalent insights on given matters, allowing topics and concerns to be addressed more proficiently. Groups also must ensure that they are tapping both internal and external knowledge sources, acquiring helpful insights, regardless of their origin, to aid them in addressing whatever tasks await their attention [35]. These and related facets of organizational learning clearly must be incorporated into group operations in order to achieve maximum impact. Chapter 11 explores this topic comprehensively.

12.6.7   *Strong Accountability*

A strong sense of accountability must pervade groups in their entirety if they are to realize top performance. This stands to reason as all groups and the individuals making up their membership are vital components required for the successful delivery of health and medicine. **Accountability** specifically refers to a state of being accountable, that is, responsible, for one's actions and resulting performance. If group members each hold themselves accountable for their actions, the group itself will be an accountable entity, positioned to successfully accomplish its own mission and contribute positively to the greater mission of the organization [1, 26]. When low or nonexistent levels of accountability manifest in groups, careless attitudes and actions will prevail. **Social loafing**—a phenomenon where individuals exert less effort in group settings than they would if working alone, relying on their peers to pick up the slack—is a particular threat, diminishing group potential [2, 23]. Strong accountability can be enhanced by being particularly vigilant in staffing initiatives, hiring capable individuals and clearly communicating expectations that employees must take personal responsibility for their actions. Socialization systems, such as employee orientation, onboarding, and mentoring, also should prominently reference the need for employees to be accountable. Systems for rewarding compliance and penalizing noncompliance also are helpful, with these and related mechanisms permitting accountability to flourish, paying dividends, accordingly.

WK Reflections: Fostering Employee Bonding Through Casual Means

Over the pages of this chapter, discussions of groups have centered primarily on formal, work-based efforts occurring within healthcare organizations. However, in pursuing such formal initiatives, one should not neglect also incorporating casual techniques which foster bonding between and among employees, strengthening groups operating within given healthcare establishments. In Chap. 1, Willis Knighton Health's methods for establishing esprit de corps are presented, notably outlining techniques used to foster the "family feel" that characterizes the institution and its culture. Many of the described initiatives represent excellent examples of casual pursuits that can be used to build employee camaraderie and foster bonding. One particularly successful selection, briefly presented in Chap. 1, deserves to be further described to illustrate the power of casual pursuits in group development.

As profiled in Chap. 1, Willis Knighton Health annually hosts WK Day, an all-day picnic and barbecue held at the Louisiana State Fair. At this event, employees and their family members are granted free admission to the fair where they enjoy free food and participate in fun games in a special tent exclusively arranged for Willis Knighton Health. They also are afforded unlimited access to rides on the midway. More than 10,000 employees and their family members routinely attend this event each year, bringing the Willis Knighton Health family together in a casual, relaxed recreational environment to foster mutual appreciation, enjoyment, and bonding.

Willis Knighton Health's executives organized WK Day as a method for meaningfully demonstrating employee appreciation. The event differs from typical forms of employee appreciation which primarily occur onsite, such as employee birthday parties and parties celebrating various holidays. It even differs from common offsite events, such as retreats which take place at locations removed from the institution, but center primarily on work-related matters. WK Day is free of any work requirement; it is a purely casual, no-obligations event. Employees can relax and simply have fun. It is this unique arrangement that gives WK Day its broad appeal and superior capability for building morale and institutional affinity. The event also has proven to be highly effective for building bridges between and among the members of the WK family, as it offers opportunities for employees to get to know each other in contexts outside of the workplace. By also permitting the family members of employees to attend the event, WK Day provides yet another avenue for staff members to more deeply understand their colleagues, advancing relationships.

The success of WK Day serves as a powerful reminder of the value of complementing formal techniques for group development with informal, casual ones. Healthcare organizations, or any institution for that matter, often steer clear of investing in events of significant magnitude which are purely recreational and removed from anything related to work, believing that such outlays have little value. However, such perspectives focus only on tangible elements, neglecting intangible benefits. In the case of WK Day, associated investments facilitate the development of meaningful relationships between and among employees, with this intangible benefit clearly producing real value in the form of enhanced employee cohesion throughout the enterprise. Some things simply cannot be achieved in work settings, necessitating approaches that, although they may not involve work, build bonds that directly impact work and improve personal and institutional productivity.

12.7   Summary and Conclusions

Given the prevalence of groups in health and medical settings, coupled with their importance in performing the work necessary for the successful delivery of patient care, healthcare providers must possess a firm understanding of collective assemblies of personnel. Group knowledge also serves as a foundation for bolstering one's understanding of organizational behavior and management, as group intelligence is a building block of many of the discipline's components. Indeed, one would be hard pressed to claim an understanding of healthcare establishments and their operation without possessing a profound knowledge of groups. In even the smallest health and medical organizations, healthcare managers are part of and interact with many different types of groups, with these being characterized by high diversity, necessitating an understanding of the group development process and qualities which yield high-performing groups. When this knowledge is put into practice in healthcare establishments and successful assimilation is achieved throughout given organizations, synergistic effects and impacts result, driving performance which benefits institutions, personnel, and patients. As such, healthcare providers must ensure that they hold associated prowess, permitting them to fully appreciate groups and realize the benefits afforded by their successful management.

Key Terms

- Accountability
- Adjourning
- Command Group
- Diversity
- Fault Lines
- Formal Group
- Forming
- Friendship Group
- Group
- Group Cohesion
- Group Dynamics
- Groupthink
- Informal Group
- Interest Group
- Lone Wolf
- Norming
- Norms
- Organizational Learning
- Performing
- Shared Leadership
- Social Loafing
- Storming
- Synergy
- Task Group
- Team
- Tuckman's Model of Group Development

Exercises

1. In your own words, define groups, discuss their prevalence in health and medicine, and detail their importance in delivering patient care.
2. Compare and contrast groups and teams. Reflect on your recent work experiences and describe several groups and teams of which you have been a member. How would you rank your group and team experiences and why?
3. Demonstrate your understanding of formal groups and informal groups by defining both types. Reflect on your current employment experience and provide examples of formal and informal groups in operation. What impacts have you observed between and among these groups? Share associated details.
4. Define the concept of diversity, discuss its prevalence in health and medicine, and describe its role, influence, and importance in groups within healthcare establishments.
5. Outline Tuckman's model of group development and provide a brief overview of each of its stages. Reflect on your current employment experience, identify several groups of which you hold membership, and indicate the developmental stage of each group. Be sure to provide associated justifications.
6. Define the concept of accountability and discuss its role and importance in group performance. What tools and techniques does your workplace use to hold its employees accountable? What tools and techniques do you personally use to ensure that you demonstrate strong accountability in the workplace?
7. Define the concept of social loafing and describe how this phenomenon can impact group performance. Have you ever observed individuals engaging in this behavior? Have you yourself ever done so? Share these and any other associated experiences regarding this concept.
8. Identify and discuss qualities which enhance group performance and discuss methods for ensuring their presence in groups within health and medical institutions. Which quality do you view to be most important and why?

References

1. Elrod, J. K. (2013). *Breadcrumbs to cheesecake*. R&R Publishers.
2. Hitt, M. A., Miller, C. C., Colella, A., & Triana, M. D. C. (2018). *Organizational behavior* (5th ed.). Wiley.
3. Decaro, P. (2010). *Small group communication synergy*. Kendall Hunt.
4. Shi, L., & Singh, D. A. (2023). *Essentials of the US health care system* (6th ed.). Jones and Bartlett.
5. McConnell, C. R. (2020). *Hospitals and health systems: What they are and how they work*. Jones and Bartlett.
6. Hansen, M. T. (2009). *Collaboration: How leaders avoid the traps, create unity, and reap big results*. Harvard Business Press.
7. Rice-Bailey, T., & Chong, F. (2023). *Interpersonal skills for group collaboration: Creating high-performance teams in the classroom and the workplace*. Routledge.
8. Sawyer, K. (2017). *Group genius: The creative power of collaboration*. Basic Books.

9. Elrod, J. K., & Fortenberry, J. L., Jr. (2018). Am I seeing things through the eyes of patients? An exercise in bolstering patient attentiveness and empathy. *BMC Health Services Research, 18*(Suppl 3), 41–44.
10. Gardnes, H. K., & Matviak, I. A. (2022). *Smarter collaboration: A new approach to breaking down barriers and transforming work*. Harvard Business Review Press.
11. Lencioni, P. (2006). *Silos, politics, and turf wars: A leadership fable about destroying the barriers that turn colleagues into competitors*. Jossey-Bass.
12. Forsyth, D. R. (2019). *Group dynamics* (7th ed.). Cengage.
13. Blau, N. (2021). *Group dynamics: Connecting through communication*. Kendall Hunt.
14. Robbins, S. P., & Judge, T. A. (2019). *Organizational behavior* (18th ed.). Pearson.
15. Griffin, R. W., Phillips, J. M., & Gully, S. M. (2020). *Organizational behavior: Managing people and organizations* (13th ed.). Cengage.
16. Schermerhorn, J. R., Jr., Hunt, J. G., & Osborn, R. N. (1998). *Basic organizational behavior* (2nd ed.). Wiley.
17. Konopaske, R., Ivancevich, J. M., & Matteson, M. T. (2018). *Organizational behavior and management* (11th ed.). McGraw-Hill.
18. U. S. Bureau of Labor Statistics. (2022). *Occupational outlook handbook*. Retrieved April 3, 2023, from https://www.bls.gov/ooh/
19. O*NET OnLine. (2023). *Health care and social assistance*. Retrieved April 3, 2023, from https://www.onetonline.org/find/industry?i=62
20. Flynn, W. J., Valentine, S. R., & Meglich, P. A. (2022). *Healthcare human resource management* (4th ed.). Cengage.
21. Kotler, P., Keller, K. L., & Chernev, A. (2022). *Marketing management* (16th ed.). Pearson.
22. McShane, S. L., & Von Glinow, M. A. (2019). *Organizational behavior* (4th ed.). McGraw-Hill.
23. Colquitt, J. A., Lepine, J. A., & Wesson, M. J. (2019). *Organizational behavior: Improving performance and commitment in the workplace* (6th ed.). McGraw-Hill.
24. Tuckman, B. W. (1965). Developmental sequence in small groups. *Psychological Bulletin, 63*(6), 384–399.
25. Tuckman, B. W., & Jensen, M. A. C. (2010). Stages of small-group development revisited. *Group Facilitation: A Research and Applications Journal, 10*, 43–48.
26. Kinicki, A., & Soignet, D. B. (2022). *Management: A practical introduction* (10th ed.). McGraw-Hill.
27. Northouse, P. G. (2022). *Leadership: Theory and practice* (9th ed.). Sage.
28. Anderson, D. L. (2019). *Organization design: Creating strategic and agile organizations*. Sage.
29. Galbraith, J. R. (2014). *Designing organizations: Strategy, structure, and process at the business unit and enterprise levels* (3rd ed.). Jossey-Bass.
30. Lumsden, G., Lumsden, D., & Wiethoff, C. (2010). *Communicating in groups and teams: Sharing leadership* (5th ed.). Wadsworth.
31. Newman, A. (2017). *Business communication: In person, in print, online* (10th ed.). Cengage.
32. Janis, I. L. (2016). Groupthink: The desperate drive for consensus at any cost. In J. M. Shafritz, J. S. Ott, & Y. S. Jang (Eds.), *Classics of organization theory* (8th ed., pp. 161–168). Cengage.
33. Senge, P. M. (2006). *The fifth discipline: The art and practice of the learning organization*. Doubleday.
34. Elrod, J. K., & Fortenberry, J. L., Jr. (2017). Centers of excellence in healthcare institutions: What they are and how to assemble them. *BMC Health Services Research, 17*(Suppl 1), 15–24.
35. Elrod, J. K., & Fortenberry, J. L., Jr. (2017). Peering beyond the walls of healthcare institutions: A catalyst for innovation. *BMC Health Services Research, 17*(Suppl 1), 35–38.

Chapter 13
Power and Politics in Health and Medicine

Learning Objectives

After examining this chapter, readers will have the ability to:

- Define power, discuss how it can be used positively and negatively, speak on its ethical neutrality, and reveal its implications in health and medical organizations.
- Compare and contrast position power and personal power, defining each and detailing how they appear in healthcare establishments.
- Define each of the five types of power—legitimate power, reward power, coercive power, expert power, and referent power—and provide examples of each type in health and medical settings.
- Provide an overview of the strategic contingencies theory of power and discuss how the situational factors of uncertainty, substitutability, and centrality impact power.
- Identify and discuss three common ways that individuals react to attempts to influence them, indicate which responses are within the zone of indifference, and describe methods for using power in a manner to foster productive reactions.
- Define organizational politics, identify common tactics used by those engaged in such, and discuss approaches for minimizing political gamesmanship in healthcare establishments.

WK Reflections: Ensuring the Responsible Use of Power

Few errors made in healthcare establishments are as great as that of giving power to individuals who use it inappropriately. Inappropriate use of power ranges from innocent mistakes made by novice managers to outright, conscious abuse of power by anyone holding a position of authority. Regardless

J. K. Elrod, J. L. Fortenberry, Jr., *Organizational Behavior and Management in Health and Medicine*, https://doi.org/10.1007/978-3-031-61823-9_13

of form and magnitude, the consequences of misuse of power can be catastrophic, warranting vigilance on the part of healthcare providers to ensure its proper application by each and every individual holding authority within given institutions. Power is a tool and, just as with any implement, it can be used for good or for evil. When it is used for good, power provides a critical ingredient for directing attention and efforts in a manner that produces work and related desired outcomes. When it is used for evil, power produces malignancies within organizations which undermine institutional missions and very often harm completely innocent parties, ultimately positioning establishments for hardship. Given the obvious detriments associated with misuse, what can healthcare organizations do to ensure that power is used appropriately within the halls of medicine? The answer rests with ensuring that all individuals holding positions of authority in given establishments follow good managerial practices.

Across prior pages of this text, many techniques have been presented which can be helpful for ensuring that power is used responsibly within healthcare organizations. Chapter 7 contains a treasure trove of information relevant to the prudent use of power. Applicability of this chapter is somewhat obvious, as abuses of power constitute ethical violations. From that chapter, readers will recall the components which are required in any comprehensive ethics program, namely, a formal code of conduct, staffing practices which emphasize ethics, ethics training programs, and systems of accountability and control which foster ethical behaviors. Collectively, these mechanisms are capable of addressing most any ethical dilemma encountered in healthcare institutions, including those involving the use of power. Falling under the auspices of healthcare institutions to devise and implement, they provide a framework which can be used by healthcare organizations to ensure ethical operation, with this also extending to the application of power [1–7].

Of course, there also are useful guiding principles that managers can consult to help them ensure that power is kept in check. Chapter 1 itemizes Henri Fayol's 14 general principles of management, namely, division of work, authority and responsibility, discipline, unity of command, unity of direction, subordination of individual interest to the general interest, remuneration of personnel, centralization, scalar chain (line of authority), order, equity, stability of tenure of personnel, initiative, and esprit de corps [8]. Five of these—authority and responsibility, discipline, subordination of individual interest to the general interest, equity, and esprit de corps—have particularly direct implications for power and its proper use in organizations.

Recall from Chap. 1 that the principle of authority and responsibility emphasizes the need for managers to be accountable for their actions and associated outcomes, with this naturally precluding abuse on any front, including the application of power. The principle of discipline conveys the need for managers to conduct themselves in a manner consistent with the wishes of their organization. This means that managers must comply with institutional policy, notably including associated codes of conduct which routinely include statements prohibiting unethical activities of any kind. The principle of subordination of individual interest to the general interest conveys that the interests of one employee or a small group of employees should not take precedent over the mission being pursued by the establishment. As abuses of power often stem from self-centered thoughts and actions, this principle can help managers to keep their priorities straight, guarding themselves against any form of temptation to pursue greedy, egotistical, or otherwise selfish and inappropriate avenues. The principle of equity concerns efforts to ensure fairness and impartiality in the workplace. The abuse of power naturally conflicts with this principle, making adherence to the principle of equity a helpful defense against negative mindsets and practices. Finally, the principle of esprit de corps involves building a sense of unity between and among the ranks, fostering teamwork that allows the workforce to direct efforts in concerted fashion toward the achievement of designated goals and objectives. Fostering teamwork obviously precludes playing employees against each other, taking credit for ideas developed by someone else, supervising others in a harassing and intimidating manner, engaging in political gamesmanship, and like offenses that often emerge when power is exploited. Keeping these principles at the forefront of one's mind can be most helpful in efforts to ensure that power is being used responsibly [8].

With the methods expressed in these passages being incorporated into operations, healthcare organizations are well positioned to ensure that their personnel use power responsibly. While these techniques provide an excellent foundation for power management, additional benefits are possible through prudent managerial applications. Excellent communication to ensure well-informed personnel, a productive organizational culture which fosters professionalism, capable motivators to induce desired actions and behaviors, proper training to educate employees on correct practices, and related investments all aid in ensuring the proper application of power across establishments. Note that this is a joint effort between healthcare organizations and their employees. Healthcare organizations are responsible for establishing and implementing a sound ethical framework, complete with prudent accountability safeguards, and employees are responsible for ensuring their compliance, reminding themselves regularly of the principles which lead to success. Through this tandem effort, power within given healthcare establishments will be poised to be used in a productive and proper manner, free of misuse and abuse.

13.1 Background

When visiting most any modern healthcare establishment, one is hard pressed not to be awed by the sights and scenes observed while walking around and through them. Among other things, one typically sees carefully manicured grounds, modern architecture, attractive service environments, state-of-the-art technologies, and, perhaps most notably, dedicated staff members responsible for attending to the wants and needs of patients. Monumental efforts are required to effect such complex operations, necessitating a nearly infinite array of organizational activities and events [1, 9–12]. Even individuals possessing only a rudimentary knowledge of business can envision some of the required tasks. Missions must be developed and organizational structures devised, supplying an operational framework. Financing must be arranged and budgets prepared to ensure well-resourced pursuits. Capable staff members must be hired and scheduled properly to deliver comprehensive patient care. Customers must be encouraged to forward their patronage, becoming patients of given establishments [13–20]. However, underlying these commonly recognized endeavors, and in fact, supporting each and every one of them, is a more obscure but profoundly critical component of organizational behavior and management: power.

In many respects, power can be viewed as the mainstay of a healthcare organization, supporting virtually every initiative. While power sometimes is visible, observed through overt actions such as prominently expressed commands echoing from managers to subordinates, it more often than not is invisible, being understood so well by personnel that visible actions are not necessary. Regardless of form, power is an ever-present force inhabiting all healthcare establishments. Through power, healthcare organizations achieve order. Without it, chaos would reign [1, 21, 22]. Given this, it is imperative for healthcare providers to gain a detailed understanding of power, including its various types, situational factors influencing its accumulation, common responses when power is wielded, nuances of organizational politics, and the like in order to use power effectively within their given institutions. This chapter addresses power and its many facets, shedding light on this obscure but vital component of organizational behavior and management.

13.2 Defining Power

Power is defined as the ability to influence the thoughts, actions, and behaviors of others, permitting the achievement of desired outcomes, even in the face of resistance [22, 23]. It is a subject of great familiarity to most anyone, being encountered at a very early age, perhaps most notably through disciplinary processes occurring during childhood. One's familiarity with power does not end there, however, as it is a commonly used and observed manifestation across one's lifetime on both personal and professional fronts [24]. Its presence is especially prominent in health and medical organizations where operations could not be conducted successfully in its absence. Whether directly observed or not, it underpins the entirety of managerial processes and procedures and is a foundation of leadership. Words closely related to power include authority, domination, influence, force, and control [23]. Although these terms technically are distinctive, they very often are used interchangeably in practice. They all essentially refer to compelling another party to act in a prescribed manner, permitting achievement of the goals and objectives of the power-wielding party.

Power very often carries negative connotations, with some seeing it exclusively as an instrument of coercion, exploitation, manipulation, and the like. As such, power is somewhat of a controversial topic, making for difficult discussion [24]. Scholar Rosabeth Moss Kanter, in fact, described power as "America's last dirty word," expressing that it is easier to talk about most any topic, even controversial ones, than it is to discuss power [25, p. 274]. Power certainly can be used caustically and it is notoriously able to corrupt the undisciplined. Lord Acton's often quoted statement, "power tends to corrupt, and absolute power corrupts absolutely," certainly holds true [26, p. 465]. However, power also has another side, one that is positive and aimed at social development. Renowned author and researcher David McClelland aptly termed this distinction **the two faces of power**, one positive (which he termed *social*) that sees power being used to foster general good and the other negative (which he termed *egoistic*) that sees power being used for personal gain [27]. Understanding this balanced perspective is essential if healthcare managers are to make the most of power. In that it can be used for good or bad purposes, power is considered to be **ethically neutral**. Its impact—positive or negative—rests with the motives of its users [23]. This adds yet another justification for ensuring that those in positions of authority in health and medicine are of good character, as power in the hands of individuals without such high standards can be damaging, harming employee morale, organizational productivity, and, ultimately, patient care.

13.3 Types of Power

Power emerges from a variety of sources, with five bases or types being identified, namely, legitimate power, reward power, coercive power, expert power, and referent power [28]. They appear with regularity in health and medical settings. An individual may hold each of these types of power and the most successful managers typically do [29]. The first three types—legitimate, reward, and coercive—can be categorized into a broad group known as **position power**, as they each are derived from holding a formal position of responsibility (e.g., corporate officer, manager, supervisor), granting an individual the legitimate authority to issue directives to others, expect compliance, and reward or penalize actions [30]. Decision-making authority also rests with those holding position power, bolstering their associated influence. Their control over money, information, and other resources further reinforces their authority [31].

The last two types of power—expert and referent—can be categorized into a broad group known as **personal power**, as they each stem from possessing appealing characteristics or attributes, compelling the admiration, respect, and followership of others. Personal power is not tied to a formal position of responsibility. Unique knowledge, personal charisma, inherent leadership ability, and more can serve as the foundation of personal power, with these characteristics coming from within oneself. As such, even individuals who do not hold formal managerial authority can possess this type of power [30]. To better understand the broad categories of position power and personal power, the five types of power making up these categories must be more closely explored.

13.3.1 Legitimate Power

Individuals holding formal managerial positions in organizations, permitting them the authority to guide and direct others within their given establishments, are said to possess **legitimate power** [28]. It usually is the first type of power that comes to mind when one thinks about authority and its underpinnings [26]. Its impact on organizational operations is paramount, with legitimate power typically being considered to be the most important source of power in establishments [32]. Legitimate power is occasionally referred to as **formal authority**, with its holders possessing official titles and occupying designated places in their given institutions' organizational charts [29].

A hospital CEO, director of nursing, laboratory manager, and dietary supervisor each possess legitimate power, courtesy of the managerial roles they occupy. Typically, the higher someone is in the chain of command, the greater their legitimate power [29]. Organizational values dictate that holders of legitimate power have a valid or legitimate right to influence subordinates and that these subordinates, in turn, have an obligation to comply with their requests. The acknowledgment of legitimate power by organizational members stems from three things: cultural norms which stipulate that some possess the right to command others, acceptance of institutional social structures necessitating respecting the organizational hierarchy, and designations by governing boards, CEOs, and other legitimizing agents endowing particular individuals with oversight authority [28].

13.3.2 Reward Power

Power derived from one's ability to issue rewards and related incentives, such as pay, promotions, awards, preferred work schedules, and the like, is known as **reward power**. This type of power is possessed by managers as a result of their formal authority within their respective organizations, making it an extension of legitimate power [28]. Compliance is motivated by the positive benefits available to those eligible to receive associated rewards, giving power to the individual offering the incentives [33]. Consider, for example, the impact of a hospital's offer to send a limited number of top-performing LPNs to an LPN-to-RN training program at no expense to the award recipients. With level of performance determining the winners of this opportunity, the director of nursing and related nurse managers will carry significant power as their associated assessments will determine the award recipients. This, in turn, will influence the behavior of LPNs who are interested in the opportunity in a manner desired by the hospital, namely, to deliver their very best as they go about attending to their duties and responsibilities.

The motivational impact of rewards depends on two things. The first one is magnitude of the reward. More prominent rewards (e.g., an extra vacation day for working a difficult-to-fill shift) will have greater impact potential than less prominent ones (e.g., a voucher for a free meal at the hospital's cafeteria). The second one pertains to the degree of certainty held by subordinates that their managers can and will actually deliver given rewards. If the targets of a reward have confidence that a particular incentive will be awarded if the requirements for receipt are fulfilled, it will be motivating, giving power to the offering party. If not, the given reward will not yield power [28]. Importantly, rewards offered must have value to their targets. This necessitates that managers desirous of compelling particular behaviors via rewards must understand what their subordinates value, ensuring that the rewards offered are motivating to them. In the absence of this, the incentives will have no impact, failing to induce desired actions [31].

13.3.3 Coercive Power

Power stemming from one's ability to punish is referred to as **coercive power**. Coercive power essentially is the antithesis of reward power, relying on threats, undesirable consequences, and other discouragements to prompt particular behaviors. Reprimanding a staff nurse for arriving late, demoting a dietary manager for a lapsed certification, terminating a hospital vice president for insubordination, and the like are common actions resulting from the use of punitive tools in healthcare institutions. The threat of penalties associated with noncompliance serves as a powerful incentive for ensuring compliance. As with reward power, coercive power is held by managers because of their formal, legitimate authority within their given institutions. The strength of coercive power is dependent on the magnitude of the punishments that managers have at their disposal and further influenced by the probability, as perceived by subordinates, that managers can and will actually inflict such punishments [28]. With coercive power, fear is the primary motivator of compliance [29]. Care must be taken when deploying this type of power, however, as its regular use can create environments characterized by hostility, distrust, and diminished morale, negatively impacting performance. As such, coercive power must be used very conservatively in organizations [29, 30].

13.3.4 Expert Power

Power derived from one's special expertise, technical knowledge, or related intellectual insights and abilities is referred to as **expert power** [28]. Individuals possessing proficiencies that are critical for the operational success of their organizations are positively positioned to influence those who are in need of that expertise [29]. Consider the classic example of the technologically savvy admissions clerk who aids her less capable peers within the patient accounts department whenever they encounter difficulties setting up their smartphones, installing software on their computers, using the latest video technologies, and so on. Holding and making use of this much needed expertise gives her power within her work group which she otherwise would not possess. As expert power is based on an individual's acumen, it is considered to be personal power and, as such, it can be possessed by anyone. In fact, acquisition of this type of power is completely at the discretion of the individual. Those interested in doing so would first identify proficiencies that are in high demand within their given organizations. Then, they would seek to gain the associated expertise through formal programs of study, workforce development opportunities, personal study, and the like, affording them knowledge for use—and associated power accumulation—within their establishments [30].

Individuals respond to expert power in much the same manner as they do legitimate power, namely, by following the directives communicated, indicating the great deference that is given to experts [32]. This power, however, can be fleeting. If others in a work group acquire acumen similar to that of an individual who previously possessed this knowledge exclusively, associated power held by that person will diminish [34]. Expert power also is confined to the areas in which one's expertise applies, limiting this form of power [28]. In the example provided earlier regarding power acquired by the technologically savvy admissions clerk, for obvious reasons, the scope of her power rests with matters tied to the use of technologies in the workplace. Transference of this particular power source to unrelated areas generally is not possible.

13.3.5 Referent Power

Individuals who hold influence over others on the basis of admiration, kinship, loyalty, attraction, respect, and similar qualities are said to possess **referent power**. Those with referent power are able to convince and compel others to support and follow them, with followers being moved by affinity and relatedness, motivating desires to identify with and engage the person holding this type of power [28]. The legendary health system CEO who makes all the right decisions, the gifted physician who possesses the perfect bedside manner, the compassionate nurse who exhibits true concern for patients, the devout hospital chaplain who eloquently provides spiritual guidance and always remembers everybody's name, and similar appealing figures serve as excellent examples of individuals possessing referent power. Every healthcare institution has them and they are highly cherished, courtesy of their appealing personal qualities.

The basis of referent power rests with one's charisma [31]. The term **charisma**, derived from the Greek word meaning "gift," refers to highly alluring qualities which are possessed by an individual, characterizing the person and affording him or her with profound abilities to influence others. Confidence, optimism, devotion, vision, enthusiasm, commitment, and the like are qualities often associated with the charismatic [33, 34]. Although charisma is routinely viewed to be a trait bestowed upon one at birth, opportunities are possible for anyone to build charismatic skills through training, reflection, and related personal development activities. As such, referent power can be possessed by most anyone in organizations, making it a form of personal power [33]. Referent power is considered to be the most resilient form of power in that once it is acquired, it is difficult to lose. Unlike expert power, which applies only to particular areas tied to the associated expertise, referent power can be used more universally, directing influence across multiple areas within organizations [34].

13.4 Contingencies of Power

The amount of power possessed by parties in organizations is contingent on situational factors associated with uncertainty, substitutability, and centrality, with this being known as the **strategic contingencies theory of power** [35]. The first factor, **uncertainty**, is experienced often in healthcare organizations. Patient volume might be waning, courtesy of a new competitor entering the market, leading to uncertainty. Supply chain issues for critical surgical equipment might be encountered, hampering access and threatening scheduled medical procedures. Disputes over pay for nurses or other critical staff members might threaten walk-outs capable of crippling operations. Such environments of uncertainty must be navigated carefully, requiring keen skills and abilities, and the parties which have the will and the way to successfully address these difficult situations understandably will accumulate power, courtesy of their associated acumen.

The second factor, **substitutability**, concerns how easy it is for an organization to replace the production and output of a given party. The more difficult it is to do so, the greater the power held by that individual or work group [35]. Consider the case of a long-tenured hospital administrator who possesses decades of experience within a given institution. The administrator's lengthy history and experience would produce a level of knowledge unmatched and virtually irreplaceable, bolstering associated power held by this person. The same would be true of a physician practicing a rare medical specialty such as pediatric neurosurgery. Within his medical center, the physician will carry a high degree of power, given that substitutes for his services are highly limited and qualified candidates are very difficult to find. Substitutability also pertains to work groups. If the production of a particular department can be performed by another department or outsourced to external entities, its power is diminished as other options for provision of its services exist. If, however, substitutes do not exist or are prohibitive to acquire, power of the work group is bolstered.

The last factor, **centrality**, concerns the relative contributions provided by parties to the final output produced by an organization. The greater the contribution, the greater the power [35]. In a hospital, the nursing department makes a profound contribution to the core services provided by the institution. Without its services, hospital operations would cease. Contrast this with the hospital's marketing department. Though critical, if an event shuttered this department temporarily, hospital operations could continue unfettered. With the nursing department being more central to the hospital's production than that of the marketing department, the nursing department will carry more power. Similarly, a medical center's physicians, whose production is integral to the patient experience, would hold more power than the medical center's grant writers, whose efforts are less vital for delivering the core product provided by the establishment.

Uncertainty, substitutability, and centrality influence the amount of power held by parties in health and medical organizations, virtually guaranteeing variability of power across establishments. An awareness of the strategic contingencies theory of power is helpful in understanding the latitude of authority possessed by individuals and work groups [35]. Such knowledge can aid healthcare institutions in organization design, workforce planning, negotiation, and related activities.

13.5   Reactions to Power

Power wielders—typically managers in organizational settings—only represent part of the power equation. The targets of power—typically subordinates—also must be considered in order to fully grasp the concept of power. One particularly must understand how individuals react to attempts to influence them, with three ways—resistance, compliance, and commitment—being common courses. Those responding with **resistance** are confrontational, questioning the authority of those issuing directives and even opposing them. This can be prompted by many things, ranging from genuine concern on the part of employees to rebellion for the sake of rebellion. It also can be prompted by abuses of power by managers. Another reaction to power is that of **compliance**, where employees obey issued decrees, endeavoring to meet expectations, but they offer nothing more [36, 37]. This reaction falls within what is known as the **zone of indifference**, where employees accept directives from superiors without questioning or challenging their authority [31]. The last reaction option—**commitment**—also falls within the zone of indifference. Here, those subject to power and influence react by committing to the directives issued, opting to give their very best to ensure that expectations are not only met, but exceeded [36, 37]. This represents the ideal reaction to power that healthcare providers wish to see in their workforces.

Quite obviously, healthcare managers desire directives issued to be within the zone of indifference, compelling subordinates to pursue their work satisfactorily, ideally in a committed manner. Judicious, responsible use of power, deployed in a constructive rather than punitive manner, offers the best avenue for realizing this outcome. This involves using the positive face of power, shunning the negative one that can invoke resentment and resistance. Consideration also should be given to distributing at least some power to subordinates, granting them a voice in how work is conducted. Known as **empowerment**, this particular approach can aid in reducing resistance as employees have a say in operations, reducing feelings of animosity that often come with powerlessness [30]. Research indicates that empowerment positively impacts employees, increasing job satisfaction, elevating organizational commitment, bolstering performance, reducing turnover, and diminishing employee stress, with these attributes collectively driving institutional productivity [26]. These and related developmental efforts can help to ensure that employees remain in the zone of indifference, permitting healthcare operations to proceed harmoniously and productively.

WK Reflections: A Framework for Fostering Empowerment

Willis Knighton Health has worked diligently to establish an organization which is well known for empowering its employees. Over the years, the institution has crafted a method for fostering empowerment, consisting of three primary steps: developing an understanding of employees to assess their abilities and ambitions, providing adequate support to promote empowerment success, and maintaining patience and exercising tolerance as newly empowered employees learn the ropes. The first step—developing an understanding of employees to assess their abilities and ambitions—is essential as managers must determine who from among their subordinates has the potential or is currently capable of serving in an empowered capacity. On identification, managers then must investigate whether these employees possess the desire to do so. If employees possess "the will and the way," then the first hurdle has been cleared successfully.

The second step—providing adequate support to promote empowerment success—requires that managers provide sufficient resources to those employees who have demonstrated the ability and desire to operate as empowered agents. Two investments are imperative here. The first concerns investments in the personal development of the given candidate, and the second concerns investments in mentoring the individual. A newly empowered employee faces new and different challenges for which they may not be adequately prepared to pursue. In such cases, healthcare organizations must educate the employees, either by internal workforce development initiatives or external educational opportunities. Proper mentoring is also essential, permitting employees to ask questions, get advice, and address any other concern with an experienced manager. With adequate resources dedicated to the newly empowered employee, the second step of the process is complete.

The third and final step—maintaining patience and exercising tolerance as newly empowered employees learn the ropes—references an often over-looked ingredient which fosters empowerment success. Empowerment natu-rally involves **delegation**—turning over the authority for accomplishing particular tasks to others—with this sometimes proving to be challenging to those managers relinquishing this authority. Newly empowered employees typically are inexperienced. A learning curve should be expected, with multi-ple attempts at delegated work often being needed in order to get things right, at least until experience and resulting confidence are built. Patience obviously is required in such situations. In addition to patience, a healthy dose of tolerance is required. As individuals rarely perform tasks in the exact same fashion, the stage is set in delegation for managers to be disenchanted with the methods used by newly empowered employees simply due to variation in task accomplishment. Managers must understand that approaches will vary and that some decisions that are made might not be identical to those that the manager would make. As long as efforts are within the range of accep-tance, delegating managers must exercise tolerance and permit empowered individuals to carry out assignments in the manner that they see fit, even if it varies from the approaches preferred by delegators. Doing so will bolster empowerment success.

Healthcare institutions desirous of fostering empowerment are encour-aged to incorporate the three steps which Willis Knighton Health has found to be helpful. Through this, the benefits itemized earlier in the chapter very much can be realized with concerted effort. Willis Knighton Health has also found operationalization of the framework to be particularly helpful for devel-oping junior managers in preparation for senior roles within the institution, making it useful for succession planning. Often times, health and medical establishments seek to empower employees through informal means, but this tends to foster inconsistency. Adherence with the simple guidance of the recommended framework will ensure formality, promoting consistency over time, amplifying the ability of healthcare organizations to successfully empower their employees.

13.6 Organizational Politics

A discussion of power in health and medicine would be incomplete without direct-ing attention toward organizational politics. The concept of **organizational politics** references a range of activities and behaviors taken in an effort to advance one's own interests with little or no regard for the interests of the greater organization. As political overtures, these deeds and actions are not part of one's formal duties and responsibilities, but they do have the capability of impacting work and other aspects of organizations. Political activities and behaviors can be initiated solely by an individual, as in the case of a medical clinic administrator claiming ownership of an idea that actually had been envisioned and advanced by a subordinate. Very often, though, political gamesmanship occurs at the hands of **coalitions**, groups of individuals who band together to drive or otherwise promote a particular cause of interest to its members [34]. A medical center's decision to change employee benefits might, for example, give rise to a coalition of physicians, nurses, and other employees desirous of blocking the change. The aim of organizational politics can prove to be beneficial or detrimental to institutions, with this being dependent on the desires of those engaged in political gamesmanship and whether these happen to coincide with or oppose institutional missions.

Common tactics used by those engaged in organizational politics include building networks of colleagues to support personal causes, lobbying power brokers in the institution to support private aspirations, bending rules or bypassing them altogether to remove obstructions to personal aims, promoting one's own skills and accomplishments but not doing the same for others, praising others disingenuously to gain buy-in for personal aims, and attacking or blaming others even if the fault rests with oneself [38]. Each of these tactics reveals in varying ways the self-centeredness that is inherent in organizational politics. Very often, those engaged in political behavior try to disguise their motives, taking great care to make selfish gestures appear to be altruistic, although many are not fooled by such tactics.

While some may view political efforts to be innocent, in reality they are not, primarily due to their distracting qualities which divert attention away from institutional missions, diminishing organizational performance. When organizational politics run rampant, dedicated employees often feel threatened, believing, for example, that they will be overshadowed by those engaged in political gamesmanship, potentially harming their chances of receiving premium work assignments, promotions, salary increases, and other benefits. This can increase stress levels, diminish morale, and reduce job satisfaction. It also can create scenarios where committed employees believe that they are left with no other option than to respond in kind, further politicizing the workplace [26].

So how can a healthcare establishment minimize the impact and occurrence of organizational politics? The first strategy entails establishing order in the workplace, ensuring that clear policies govern all aspects of operation. Vague guidelines offer opportunities for flexible, self-serving interpretations, opening the door for rampant organizational politics. Political aspirations often can be foiled by detailed policy frameworks. A second strategy involves efforts to reduce uncertainty at every available opportunity. When employees face uncertainty, such as looming layoffs, forthcoming mergers, the retirement of a beloved CEO, or any other form of change, many will react politically, jockeying for position for purposes of self-preservation [26, 32]. Uncertainty is best addressed by communicating accurately and robustly with employees, ensuring that they are kept apprised of the latest information, especially when threatening change looms. Minimally, this will help prevent rumors from circulating, reducing the likelihood of employees filling informational gaps on their own, creating disinformation and magnifying already stressful situations.

Resource scarcity also has been known to fuel organizational politics. When limited pools of resources exist, parties often will resort to political gamesmanship in a bid to secure as much as possible, even if broader distribution would be more beneficial. This is one of the most problematic sources of organizational politics to address, as resource limitations often are difficult and sometimes impossible to remedy. If resources cannot be increased, reducing competition for them, the best approach is to ensure transparency in their distribution, justifying decisions, accordingly. Knowledge of how and why resource allocation decisions were made can go a long way toward alleviating angst in the workplace, reducing the likelihood of political responses. A final strategy for reducing organizational politics involves creating an environment where political gamesmanship is not tolerated. This begins with top executives leading by example, reinforcing the notion that playing politics has no place within the establishment [32]. Doing so will aid healthcare organizations in ensuring that attention is directed where it belongs, namely, toward institutional missions.

13.7 Summary and Conclusions

Power is an obscure but vital component of organizational behavior and management, serving as a foundational element which supports virtually the entirety of all other components of the discipline, including leadership, motivation, organizational structure and design, conflict management, and more. At its core, power serves as an instrument of order, ensuring that institutional operations are productive and prosperous, free from the ravages of disruption and chaos. Given its importance, healthcare providers must endeavor to acquire a comprehensive understanding of power, its various facets, methods for operationalizing the concept in the workplace, and related insights. As power can be used in both positive and negative fashions, special care must be taken by the individual wielding power to be disciplined, ensuring that applications of power center on advancing institutional missions, rather than self-serving ambitions. Healthcare managers who consistently deploy the positive face of power are assets to their institutions, situated to productively influence others within their given organizations. Prowess on this important front should be considered mandatory for anyone holding positions of authority in health and medicine.

Key Terms

- Centrality
- Charisma
- Coalition

- Coercive Power
- Commitment
- Compliance
- Delegation
- Empowerment
- Ethical Neutrality
- Expert Power
- Formal Authority
- Legitimate Power
- Organizational Politics
- Personal Power
- Position Power
- Power
- Referent Power
- Resistance
- Reward Power
- Strategic Contingencies Theory of Power
- Substitutability
- The Two Faces of Power
- Uncertainty
- Zone of Indifference

Exercises

1. In your own words, define power, discuss how it can be used positively and negatively, speak on its ethical neutrality, and discuss its implications in health and medical organizations.
2. Compare and contrast position power and personal power. Reflect on your recent work experiences and provide examples that you have observed which illustrate both of these broad categories of power.
3. Define each of the five types of power: legitimate power, reward power, coercive power, expert power, and referent power. Reflect on your recent work experiences and provide examples illustrating each type of power as you have observed it in practice. Which type do you personally rely on most and why?
4. Provide an overview of the strategic contingencies theory of power and discuss its implications in healthcare organizations. Think deeply about a current work experience and describe your work group's power base through the lens of each of the three situational factors of uncertainty, substitutability, and centrality. Which of the three most contributes to the power held by your work group and why?
5. Discuss how individuals might react to attempts to influence them, noting the three possibilities outlined in the chapter and indicating which reactions are

within the zone of indifference. Describe two workplace situations, one where directives issued to you fell outside of the zone of indifference and the other where directives issued to you fell inside of the zone of indifference. For the situation falling outside of the zone of indifference, what steps could your manager have taken to avoid this to ensure your acceptance of the issued directives?

6. Explain the concept of empowerment. Think back on your work experiences and describe a situation in which you felt empowered and a situation in which you felt powerless. For each experience, what was the outcome and how did it advance your personal and professional development?

7. Define and discuss the topic of organizational politics. How would you characterize the level of organizational politics in your workplace? Is it low, medium, or high? What political tactics have you observed and how has your organization responded to them? If you could change anything regarding the political nature of your establishment, what would it be and why?

8. Reflect on the insights you have gained on the topic of power, think deeply about how you plan to use it going forward as a healthcare executive, and prepare a brief narrative sharing your associated aspirations and expectations.

References

1. Elrod, J. K. (2013). *Breadcrumbs to cheesecake*. R&R Publishers.
2. Schermerhorn, J. R., Jr., & Bachrach, D. G. (2015). *Management* (13th ed.). Wiley.
3. Kinicki, A., & Soignet, D. B. (2022). *Management: A practical introduction* (10th ed.). McGraw-Hill.
4. Robbins, S. P., & Coulter, M. (2021). *Management* (15th ed.). Pearson.
5. Stanwick, P. A., & Stanwick, S. D. (2016). *Understanding business ethics* (3rd ed.). Sage.
6. Marcus, A. A., & Hargrave, T. J. (2021). *Managing business ethics: Making ethical decisions*. Sage.
7. Morrison, E. E. (2020). *Ethics in health administration: A practical approach for decision makers* (4th ed.). Jones and Bartlett.
8. Fayol, H. (2016). General principles of management. In J. M. Shafritz, J. S. Ott, & Y. S. Jang (Eds.), *Classics of organization theory* (8th ed., pp. 53–65). Cengage.
9. Shi, L., & Singh, D. A. (2023). *Essentials of the US health care system* (6th ed.). Jones and Bartlett.
10. McConnell, C. R. (2020). *Hospitals and health systems: What they are and how they work*. Jones and Bartlett.
11. Walston, S. L., & Johnson, K. L. (2021). *Healthcare in the United States: Clinical, financial, and operational dimensions*. Health Administration Press.
12. Wilensky, S. E., & Teitelbaum, J. B. (2023). *Essentials of health policy and law* (5th ed.). Jones and Bartlett.
13. Ginter, P. M., Duncan, W. J., & Swayne, L. E. (2013). *Strategic management of health care organizations* (7th ed.). Jossey-Bass.
14. Hillestad, S. G., & Berkowitz, E. N. (2020). *Health care market strategy: From planning to action* (5th ed.). Jones and Bartlett.
15. Reiter, K. L., & Song, P. H. (2021). *Gapenski's healthcare finance: An introduction to accounting and financial management* (7th ed.). Health Administration Press.

16. Cleverley, W. O., & Cleverly, J. O. (2017). *Essentials of health care finance* (8th ed.). Jones and Bartlett.
17. Flynn, W. J., Valentine, S. R., & Meglich, P. A. (2022). *Healthcare human resource management* (4th ed.). Cengage.
18. Niles, N. J. (2020). *Basic concepts of health care human resource management* (2nd ed.). Jones and Bartlett.
19. Kotler, P., Stevens, R. J., & Shalowitz, J. (2021). *Strategic marketing for health care organizations: Building a customer-driven health system* (2nd ed.). Wiley.
20. Fortenberry, J. L., Jr. (2010). *Health care marketing: Tools and techniques* (3rd ed.). Jones and Bartlett.
21. Clegg, S. R., Courpasson, D., & Phillips, N. (2006). *Power and organizations*. Sage.
22. Pfeffer, J. (1992). *Managing with power: Politics and influence in organizations*. Harvard Business School Press.
23. Fairholm, G. W. (2009). *Organizational power politics: Tactics in organizational leadership* (2nd ed.). Praeger.
24. Shafritz, J. M., Ott, J. S., & Jang, Y. S. (Eds.). (2016). *Classics of organization theory* (8th ed.). Cengage.
25. Kanter, R. M. (2016). Power failure in management circuits. In J. M. Shafritz, J. S. Ott, & Y. S. Jang (Eds.), *Classics of organization theory* (8th ed., pp. 274–283). Cengage.
26. Kinicki, A., & Fugate, M. (2018). *Organizational behavior: A practical, problem-solving approach* (2nd ed.). McGraw-Hill.
27. McClelland, D. C. (1970). The two faces of power. *Journal of International Affairs, 24*(1), 29–47.
28. French, J. R. P., Jr., & Raven, B. (2016). The bases of social power. In J. M. Shafritz, J. S. Ott, & Y. S. Jang (Eds.), *Classics of organization theory* (8th ed., pp. 251–260). Cengage.
29. Colquitt, J. A., Lepine, J. A., & Wesson, M. J. (2019). *Organizational behavior: Improving performance and commitment in the workplace* (6th ed.). McGraw-Hill.
30. Griffin, R. W., Phillips, J. M., & Gully, S. M. (2020). *Organizational behavior: Managing people and organizations* (13th ed.). Cengage.
31. Konopaske, R., Ivancevich, J. M., & Matteson, M. T. (2018). *Organizational behavior and management* (11th ed.). McGraw-Hill.
32. McShane, S. L., & Von Glinow, M. A. (2019). *Organizational behavior* (4th ed.). McGraw-Hill.
33. Robbins, S. P., & Judge, T. A. (2019). *Organizational behavior* (18th ed.). Pearson.
34. Hitt, M. A., Miller, C. C., Colella, A., & Triana, M. D. C. (2018). *Organizational behavior* (5th ed.). Wiley.
35. Hickson, D. J., Hinings, C. R., Lee, C. A., Schneck, R. E., & Pennings, J. M. (1971). A strategic contingencies' theory of intraorganizational power. *Administrative Science Quarterly, 16*(2), 216–229.
36. Yukl, G. A., & Gardner, W. L. I. I. I. (2020). *Leadership in organizations* (9th ed.). Pearson.
37. Falbe, C. M., & Yukl, G. (1992). Consequences for managers of using single influence tactics and combinations of tactics. *Academy of Management Journal, 35*(3), 638–652.
38. Allen, R. W., Madison, D. L., Porter, L. W., Renwick, P. A., & Mayes, B. T. (1979). Organizational politics. *California Management Review, 22*(1), 77–83.

Chapter 14
Conflict and Negotiation in Health and Medicine

Learning Objectives

After examining this chapter, readers will have the ability to:

- Define conflict, discuss its prevalence in health and medicine, and speak on the need for it to be addressed in a timely and effective manner.
- Define conflict management and discuss the necessity for healthcare establishments to gain associated proficiencies.
- Discuss functional and dysfunctional conflict and supply examples of how conflict can help and hurt productivity in healthcare organizations.
- Compare and contrast task conflict and relationship conflict, noting examples of each type in health and medical settings.
- Identify and define typical sources of conflict and common responses to conflict in health and medicine.
- Define negotiation, discuss its primary types, and provide a general overview of the negotiation process.
- Understand the value of strategic frameworks in the management of conflict in healthcare institutions.

WK Reflections: Managerial Skills for Addressing Conflict

The successful management of conflict within healthcare organizations requires managerial excellence on many fronts. As the pages of this chapter will reveal, conflict can be quite difficult to address, given the many forms that it can take in healthcare organizations, necessitating extreme managerial prowess. Conflict management skills develop throughout the work lives of managers, courtesy of their experiences handling instances of discord in the workplace. Focused training efforts centered on skill building also are capable of bolstering one's ability to gain conflict management proficiencies. While a

J. K. Elrod, J. L. Fortenberry, Jr., *Organizational Behavior and Management in Health and Medicine*, https://doi.org/10.1007/978-3-031-61823-9_14

variety of managerial competencies are required, from Willis Knighton Health's observations over many decades, five have a particularly heavy influence on one's ability to successfully manage conflict. Top managerial skills for address-ing conflict include foundational knowledge, analytical skills, objectivity, interpersonal communication skills, and patience.

Foundational knowledge refers to intelligence regarding institutional policies and procedures governing the operations of a healthcare organiza-tion. Key sources include the mission statement, strategic plan, code of con-duct, personnel handbook, and similar documents of given establishments. Institutional policies provide guidance on multiple fronts, with these, in turn, helping to guide conflict management efforts. Assume, for example, that two factions of hospital managers have emerged, with the parties calling for the hospital to pursue different courses of action. Resolving this conflict obviously would require possessing a thorough knowledge of the mission and strategic plan of the establishment as this will help to determine the compliance of the two courses of action. This alone might resolve the matter if, for example, one of the pathways deviated from the core tenets of the institution. Regardless, efforts to bring the parties together would necessitate excellent foundational knowledge. By possessing such knowledge, managers are aided in their assessments of conflict scenarios, making them better equipped to handle associated matters. As such, healthcare institutions must ensure that work-force development efforts include clear conveyance of critical foundational information and managerial employees must endeavor to commit this infor-mation to memory for immediate recall and use in practice.

Analytical skills refer to abilities to study situations, make sense of things, and formulate steps to address inquiries at hand. Specifically, a range of research techniques are called upon to draw conclusions. Commonly used analytical skills include research design, data acquisition, data analysis, and critical thinking. Conflict in healthcare organizations often is difficult to deci-pher, with face value assessments typically being highly unreliable. Opposing interests naturally set the stage for those holding given interests to paint them in the best light possible, with this sometimes leading to inaccurate por-trayals. The truth is needed, necessitating digging deeper to identify root causes that show definitively what actually is occurring between opposing sides. By deploying a capable analytical skill set, managers will be equipped to conduct proper investigations to glean accurate portrayals of conflict scenar-ios, setting the stage for their resolution.

Objectivity refers to the ability to maintain an unbiased perspective when analyzing and evaluating situations. Associated judgments are based on actual facts, rather than one's particular feelings on the matter. This can be challenging for many. Everyone has personal tastes, preferences, and perspec-tives. Further, through the process of work, friendships often develop. These and similar influences can lead to favoritism which erodes one's ability to maintain objectivity in associated assessments. The best counter to falling into subjectivity is that of maintaining self-awareness, questioning thoughts and actions throughout the conflict resolution process to help ensure unbiased treatment. It sometimes can be helpful to role-play by assuming the position of an outside party completely free of any associated interests, working to see the situation from that particular perspective. How might this outside party view the decision that is about to be made? Would this party view the decision to be biased toward one side or the other? This "outsider perspective" can help to bolster objectivity in one's conflict resolution efforts.

Interpersonal communication skills refer to abilities to proficiently engage in productive dialogues with individuals. This requires capabilities in both verbal and nonverbal communication. **Verbal communication** makes use of written or spoken words to interact with others. **Nonverbal communication** makes use of physical manifestations, such as eye contact, facial expressions, body posture, vocal tone, head movements, hand gestures, touch, spatial distance from addressee, and other behaviors, to convey meaning to others. Notable interpersonal skills that can help in conflict resolution include communicating accurately and respectfully, engaging in **active listening** by focusing on both verbal and nonverbal conveyances, demonstrating empathy in interactions, and maintaining composure in stressful situations. Healthcare institutions can aid managerial employees in developing these skills by holding workforce training initiatives and other educational opportunities to shore up associated abilities, with these aiding in building conflict resolution prowess.

Patience refers to the ability to maintain composure and restraint in the face of trying obstacles and challenges. Time usually is required to properly diagnose conflict and formulate associated remedies, and this demands patience. Such temporal requirements can be very frustrating for those who want to resolve conflict scenarios immediately on their presentation. For very simple matters, this approach might be possible, but for those of greater complexity, it is unrealistic and can even be reckless. Emergency situations calling for immediate action indeed may occur from time to time, but even in those scenarios, investigations can be fast-tracked to demonstrate an acceptable level of due diligence, with this still calling for patience. Managers should enter the conflict resolution process with a mindset that they will work diligently toward resolution, making judicious use of whatever time is available to perform their assessments and formulate pathways forward, with an understanding that patience throughout the process is essential.

By developing the noted managerial competencies, healthcare managers can expect to be more proficient in their efforts to diagnose and resolve conflict occurring in the workplace. As work experience and formal training accrue, these competencies will continue to advance, with healthcare managers gaining confidence in their conflict management abilities. Building associated skills indeed is a career-long process. Conflict management prowess is highly valued in healthcare establishments, given the frequency of conflict experienced in organizational life. The value of associated skills will become readily apparent as one reads through this chapter, learning about conflict and conflict management in health and medicine.

14.1 Background

The mere word conflict typically strikes fear in the hearts and minds of those serving in managerial positions in health and medical organizations. This stands to reason as disagreements, quarrels, and other forms of discord within the halls of medicine often are harmful to institutional operations. Opportunities for conflict can occur on virtually any front, as the following examples indicate. A physician group disagrees with hospital administrators regarding weekend coverage requirements. The directors of nursing and laboratory services cannot come to terms regarding the implementation of a patient care protocol. An imaging department director views the price quote received from a manufacturer for a new MRI unit to be unacceptable. The respiratory therapy department is dissatisfied that its pay rates are not identical to those of nursing services. An HR officer's ego prevents him from working collegially with the greater department. The nursing department is at odds with dietary services regarding the timely delivery of patient meals. Productivity indeed is a prerequisite for success and conflict very often is the enemy, placing stumbling blocks along the avenues leading to mission fulfillment [1–6].

Healthcare establishments certainly present as potential tinderboxes of conflict. The workforce is highly diverse, creating natural opportunities for differentiated viewpoints to emerge. Wide variations in education levels and incomes alone diminish propensities for personnel to see eye-to-eye, exacerbating tensions between and among them. Further, duties and responsibilities held by this diverse workforce are highly specialized, fostering the development of silos where employees focus predominantly on their own piece of the healthcare delivery puzzle, rather than the entirety of the patient care process, amplifying opportunities for the emergence of disharmony [7–11]. Professional societies, unique to specific occupational disciplines, further build walls originating in academic training programs, socializing students of medicine, nursing, business, and other specialties to view themselves and others in particular manners [12]. Further, healthcare establishments interact extensively with external parties, notably including patients, vendors, politicians, and more, creating the potential for disagreements on myriad fronts, setting the stage for rampant conflict [13, 14].

Despite the widespread potential for conflict, health and medical organizations need not become flashpoints of chaos. Healthcare providers simply must endeavor to gain competencies in properly managing conflict. Conflict actually is a multifaceted concept, fully deserving of active management within health and medicine. Its dimensionality is surprising and its impact is profound. Foundations of conflict, including its formal definition and impact on organizational performance, must clearly be understood. Types of conflict, associated sources, and related insights must also be firmly within the intellectual grasp of healthcare providers. This knowledge ultimately permits health and medical institutions to respond to conflict in a manner that fosters productivity. This particular chapter explores the concept of conflict and its management, permitting healthcare providers to understand associated fundamentals and put them into practice to ensure harmony and realize enhanced performance.

14.2   Defining Conflict

Conflict is defined as a state of incompatibility arising when one party perceives that its interests are being negatively impacted by another. It exists in most any social setting and is especially prevalent in work environments where individuals possessing different backgrounds and abilities are brought together to achieve a common goal [15]. Conflict can occur between two people (i.e., **dyadic conflict**), within a group (i.e., **intragroup conflict**), or between groups (i.e., **intergroup conflict**) [16]. Importantly, conflict is based on perception, which can be real or imagined [17]. Regardless, the impact on those who view themselves to be reduced by others in some shape, form, or fashion is real and meaningful to them, making it something that must be addressed in organizational life. And addressed, conflict must be. It rarely resolves itself, but often intensifies, creating further divides. If not dealt with, small issues can quickly become big issues, crippling otherwise productive operations [18].

Conflict in organizations emerges when an initiator of some sort appears, creating discord felt by one or more parties. When the affected party cannot resolve matters internally, these feelings enter the realm of the observable, being projected outwardly through words and actions, typically directed toward the party viewed to be the instigator of the conflict. Emotion often takes over the process, escalating the conflict further, intensifying associated expressions and mannerisms. Outcomes of conflict eventually emerge, with these either being positive or negative [19]. To ensure that conflict is minimized and, when experienced, steered toward productive outcomes, institutions engage in **conflict management**, a systematic management process involving the direction of formal efforts toward addressing matters of conflict emerging in institutions. The process of managing conflict indeed is managerial in nature, making conflict management a good descriptor. As organizations are social systems, what occurs in individual life is brought into organizational life, with conflict being one. It cannot be eliminated, but it can be managed [20, 21].

14.3   Types of Conflict

Conflict can be divided into two general types: task conflict and relationship conflict. **Task conflict** refers to conflict which centers on the content of the work at hand, including its goals and objectives and processes for completion. Notably, human factors are omitted in this type of conflict, permitting the focus to rest on operational matters, unfettered by things such as personality differences, jealousy, and related personal factors [19]. Consider a scenario involving a multihospital system's debate regarding the placement of its human resource management function. Some executives believe that HR should be centralized at a single location serving the entire system, affording cost efficiency and control. Others, however, believe that a personnel office should be established at each site, maximizing access and flexibility. Given two opposing perspectives, associated discussions and debates ensue. Assuming that the executives focus exclusively on the merits of the prevailing "centralization versus decentralization" question, the associated conflict would be considered to be task oriented, as it is dealing with an operational matter isolated from any chaos associated with personal factors.

Task conflict typically is productive, benefiting healthcare organizations. The notion that conflict can be helpful might come as a surprise to many, but at least in limited amounts and defined circumstances, it actually can prove to be enhancing. Many times, discussions and debates on work matters can lead to improved outcomes that would not have been possible if one perspective or another emerged unchallenged. Conflict in these cases forces parties to work through disagreement in such a manner as to reveal a superior pathway [22]. When conflict takes this form, it is referred to as **functional conflict** or **constructive conflict** [19]. Achieving such, however, requires a delicate balancing act, as the threshold for productive conflict is narrow and often unpredictable. It is not always possible. Sometimes task conflict veers into unproductive realms, constituting **dysfunctional conflict**. This is especially the case when personal factors creep into operational matters under consideration, diverting attention from work matters to relationship matters.

Relationship conflict refers to conflict which centers on personal issues between and among individuals. It has nothing to do with the merits of any substantive, operational matter, centering instead on personality differences, individual rivalry, jealousy, and the like [19]. This sort of conflict is almost always dysfunctional. As it focuses on superficial, personal matters rather than meaningful operational concerns, it diminishes productivity [16]. Unfortunately, relationship conflict happens to be quite common in health and medicine. Consider, for example, a medical clinic's employment of two individuals who simply do not get along with each other for reasons beyond any work-related matter. Perhaps they know each other in their given communities, do not like each other for whatever reason in that particular context, and carry that conflict into the work environment, harming workplace productivity.

Relationship conflict can be muddled with task conflict, presenting especially complicated situations. Continuing the multihospital system dilemma noted earlier, the task conflict described could also feature relationship conflict. Assume, for example, that the "centralization versus decentralization" issue emerged primarily because two factions within the institution historically have disliked each other "just because" and turned every decision into a debate even when doing so had no associated merit. It might, for example, be well understood that centralization afforded the best outcomes, but simply due to personal differences, factions took opposing sides. Whether in pure or hybrid form, relationship conflict must be dealt with carefully, given its inherent dysfunctional characteristics and deviation of focus from operational matters.

14.4 Sources of Conflict

Conflict occurs for many reasons, with several sources being frequent originators. These include interpersonal differences, differing goals, differing values, task interdependence, resource constraints, poor communication, and change [23]. Due to debilitating effects which commonly follow the appearance of conflict, possessing an awareness of its sources is essential. With such knowledge, healthcare providers can better diagnose strife and other contentious situations occurring in the workplace. This is very important as the actual source of conflict can be deceptive, appearing to emanate from one thing, when in actuality, it stems from another. The better one understands sources of conflict, the more likely one will be able to identify its actual root cause and address it productively.

14.4.1 Interpersonal Differences

Interpersonal differences represent a chief source of conflict. Varied personalities, aspirations, and motivations notably fuel relationship conflict, as profiled earlier, centered firmly on personal matters, rather than those associated with work [23]. Interpersonal differences are especially trying sources of conflict, as the characteristics and desires of individuals often are rigid, if not firmly fixed. As health and medical organizations draw people from all walks of life, healthcare providers can expect an especially broad array of differences between and among staff members, escalating the potential for conflict to occur on this front. Such conflict has the potential to reveal itself in virtually any scenario and on any facet imaginable in health and medicine. Conflict stemming from age differences, for example, is particularly pronounced in health and medical settings simply due to the industry's attraction of employees from across the age continuum. Consider, for example, a nurse nearing retirement who views young nursing graduates to "have it easy" compared to that which she had to endure when becoming a nurse decades earlier. This view likely will not be shared by the younger nurses who surely have also sacrificed in their career pursuits, setting the stage for the emergence of friction. However, age is just one of a seemingly infinite number of interpersonal differences which can provoke discord between and among individuals.

14.4.2 Differing Goals

When parties in work relationships possess different goals, conflict is inevitable. In cases where conflict emerges from this source, the goals held by one party—whether related to a task at hand or the process for accomplishing the task—are opposed to the goals of the other party, generating friction. This is a classic initiator of strife in daily organizational life. Two parties simply have goals that are not harmonious [23]. Examples in health and medicine are rich and varied. A medical clinic's leadership team is composed of two factions—one favoring outsourcing operations at every opportunity and the other preferring to maintain everything in-house—creating a divide whenever pertinent decisions are at hand, such as whether to allow a laboratory management company to oversee onsite lab operations or retain in-house oversight. A hospital's medical staff disagrees about approaches to medicine, with some physicians favoring a traditional approach and others preferring a holistic approach. Marketing executives at a home health agency favor different approaches to marketing communications, with some preferring the use of advertising as the core communicative method and others favoring personal selling, creating contention whenever marketing communications campaigns are being formulated. Clashes on the basis of differing goals range from being patently simple to enormously complex, with their frequency in the workplace representing an ongoing conflict management challenge.

14.4.3 Differing Values

Values, when defined at the level of the individual, are personal philosophies and perspectives which are acquired over time as a result of one's identity and life experiences. They differ between and among individuals, with perspectives of what is right and wrong, good and bad, and fair and unfair often being the source of conflict [23]. Conflict emanating from this particular source is very pronounced in health and medicine, as associated pursuits invariably have values underpinnings. Each and every day, healthcare providers make choices that have vast implications for health and wellness on both individual and community levels. Consider a scenario where some members of a medical center's governing board desire robust expenditures for the delivery of charitable care in the community while others favor more restrictive expenditures. One side effectively is embracing values espousing altruism, while the other side desires values centering on profit maximization. Quite obviously, if the respective factions on the governing board are steadfast, the stage is set for a protracted battle, given the vastly different mindsets associated with resource allocation. Similarly, consider a scenario where two dietary supervisors possess different values regarding how to motivate dietary aides, with one relying on threats and other forms of punishment to evoke compliance and the other preferring education, counseling, and incentives to motivate proper work behaviors. Quite obviously, the two supervisors possess vastly different mindsets, driving a wedge between them whenever the given topic is broached. These sorts of situations play out regularly across all levels within healthcare organizations.

14.4.4   Task Interdependence

Whenever one's work depends on that of another, opportunities for conflict emerge. **Division of labor**, which divides jobs into narrowly defined areas permitting specialization, practically guarantees task interdependence in most any complex work environment [23]. This is especially the case in health and medicine, given the extreme specialization characterizing service delivery pursuits. Challenges abound as employees strive to deliver their part of the service experience at the exact time that it is needed by other parties. Sometimes employees performing their given specialties must work in tandem with others, as in the case of a surgical team attending to a patient in an operating room. At other times, employees of one specialty must wait for others to complete their work before they may proceed with their own work, as in the case of clinical employees who must wait for admissions personnel to receive patients before the care experience may begin. Every link in the chain of production is critical, with each being dependent on the other. A weakness or failure in even a single link can have repercussions across multiple links, resulting in a diminished patient experience. Given such intensive task interdependence, the potential for conflict to develop in health and medicine is profound.

14.4.5   Resource Constraints

Resource constraints serve as another prevalent source of conflict. Scarce resources in an organization result in employees clamoring to get what they perceive to be their fair share. When they feel shortchanged, conflict can emerge. Regardless of how prosperous given institutions happen to be, resources available for distribution, whether in the form of time or money, are finite. Decisions must be made dictating the allocation of these limited resources [23]. As resources are finite and wants are insatiable, a zero-sum game effectively is continually played out in the halls of medicine. The concept of **zero-sum** means that one party's gains represent another party's losses. This contrasts sharply with **win-win** scenarios where all parties have their needs met. In situations where there are winners and losers, conflict is inevitable.

Consider a scenario involving a rehabilitation company's issuance of pay increases for its physical, occupational, and speech therapists at a time when the market was witnessing a severe shortage of physical therapists. Given this shortage and its drastic impact on salary rates, the decision was made to give the company's physical therapists a larger percentage increase than that issued to its occupational and speech therapists. This permitted the establishment to bolster its ability to retain its physical therapists in a challenging market. The wage increase difference eventually was leaked to others in the company, quite obviously offending its occupational and speech therapists who felt shortchanged.

Temporal resource limitations, too, can be at the center of conflict. Consider a scenario involving a hospital administrator's efforts to mentor the institution's recently hired group of junior managers. As much as the administrator desired otherwise, time limitations forced him to be selective in who he mentored because his schedule simply did not allow equal attention to be directed toward all, resulting in some feeling left out. These and scores of similar scenarios are common initiators of conflict in the halls of medicine, presenting regularly due to resource limitations.

14.4.6 Poor Communication

When communication breakdowns occur, myriad problems, including those involving conflict, inevitably will emerge. Perhaps most notably, poor communication fosters uncertainty, with this being fertile ground for the propagation of conflict [23]. Communication breakdowns are all too common in health and medicine, and they cause an undue amount of strife, impacting operations. Consider a scenario where a hospital administrator informs some department directors of forthcoming systemwide layoffs, but fails to communicate the same details to other directors. Perhaps this was unintentional, with information conveyed informally to a small group of directors at a chance meeting in advance of a formal announcement to all directors. Regardless, those directors who learn that others were informed in advance of them will invariably feel dejected, creating potential rifts stemming from having been left out of the loop.

Beyond conveyance errors and omissions, difficulties on the communication front can also relate to organizational structure and design inadequacies. A hospital might, for example, demand strict adherence to its chain of command, permitting vertical communication between superiors and subordinates, but limiting horizontal communication between departments, reducing opportunities to quickly resolve issues, hastening conflict. Similarly, work processes could be poorly designed, hampering effective communication between employees. For example, two departments expected to work very closely together, such as nursing services and respiratory therapy, could be located an inordinate distance apart within a medical center, creating a barrier impeding proper dialogue and interaction. These and similar instances increase the likelihood of conflict emerging as a result of communicative hardships.

14.4.7 Change

Another source of conflict is change. Like that of poor communication, change invokes uncertainty, and when uncertainty is experienced in health and medicine, at least some will express concern and even fear, fostering the potential for conflict. These emotions often distract employees from the work at hand, prompting them to wonder how their routines will be altered, who will win and who will lose as a result of the change, and whether they will or will not be able to personally adapt to the new way of doing things [23]. Resistance to change is common and should be expected, with this engendering conflict in the workplace as employees come to terms with losing their old way of life while mustering the courage to embrace a new one [24]. Consider a scenario involving the merger of two medical clinics. While the workloads associated with addressing two patient populations—one at each establishment—likely will give assurances to clinical employees that their jobs are secure, the same is not true for many occupying administrative roles. Duplication of jobs in areas such as human resources, finance, marketing, and information systems undoubtedly will result from the merger, generating many unknowns regarding who will retain their positions in the aftermath of the union. Beyond that, across both facilities, employees naturally will be concerned with how the merger will impact their work routines, hours of service, compensation and benefits, and much more. Collegiality, morale, and performance often dwindle in such situations. Infighting also can be triggered as employees jockey for position. Change indeed raises many emotions, with conflict being a common result.

14.5 Responses to Conflict

As conflict has many potential sources, its presence is virtually guaranteed in health and medical organizations. And whenever conflict appears, the parties involved in these instances of disagreement and discord respond in a manner consistent with their assessment of the situation and their given aims and desired outcomes. As such, responses vary based on the situation encountered and the desires of those addressing the matter at hand. These responses, however, tend to take one of the following general forms: competing, accommodating, avoiding, compromising, or collaborating [25, 26].

14.5.1 Competing Response to Conflict

A **competing response to conflict** essentially is an all-or-nothing approach where one party seeks victory at the expense of the other party. It is a dominating and forceful method of resolving conflict, typically used in situations where opponents are noncompetitive and vulnerable or in cases when urgency requires immediate resolution. It also is used when unpopular actions must be pursued [25]. For success, parties using this approach must possess sufficient power to effectively strong-arm their will on the opposing party [27]. Consider the case of a medical clinic which, due to a competitor introducing weekend hours of operation, decided to do the same, with this upsetting staff members whose forthcoming schedules now required weekend work obligations. This naturally created conflict between the medical clinic's leadership team and its staff members, but the decision ultimately stood as failing to offer equivalent hours of operation would threaten viability. The leadership team, as officers of the medical clinic, possessed the power and authority to overrule any dissent, permitting use of the competing response to resolve the matter.

14.5.2 Accommodating Response to Conflict

An **accommodating response to conflict** involves one party conceding its preference in order for the other party to have its desire met. This approach is the opposite of the competing response. With one party forgoing its own desire in a conflict, the other side effectively is accommodated, resolving the matter [25]. While an accommodating response could be considered to be "giving in," very often this is not the case. This response might be used as a means of fostering positive future dialogues with the party being accommodated, especially if forthcoming contentious interactions are anticipated. It also might be used simply as a gesture of goodwill from one party to the other [27]. Consider the case of a group of medical center executives working to plan the establishment's weekend executive on-call schedule. This particular medical center required members of the executive team to rotate on-call duties each weekend, permitting critical issues concerning administrative matters to be addressed in a timely fashion. One weekend was particularly desirable to have off because a popular community festival would be taking place at that time, attracting the citizenry en masse to the event. None of the executives desired being assigned that weekend for on-call duty, but one decided to step forward and accept the assignment in order to allow his peers to enjoy the festival weekend, free of any institutional obligations. This person's actions represented an accommodating response.

14.5.3 Avoiding Response to Conflict

An **avoiding response to conflict** is one where both parties delay addressing the matter, opting instead to deal with the conflict at a later time. This approach can be helpful in situations where tensions are high and a cooling-off period is needed. Such delays are also useful when an acceptable solution cannot be identified, prompting patience until a sensible pathway is revealed. Avoidance also can occur when parties face a decision that no one wants to make [25]. This type of response is sometimes practical, but it is often overused, as the number of situations where avoidance indeed is prudent is limited [27]. Consider a scenario involving a hospital facing a workforce reduction, with senior management calling on several directors to downsize their departments. Such layoffs are always difficult, often prompting stalling tactics—an avoidance response—in hopes that circumstances will change, permitting all staff members to remain employed. Often times, this sort of response simply postpones the inevitable, but certainly there are situations where avoidance responses prove beneficial, making it an essential conflict response option to understand and use when necessary.

14.5.4 Compromising Response to Conflict

A **compromising response to conflict** is one where both parties in a particular conflict seek to meet in the middle, identifying a solution which allows both sides a portion of what they ideally wanted. It is a time-honored approach to resolving conflict and often is the first to come to mind when considering methods of resolution. The compromising response is particularly useful in situations where parties are of roughly equivalent power, creating the potential for protracted stalemates unless they accept concessions of some sort. It also is useful when resources are limited and cannot accommodate the wishes of all. In such cases, receiving something is better than receiving nothing, partially appeasing the desires of both parties [25]. There are no distinct winners or losers with this approach [27]. Consider a situation where an experienced and highly valued medical records technician tendered her resignation, ending her lengthy employment at a hospital. On receipt of her resignation notice, the employee's supervisor sought to change her mind, but she was committed to departing, as she recently had given birth and wanted to be a stay-at-home mom. Seeking to find a middle ground, her supervisor conferred with others higher in the chain of command and gained authorization to permit the medical records technician to continue her employment remotely. This allowed her to continue to be of service to the hospital, while permitting her to remain at home to care for her child. In this case, both parties made concessions to arrive at a solution acceptable to all, typifying the compromising response.

14.5.5 Collaborating Response to Conflict

A **collaborating response to conflict** is one where both parties in a particular conflict search for a solution that allows both sides to have their desires fully met. Such an approach requires both parties to work together to arrive at a mutually beneficial solution [25]. Consider a situation where two department directors needed access to a hospital's conference room for purposes of holding a luncheon to discuss recent corporate developments. Both parties desired booking the venue for a 2-hour block beginning at Noon on the exact same date. On noticing the conflict, the two directors conferred, examining the materials they planned to share with staff members. In doing so, they realized that the materials were virtually identical, prompting them to offer the luncheon collaboratively, combining the staffs of both departments. While initially, the situation appeared to permit only one department director the access desired, collaboration allowed both department directors—and their respective employees—to fully benefit. Collaborating represents the ideal form of conflict resolution, as the parties involved in such each emerge victoriously. Such win-win scenarios, however, are not always possible as circumstances and situations might warrant different responses. Still, collaboration should be sought at each and every available opportunity.

14.6 Resolving Conflict Through Negotiation

In many cases, conflict resolution occurs through the process of **negotiation**, defined as an interaction between parties where both sides endeavor to reach an agreement concerning a particular matter or concern. It is through the process of negotiation that responses to conflict are forwarded with the intention of resolving associated issues. The process often is depicted as being highly formal, and many times, that is the case, but it is not at all uncommon for negotiations to occur on an informal basis. Some conflict scenarios, of course, are not suitable for negotiations. Conflict between two employees on a personal, nonwork-related matter would serve as an excellent example of this, with this scenario being best suited for counseling or the disciplinary process. When the right circumstances appear, however, negotiation is a powerful tool for conflict resolution [17, 19, 20, 28].

Negotiations are often viewed to be single events, occurring at a particular point in time, and very often, that is an accurate perspective. However, they also can occur over time, involving multiple interactions. Complexity of the matters under consideration in a negotiation is a chief driver of the temporal requirements of such, with greater complexity typically requiring greater time, heightened formality, and increased interactions [28]. A laboratory technician appealing to her supervisor for a work schedule adjustment, for example, will be less rigorous than, say, a pharmacy director negotiating with a manufacturer over the price of a new automated medication dispensing system. Likewise, the complexity associated with a proposed hospital merger would necessitate forwarding extremely extensive efforts before an agreement could be struck.

There are two primary types of negotiation: distributive negotiation and integrative negotiation [28]. **Distributive negotiation** treats the matters under consideration as a **fixed pie**, meaning that parties are negotiating over what they consider to be a limited pool of resources, a characteristic that amplifies opportunities for conflict, as described earlier. This zero-sum, win-loss perspective stands in sharp contrast to the win-win perspective of **integrative negotiation** which treats the matters under consideration to be an **expandable pie**, permitting opportunities for mutual gains to occur. Distributive approaches are more likely to occur when negotiations involve single issues, as little to no leeway is available when sole items are under consideration. Integrative negotiations are more likely to occur when multiple issues are under consideration. As the importance of issues under consideration often varies for negotiating parties, opportunities exist for tradeoffs to occur, offering the potential for both parties to walk away from the negotiating table being satisfied [19].

The process for conducting formal negotiations can take many forms, but a common rendition entails four steps: preparation, exchanging information, bargaining, and closing and commitment. **Preparation** arguably is the most important step, whereby parties review the matter up for negotiation, envision desired outcomes, determine their positions, and investigate the motives and approaches of the opposition. Importantly, this stage requires parties to determine their **BATNA** or **Best Alternative to a Negotiated Agreement**. A BATNA essentially is the most ideal outcome possible in the absence of a negotiated agreement. If that particular outcome is better than the deal proposed in the negotiation, it is best to withdraw and instead pursue the BATNA, making knowledge of one's BATNA an essential tool for evaluating offers [20]. Knowledge of one's BATNA also helps to determine one's **ZOPA** or **Zone of Possible Agreement**, which indicates the options a negotiating party is willing to accept [17]. The preparation stage is followed by **exchanging information** between negotiating parties, a nonconfrontational phase where each party states its position, noting associated justifications. Many inquiries are forwarded here as a means of generating a comprehensive awareness of parties and their given positions. **Bargaining**, the stage most associated with the negotiation process, follows the exchange of information. This stage involves the parties actively dialoguing on each point of the negotiation, with the goal being to strike a deal deemed to be satisfactory to both parties. The bargaining stage is sometimes referred to as the **haggling** stage as it involves parties bouncing offers back and forth between each other, working to find common ground. The **closing and commitment** stage follows, where parties, assuming successful interactions, formalize the agreement negotiated in the bargaining stage, bringing the negotiation process to a close [20].

14.7 Managing Conflict

Since conflict emerges from myriad sources in a nearly infinite array of situations, prompting a range of responses based on the unique aims of those affected by the conflict, pat formulas for its management are difficult to formulate. However, there are useful general avenues which can aid healthcare institutions in the proper management of any conflict experienced. One of the most prudent methods for conflict management centers on the **strategic framework** of a healthcare establishment. This framework presents the strategy tenets governing the institution and its operation. Its content forms the basis of foundational knowledge discussed earlier in the chapter. Chief elements of this framework are mission, vision, and values statements, documents as described in Chap. 6 which most any progressive healthcare establishment will have readily on hand. Well-developed frameworks also feature **codes of conduct**, described in detail in Chap. 7, dictating among other things the institution's expectations of its workforce, specifically relating to how personnel conduct themselves and carry out their duties and responsibilities. Healthcare institutions which have timely, accurate, and comprehensive strategic frameworks and steadfastly rely on them for operational insights and guidance, in turn, possess a capable conflict management resource [14, 29–32].

Strategic frameworks specifically provide guidance regarding the values and mindsets deemed to be acceptable by given healthcare institutions, helping to defuse conflict on interpersonal fronts and that stemming from differing goals and values. With a clear understanding of institutionally sanctioned perspectives and views, employees are aided in keeping any deviations of thought that they personally may hold in check in the workplace, ensuring that they do not interject mindsets and attitudes opposed to institutional expectations into their work routines. Even conflict occurring as a result of task interdependence issues can be managed more effectively through the lens of a healthcare provider's strategic tenets, as very often, this conflict stems from the development of **silos** of thought and action. Such isolated perspectives typically violate common strategic notions that employees are to work collegially toward mission accomplishment, with this essentially mandating concern for operations beyond one's own responsibilities [1, 12, 33]. Modern strategic frameworks also typically include prominent mandates for communicating well with staff members, stemming the potential for conflict occurring due to communication failures. Excellent communication also notably reduces uncertainty, diminishing one of the most negative effects of conflict [23]. Resource constraints often are the wildcard, as they typically are impenetrable, but strategic tenets also can be helpful in many of these cases. Resource allocation decisions certainly can be informed by strategic frameworks which often stipulate priorities, providing justifications for actions, helping to curb the emergence of conflict.

While strategic frameworks will not settle all conflict, such tenets certainly can be helpful in resolving some, making them a key asset for conflict management. For issues that remain unresolved, notably those conflicts which result in stalemates, healthcare institutions should develop protocols for addressing these matters. A popular method for doing this simply entails mandating that employees report any unresolvable conflict to the next highest level of authority in the chain of command for resolution. Depending on the nature of the conflict encountered, it might be allowed to proceed, assuming it is of the functional kind and expected to lead to enhanced outcomes. Dysfunctional conflict, however, must be addressed aggressively; stamped out quickly to extinguish its debilitating effects. Doing so often calls for the issuance of administrative directives requiring embattled parties to take certain actions (e.g., pursue a particular pathway, abandon an alternative). Disciplinary actions also might be called for in worst-case scenarios if dysfunctional conflict continues [1].

Each healthcare institution ultimately must decide for itself how best to handle conflict. Regardless of the approach selected, a prudent strategic framework and associated protocols for breaking stalemates and other forms of unhelpful conflict certainly represent excellent avenues for fostering collegiality. In time, healthcare providers will see their given approaches for handling conflict become part of organizational culture, providing a guidance mechanism for handling discord that is understood by current employees and transferred to newcomers through socialization, permitting operations to proceed productively, unburdened by conflict.

WK Reflections: A Helpful Tip for Fact-Finding

As illustrated by the content of this chapter, conflict management generally involves significant fact-finding efforts. Sometimes fact-finding goes well; other times it is more challenging. Much depends on institutional protocols for handling conflict-related data collection. When instances of conflict present themselves, Willis Knighton Health historically has relied on bringing the embattled parties together in a fact-finding session guided by a supervisor. If, for example, a manager and his or her subordinate are embroiled in a conflict which cannot be resolved between the two, the manager's supervisor will bring both parties together to hear their respective accounts and work toward resolution. In cases where two employees are in a conflict which they cannot resolve between themselves, the staff members' supervisor will oversee the fact-finding session. Sometimes the conflict is allowed to continue if it functional, but if it is dysfunctional, it will be addressed immediately.

With this approach, since each individual shares his or her side of the story in full view of the opposing party, the supervisor has a much easier time collecting accurate information which will ultimately reveal the truth of what actually is occurring in the workplace. Importantly, conflicting perspectives can be immediately probed with both parties present, expediting what would take significantly more time if handled separately. Some cases simply would have no hope of being resolved without direct and simultaneous multiparty engagement. Further, the presence of the opposing party encourages accuracy in reporting, given that misrepresentations can be immediately rebutted. This particular method of handling conflict will not work in all cases of conflict, for example, when the matter involves an egregious allegation, such as abuse of power. For routine matters, however, it has proven to be quite effective in expediting and enhancing fact-finding which ultimately aids in conflict resolution. While this approach might seem obvious, resolution efforts sometimes are relegated to informality, plagued by biases, handled by the inexperienced, or hampered by other factors, leading to incomplete information for making critical conflict-related decisions. A proper fact-finding protocol will help to ensure thorough investigations and rich information, facilitating conflict resolution.

14.8   Summary and Conclusions

Conflict is a common and enduring feature of health and medical organizations, requiring vigilance in its evaluation and management. Healthcare providers must endeavor to resolve conflict efficiently and effectively, carefully handling its functional variants and eradicating its dysfunctional kinds, allowing operations to thrive. This necessitates developing a thorough foundation of knowledge regarding conflict, its various types, common responses to conflict, and its typical sources. It also requires designing and maintaining productive strategic frameworks and protocols for managing stalemates and other forms of contention occurring in the halls of medicine. Knowledge of conflict and conflict management skill sets must be possessed by more than those occupying the upper echelons of health and medical organizations. Such proficiencies must also be held by those lower in organizational hierarchies, as conflict touches the entirety of institutions. By fielding healthcare organizations featuring staff members skilled in addressing conflict, the stage is set for operations to flourish, affording lasting benefits for all.

Key Terms

- Accommodating Response to Conflict
- Active Listening
- Analytical Skills
- Avoiding Response to Conflict
- Bargaining
- BATNA
- Best Alternative to a Negotiated Agreement
- Closing and Commitment
- Code of Conduct
- Collaborating Response to Conflict
- Competing Response to Conflict
- Compromising Response to Conflict
- Conflict
- Conflict Management
- Constructive Conflict
- Distributive Negotiation
- Division of Labor
- Dyadic Conflict
- Dysfunctional Conflict
- Exchanging Information
- Expandable Pie
- Fixed Pie
- Foundational Knowledge

- Functional Conflict
- Haggling
- Integrative Negotiation
- Intergroup Conflict
- Interpersonal Communication Skills
- Intragroup Conflict
- Negotiation
- Nonverbal Communication
- Objectivity
- Patience
- Preparation
- Relationship Conflict
- Silo
- Strategic Framework
- Task Conflict
- Values
- Verbal Communication
- Win-Win
- Zero-Sum
- Zone of Possible Agreement
- ZOPA

Exercises

1. In your own words, define conflict, discuss its prevalence in health and medicine, and speak on the need for it to be addressed in a timely and effective manner.
2. Define conflict management and discuss the necessity for healthcare establishments to gain proficiencies in this important area. How would you characterize the conflict management acumen of your current employer? How would you characterize your own conflict management abilities?
3. Define functional conflict and dysfunctional conflict. Think deeply about your current and prior work experiences. Provide examples where you have observed conflict to be helpful to your organization and hurtful to your organization.
4. Compare and contrast task conflict and relationship conflict. Reflect on your recent work experiences and provide examples that you have observed which illustrate both of these types of conflict.
5. Identify and define the seven common sources of conflict, as profiled in the chapter. Which source have you observed the most in your work experiences? Which source have you observed the least? Share associated details.
6. Identify and define the five responses to conflict, as profiled in the chapter, and provide insights regarding their use in resolving contentious situations in health and medicine. Select two of these responses and provide examples of situations in which you put them into use.

7. Explain the concept of zero-sum. Think back on your experiences and describe a situation where resolving a conflict involved winners and losers. In retrospect, could any improvements have been made to allow both parties to win?
8. Explain the concept of win-win. Think back on your experiences and describe a situation where a particular conflict was resolved in a manner which permitted both parties to win. How was this win-win achieved?

References

1. Elrod, J. K. (2013). *Breadcrumbs to cheesecake*. R&R Publishers.
2. Rahim, M. A. (2023). *Managing conflict in organizations* (5th ed.). Routledge.
3. Robbins, S. P., & Coulter, M. (2021). *Management* (15th ed.). Pearson.
4. Coleman, P. T., Deutsch, M., & Marcus, E. C. (Eds.). (2014). *The handbook of conflict resolution: Theory and practice* (3rd ed.). Jossey-Bass.
5. Corvette, B. A. B. (2006). *Conflict management: A practical guide to developing negotiation strategies*. Pearson.
6. Shafritz, J. M., Ott, J. S., & Jang, Y. S. (Eds.). (2016). *Classics of organization theory* (8th ed.). Cengage.
7. U. S. Bureau of Labor Statistics. (2022). *Occupational outlook handbook*. Retrieved April 3, 2023, from https://www.bls.gov/ooh/
8. O*NET OnLine. (2023). *Health care and social assistance*. Retrieved April 3, 2023, from https://www.onetonline.org/find/industry?i=62
9. McConnell, C. R. (2020). *Hospitals and health systems: What they are and how they work*. Jones and Bartlett.
10. Shi, L., & Singh, D. A. (2023). *Essentials of the US health care system* (6th ed.). Jones and Bartlett.
11. Flynn, W. J., Valentine, S. R., & Meglich, P. A. (2022). *Healthcare human resource management* (4th ed.). Cengage.
12. Elrod, J. K., & Fortenberry, J. L., Jr. (2017). Peering beyond the walls of healthcare institutions: A catalyst for innovation. *BMC Health Services Research, 17*(Suppl 1), 35–38.
13. Kotler, P., Keller, K. L., & Chernev, A. (2022). *Marketing management* (16th ed.). Pearson.
14. Fortenberry, J. L., Jr. (2010). *Health care marketing: Tools and techniques* (3rd ed.). Jones and Bartlett.
15. Raines, S. S. (2020). *Conflict management for managers: Resolving workplace, client, and policy disputes* (2nd ed.). Rowman and Littlefield.
16. Robbins, S. P., & Judge, T. A. (2019). *Organizational behavior* (18th ed.). Pearson.
17. Kinicki, A., & Fugate, M. (2018). *Organizational behavior: A practical, problem-solving approach* (2nd ed.). McGraw-Hill.
18. Liddle, D. (2017). *Managing conflict: A practical guide to resolution in the workplace*. Kogan Page.
19. McShane, S. L., & Von Glinow, M. A. (2019). *Organizational behavior* (4th ed.). McGraw-Hill.
20. Colquitt, J. A., Lepine, J. A., & Wesson, M. J. (2019). *Organizational behavior: Improving performance and commitment in the workplace* (6th ed.). McGraw-Hill.
21. Cloke, K., & Goldsmith, J. (2011). *Resolving conflicts at work: Ten strategies for everyone on the job* (3rd ed.). Jossey-Bass.
22. Gallo, A. (2017). *HBR guide to dealing with conflict*. Harvard Business Review Press.
23. Griffin, R. W., Phillips, J. M., & Gully, S. M. (2020). *Organizational behavior: Managing people and organizations* (13th ed.). Cengage.
24. Burke, W. W. (2018). *Organization change: Theory and practice* (5th ed.). Sage.

25. Hitt, M. A., Miller, C. C., Colella, A., & Triana, M. D. C. (2018). *Organizational behavior* (5th ed.). Wiley.
26. Thomas, K. W. (1992). Conflict and conflict management: Reflections and update. *Journal of Organizational Behavior, 13*(3), 265–274.
27. Konopaske, R., Ivancevich, J. M., & Matteson, M. T. (2018). *Organizational behavior and management* (11th ed.). McGraw-Hill.
28. Harvard Business Review Press. (2003). *Harvard business essentials: Guide to negotiation.* Harvard Business School Publishing.
29. Ginter, P. M., Duncan, W. J., & Swayne, L. E. (2013). *Strategic management of health care organizations* (7th ed.). Jossey-Bass.
30. Hillestad, S. G., & Berkowitz, E. N. (2020). *Health care market strategy: From planning to action* (5th ed.). Jones and Bartlett.
31. Schermerhorn, J. R., Jr., & Bachrach, D. G. (2015). *Management* (13th ed.). Wiley.
32. Collins, D. (2019). *Business ethics: Best practices for designing and managing ethical organizations* (2nd ed.). Sage.
33. Senge, P. M. (2006). *The fifth discipline: The art and practice of the learning organization.* Doubleday.

Glossary

Authority A reference to the power granted to managers by organizations giving them the right to give orders and mandate compliance.

Best Alternative to a Negotiated Agreement Abbreviated as BATNA, this essentially references the most ideal outcome possible in the absence of a negotiated agreement.

Body Language Nonverbal communicative expressions conveyed via articulation of the human form (e.g., rolling one's eyes at a ridiculous assertion, shaking one's fist when upset, jumping up and down enthusiastically on receiving news of a promotion).

Bounded Rationality A reference to decision-making in real-world applications, acknowledging that rationality in actual practice is limited and imperfect. Bounded rationality does not seek maximization in decision-making, but instead opts to satisfice, pursuing an avenue that is satisfactory or "good enough," rather than one deemed to be the best possible.

Brainstorming Group discussions aimed at generating ideas or solving problems. Ideas brought forth during brainstorming sessions typically beget more ideas as discussions proceed and multiple parties interject their thoughts and opinions, vastly increasing the prospects of generating useful perspectives concerning the topic at hand.

Budgeting One of the key activities of management; it concerns all matters of fiscal planning, accounting, and financial control within an organization.

Burnout A state of exhaustion felt by employees resulting from being bombarded by workplace stress over time, ultimately leaving them feeling overwhelmed, distressed, and demoralized.

Centralized organization An establishment which concentrates power and authority at the top of its given institutional hierarchy.

Chain of Command A reference to the lines of authority running from the very top official within an organization to the lowest ranks of the establishment.

© The Editor(s) (if applicable) and The Author(s), under exclusive license to Springer Nature Switzerland AG 2024
J. K. Elrod, J. L. Fortenberry, Jr., *Organizational Behavior and Management in Health and Medicine*, https://doi.org/10.1007/978-3-031-61823-9

Change Agent An individual who has mastered change management, proving himself or herself capable of building bridges within his or her establishment which lead people, places, and things from a current state to one that is desired.

Change Management The process of actively addressing change by guiding and directing change initiatives within an organization.

Charisma Derived from the Greek word meaning "gift," charisma refers to highly alluring qualities which are possessed by an individual, characterizing the person and affording him or her with profound abilities to influence others. Confidence, optimism, devotion, vision, enthusiasm, commitment, and the like are qualities often associated with the charismatic.

Charismatic Leadership An approach to leadership expressed by a leader with highly alluring qualities, notably including great confidence and optimism, extreme devotion to the pursuit and realization of a compelling vision, enthusiastic and inspiring communication abilities, and unyielding commitment to followers.

Coalition A group of individuals which bands together to drive or otherwise promote a particular cause of interest to its members.

Code of Conduct A directive which stipulates the ethical positions of an organization, providing guidance for employees and assurances for other parties as to the moral stance taken by the establishment.

Coercive Power Power stemming from one's ability to punish. It essentially is the antithesis of reward power, relying on threats, undesirable consequences, and other discouragements to prompt particular behaviors.

Collegiality A reference to camaraderie between and among colleagues.

Commitment A highly desired state in organizational life realized when individuals dedicate themselves to mission fulfillment, essentially becoming champions of their given organizations.

Communication The process through which two or more parties exchange information, making use of mutually understood language, symbols, and other expressions to successfully convey meaning and understanding.

Communication Barrier Any impediment that prevents the successful transmission of messages between parties.

Communication Channel A reference to a particular communication medium for transmitting a message to others. Options range from traditional forms (e.g., in-person meetings, posted letters) to technology-based variants (e.g., telephone conversations, email dialogues, text messaging, video conferencing). Selection generally is based on the objective of the communication, the content to be carried, and the channel's acceptability by both the sender and receiver.

Competitive Advantage Any attribute, capability, or quality possessed by an establishment which gives it an edge over its competitors.

Conflict A state of incompatibility arising when one party perceives that its interests are being negatively impacted by another.

Conflict Management A systematic management process involving the direction of formal efforts toward addressing matters of conflict emerging in institutions.

Coordinating One of the key activities of management; it refers to efforts to understand and address the interrelated components required of work, permitting it to be accomplished effectively.

Corporate Culture A mindset, expressed through and influenced by tangible and intangible means, which characterizes an institution and its operation. More simply, it could be described as a philosophy of operation embraced by an organization and expressed through both visual and nonvisual means. Corporate culture often is used as a parallel term for organizational culture.

Counterculture A subculture which is in conflict with the dominant culture, directly challenging the prevailing mindset within a given organization.

Creativity The ability to address problems in a novel, imaginative fashion. This involves "outside of the box" thinking that sidesteps status quo approaches in favor of new ones which have the potential to deliver enhanced outcomes.

Cross-Training A practice which permits the replication of skill sets to ensure that knowledge is possessed by more than one person.

Culture Audit An evaluation conducted to assess the characteristics and qualities of an establishment's organizational culture, permitting an understanding of its current state, affording opportunities for refinement to ensure desired performance.

Culture Gap The difference between the organizational culture desired by an establishment and the actual organizational culture exhibited within the institution.

Culture Walk A method for observing an organizational culture by literally walking through a given institution, department, or related unit, observing cultural artifacts, interactions between and among employees, dialogues between employees and customers, and the like to provide enlightenment regarding the organizational culture in operation. Culture walks essentially constitute a form of field research completed onsite in active institutional environments, making them very capable knowledge builders.

Dashboard A strategic resource which combines various sources of information into a single presentation, permitting a comprehensive portrayal which can aid in planning, decision-making, and other strategic aims.

Decentralized organization An establishment which distributes power and authority, at least to some degree, throughout its institutional hierarchy.

Decision The result of decision-making, reflecting the particular choice that was made. The alternative selected generally represents the best solution available under given circumstances, making a decision, in many respects, a matter of compromise.

Decision-Making The process of selecting a course of action from among available alternatives for purposes of addressing a particular matter or concern. It is one of the primary responsibilities held by managers, occupying a significant portion of their time, regardless of their level within institutional hierarchies.

Delegation The practice of turning over the authority for accomplishing particular tasks to subordinates for purposes of distributing work, developing employees showing potential, and engendering associated trust.

Directing One of the key activities of management; it centers on issuing general and specific orders to subordinates who, in turn, are charged with their fulfillment for purposes of achieving designated goals and objectives.

Diversity A reference for any particular composition that contains a variety of different elements, characteristics, or qualities. It handily and accurately describes the healthcare industry, with virtually every aspect of operation involving at least some level of diversity.

Division of Labor A principle of management that references the need for work to be divided in a manner to permit employees to specialize in particular areas of responsibility, thus maximizing productivity. Division of labor is also termed division of work.

Division of Work A principle of management that references the need for work to be divided in a manner to permit employees to specialize in particular areas of responsibility, thus maximizing productivity. Division of work is also termed division of labor.

Dominant Culture An organizational culture that is embraced by the majority of the members of an institution.

Dyadic Conflict Conflict occurring between two people.

Dysfunctional Conflict Conflict which is unproductive.

Emergent Strategy A strategy which has been modified from its initial (i.e., intended) form to accommodate situational changes, making it better suited for addressing a given challenge and achieving a desired result.

Empathy The ability to see things from the perspective of another person.

Empowerment A technique for reducing resistance in organizations by giving employees a say in operations, reducing potential feelings of animosity which often come with powerlessness.

Environmental Scanning The activity of studying the environment for purposes of identifying opportunities and threats, permitting them to be proactively addressed by an organization.

Esprit de Corps A principle of management which sees organizations build a sense of unity between and among the ranks, fostering teamwork that allows the workforce to direct efforts in concerted fashion toward the achievement of designated goals and objectives.

Ethics Moral principles, values, and beliefs which govern the actions and behaviors of individuals, with associated mindsets providing them with guidance regarding what is good or bad and right or wrong.

Evolutionary change A reference to change that involves incremental adjustments, with these sometimes being termed "baby steps."

Executional Excellence The ability of an organization to implement strategy proficiently.

Experience Curve A depiction of the knowledge building process, generally communicating that as learning or experience increases, performance does, as well. An experience curve is also known as a learning curve.

Expert Power Power derived from one's special expertise, technical knowledge, or related intellectual insights and abilities, permitting the individual to influence those who are in need of that expertise.

Exploitative Learning A form of learning which seeks to make better use of existing knowledge within an organization, effectively exploiting currently held resources to derive maximum benefits.

Exploratory Learning A form of learning which seeks to identify and secure new knowledge for use within an organization, permitting innovation and advancement, courtesy of these novel insights.

External Environment A reference to forces emerging from outside of an organization which have the potential to influence the given establishment and its operation. The external environment is also known as the macroenvironment.

Extrinsic Motivation Motivation derived from external influences. Individuals are compelled to action by inspiration originating from outside parties (e.g., a productivity bonus put forth by an employer, encouragement offered by a friend to seek a promotion), as opposed to internal, personal influences.

Feedback A response forwarded in reply to a given message.

Formal Communication A reference to messages which travel via official channels in organizations, generally in accordance with their established organizational hierarchies.

Functional Conflict Conflict which is productive in that it forces parties to work through disagreement in such a manner as to reveal a superior pathway. Functional conflict is also referred to as constructive conflict.

Grapevine A reference to the informal communication network in an organization.

Group A collection of two or more individuals who share one or more characteristics, goals, or purposes. Over the course of one's life, individuals are members of numerous groups. Some are joined by choice; others by circumstance. Membership may last a lifetime or it may be fleeting. One's race, education, religion, occupation, hobbies, tastes, preferences, or any other attribute or quality characterizing an individual can serve as the basis of group membership.

Group Cohesion A notable and highly desirable attribute of a group, characterized by the formation of bonds between and among its members, permitting them to pursue goals and objectives in a unified manner.

Group Dynamics A reference for the interactions and exchanges that occur between and among individuals when they are organized into groups.

Groupthink A phenomenon where group members opt to go along with a particular course of action in an effort to maintain consensus rather than engage in sufficient debate to thoroughly vet the pathway under consideration. When this occurs, the benefits that groups are capable of deriving through their diverse perspectives are diminished, reducing the potential of group decision-making.

Informal Communication A reference to messages which travel via unofficial channels within an organization.

Information Overload The provision of so much information that employees cannot process it in a productive and meaningful manner.

Insular Mindset A perspective of an organization or individual which is so intensively-focused inwardly that it crowds out attention directed toward the greater environment.

Intellectual Capital Knowledge held by an organization which is so well developed and comprehensive that it is considered to be an asset, positively influencing operations, supplying competitive advantages, and amplifying performance.

Intended Strategy The initial strategy formulated by an organization to address a challenge and achieve a desired result. It frequently is modified to accommodate situational changes, resulting in what is known as an emergent strategy.

Intergroup Conflict Conflict occurring between groups.

Internal Environment A reference to forces emerging from within an organization which have the potential to influence the given establishment and its operation. The internal environment is also known as the microenvironment.

Intragroup Conflict Conflict occurring within a group.

Intrinsic Motivation Motivation derived from internal, personal influences, as opposed to that originating from outside parties.

Intuition The ability to instinctively understand something without the application of conscious reasoning.

Jargon Specialized terminology associated with particular occupational disciplines.

Judgment A reference to the ability to draw sound conclusions after assessing and evaluating a particular matter or concern.

Knowledge Management Concerted efforts taken by organizations to build and maintain institutional intelligence and acumen.

Leader An individual who possesses one or more skills typifying leadership, compelling the followership of others.

Leadership A skill, composed of a series of appealing qualities (e.g., vision, charisma, honesty, intelligence, ambition), which permits a person to establish productive relationships with others, affording opportunities to influence them in a manner to achieve goals and objectives.

Leadership Development Program An educational offering designed to advance the leadership skills and abilities of individuals, informing and enlightening them on myriad facets of leadership which they then apply in their work lives.

Learning Curve A depiction of the knowledge building process, generally communicating that as learning or experience increases, performance does, as well. A learning curve is also known as an experience curve.

Learning Organization An institution which has successfully incorporated organizational learning into its operations.

Legitimate Power Power held by Individuals holding formal managerial positions in organizations, permitting them the authority to guide and direct others within their given establishments.

Line of Authority A principle of management which refers to the chain of command from the very top authority within an organization to the lowest ranks of the establishment. Line of authority is also termed the scalar chain.

Macroenvironment A reference to forces emerging from outside of an organization which have the potential to influence the given establishment and its operation. The macroenvironment is also known as the external environment.

Management A range of activities (i.e., planning, organizing, staffing, directing, coordinating, reporting, and budgeting) which are carried out by formally appointed individuals (e.g., chief executive officers, vice presidents, directors, managers, supervisors) for purposes of aiding organizations in realizing their missions.

Management by Walking Around An approach, abbreviated MBWA, which sees a manager engage in direct, face-to-face interactions with those under his or her supervision in their actual work settings, permitting an enlightened dialogue and enhanced understanding that can only come through direct observation and engagement. Management by Walking Around is also known as Management by Wandering Around.

Manager An individual who is responsible for the management of an organization.

Media Richness A reference to the amount of detail that a particular communication channel is capable of conveying. Generally, the more complex the communication, the richer the medium must be to properly convey the message.

Mentoring A practice involving the provision of guidance, direction, advice, and support, typically offered by a more experienced employee to a less experienced employee, for purposes of advancing knowledge and understanding.

Message A particular dispatch containing informational content for conveyance to a designated receiver.

Microenvironment A reference to forces emerging from within an organization which have the potential to influence the given establishment and its operation. The microenvironment is also known as the internal environment.

Mission The organization's purpose or reason for being, typically presented in a mission statement.

Mission Statement A document which succinctly stipulates the purpose of an organization. It is used to convey strategic priorities and other institutional characteristics. It is presented in a positive and inspiring fashion to inform and educate employees and other stakeholders about the organization and its aims.

Moral Code The moral principles, values, and beliefs which guide ethical determinations within an organization. Moral codes frequently are formalized in published codes of conduct.

Moral Manager An individual who emphasizes ethical behavior as he or she goes about engaging in the practice of management.

Motivation A state whereby an individual is compelled to pursue a goal or objective to satisfy a particular want or need. An individual described as being motivated essentially has identified something that he or she wishes to gain or possess and has decided to move toward its acquisition.

Motivation Audit An evaluation conducted to assess the state of motivation within an institution, permitting opportunities to maintain and potentially bolster noted strengths and remedy any discovered deficiencies.

Motivator A tool, technique, or incentive (e.g., compensation and benefits, bonus programs, excellent working conditions, engaging work opportunities, top quality leadership) which is deployed by an organization to compel employees to action.

Need Something required; a necessity.

Negotiation An interaction between parties where both sides endeavor to reach an agreement concerning a particular matter or concern.

Noise A term used to characterize disruptive influences which can be interjected into the communication process, distorting messages or even outright eliminating receipt by intended targets.

Nonverbal Communication Communication that makes use of physical manifestations, such as eye contact, facial expressions, body posture, vocal tone, head movements, hand gestures, touch, spatial distance from addressee, and other behaviors, to convey meaning to others.

Organization Design A component of organizational behavior and management which focuses on the process of formulating, implementing, and evaluating institutional structures, activities, and operations in a manner which facilitates the fulfillment of an organization's mission.

Organizational Behavior The formal study of human behavior in organizations.

Organizational Change The alteration of operations within an institution. It typically is prompted by circumstances and situations encountered in external and internal environments, with organizations maneuvering themselves in a manner to accommodate or adjust to these influences.

Organizational Chart A diagram which uses a series of boxes and lines to illustrate the structural arrangement of departments and people within an institution.

Organizational Climate The atmosphere or ambiance of an institution derived from the organizational culture operating within, prevailing environmental considerations, and associated influences and impacts of the workforce.

Organizational Culture A mindset, expressed through and influenced by tangible and intangible means, which characterizes an institution and its operation. More simply, it could be described as a philosophy of operation embraced by an organization and expressed through both visual and nonvisual means.

Organizational Development A component of organizational behavior and management which focuses on guiding and directing efforts that build and enhance organizational effectiveness.

Organizational Forgetting The seepage and eventual loss of institutional knowledge occurring over time as a result of employee turnover, inattentiveness, and related disruptions which ultimately break down knowledge management systems and erode organizational memory.

Organizational Learning The practice of actively acquiring, circulating, using, and retaining knowledge within an institution as a means of informing current and future pursuits, permitting enhanced performance across given establishments.

Organizational Memory A reference to institutional knowledge which is actively managed by an organization to ensure its availability on demand and retention over time.

Organizational Politics A reference for a range of activities and behaviors taken in an effort to advance one's own interests with little or no regard for the interests of the greater organization.

Organizational Structure A reference to an institution's hierarchy, depicting its chain of command, arrangement of departments, and associated reporting relationships within the organization. It is presented via a diagram known as an organizational chart.

Organizing One of the key activities of management; it concerns matters associated with the structure and design of institutions, including their various departments and work processes.

Personal Power Power derived from possessing appealing characteristics or attributes, compelling the admiration, respect, and followership of others.

Planning One of the key activities of management; it is defined as the process of thinking through and outlining the activities necessary to accomplish a particular goal or objective.

Political Gamesmanship Efforts where individuals or groups seek to elevate themselves for purposes of acquiring or maximizing power, typically at the expense of the organization.

POSDCORB An acronym, devised by Luther Gulick, which handily references the activities of management; namely, planning, organizing, staffing, directing, coordinating, reporting, and budgeting.

Position Power Power derived from holding a formal position of responsibility, granting an individual the legitimate authority to issue directives to others, expect compliance, and reward or penalize actions.

Power The ability to influence the thoughts, actions, and behaviors of others, permitting the achievement of desired outcomes, even in the face of resistance.

Problem-Solving A particular form of decision-making called upon when situations encountered are unique, requiring alternatives to be formulated and evaluated without the aid of decision rules.

Rational Decision-Making Decision-making which is characterized by its adherence to a logical process, pursued through an objective lens, influenced by complete information. The goal of rational decision-making is to maximize; that is, choose the best alternative possible.

Referent Power Power possessed by individuals who hold influence over others on the basis of admiration, kinship, loyalty, attraction, respect, and similar qualities. Those with referent power are able to convince and compel others to support and follow them, with followers being moved by affinity and relatedness, motivating desires to identify with and engage the person holding this type of power.

Reporting One of the key activities of management; a vital function requiring managers to inform their supervisors of ongoing operations, activities, and developments within their assigned work units.

Responsibility A requirement of successful managers entailing the acceptance of accountability for outcomes produced under their watch.

Revolutionary Change Comprehensive, sweeping change that profoundly alters the status quo of an organization.

Reward Power Power derived from one's ability to issue rewards and related incentives, such as pay, promotions, awards, preferred work schedules, and the like.

Risk Orientation The degree of risk an individual or institution is comfortable accepting.

Satisfice A reference for pursuing an avenue that is satisfactory or "good enough," rather than one deemed to be the best possible.

Scalar Chain A principle of management which refers to the chain of command from the very top authority within an organization to the lowest ranks of the establishment. The scalar chain is also termed line of authority.

Servant Leadership An approach to leadership whereby a leader expresses a kind of servitude toward others, routinely sacrificing his or her own privileges and conveniences for the benefit of those he or she willfully has decided to place before himself or herself, with the most notable party being subordinates. The approach essentially emphasizes that leaders are to serve their followers, with this contrasting sharply with traditional views which stress the reverse.

Silo An occurrence within an establishment where a department or other unit focuses on itself and its particular wants and needs while neglecting the wants and needs of the greater organization, compelling self-centered behaviors.

Social Loafing A phenomenon where individuals exert less effort in group settings than they would if working alone, relying on their peers to pick up the slack.

Social Responsibility An institutional philosophy and practice which challenges an organization to operate in a manner that extends benefits to the societies in which the establishment is based. For socially responsible organizations, motivations go beyond focusing on institutional concerns, incorporating also concerns for their given communities.

Socialization A process through which individuals come to realize and understand the expectations of a group, permitting them to adjust their behaviors in a manner to foster acclimation and approval.

Span of Control A reference to the number of employees a manager supervises.

Staffing One of the key activities of management; it concerns all matters associated with the personnel function of organizations, with recruitment, selection, retention, training, maintaining favorable work conditions, and the like typifying the focus of this management activity.

Stakeholder A party with vested interests in the operation and performance of a given organization (e.g., customers, vendors, board members, oversight agencies, and the citizenry of the communities in which the organization is based).

Strategic Plan A formal document, typically long-range in focus, which describes an organization comprehensively, noting its mission and vision, historical development, strengths and weaknesses, environmental characteristics, and more, outlining its strategic goals and objectives and methods for their achievement.

Strategic Planning Planning which centers on complex, often institution-wide matters, especially those with lengthy time horizons.

Strategic Thinking A talent which permits strategists to view their given organizations in an integrated, connected fashion—seeing the whole and its parts—as they go about using intuition, logic, and creativity to discover productive avenues that will lead to mission fulfillment and vision attainment.

Strategy A directed course of action which seeks to identify, pursue, and achieve a desired outcome, usually involving the securing of one or more competitive advantages. It typically is long-range in focus and dictates the overall direction of organizations for enduring periods of time.

Strategy Evaluation The final stage of the strategy process. It involves the assessment of strategies following their implementation to ascertain the degree of success achieved.

Strategy Formulation The first stage of the strategy process. Here, organizations carefully craft strategy by analyzing their environments and their capabilities, stipulating their desires, and developing goals and objectives which are anticipated to hasten achieving those desires.

Strategy Implementation The second stage of the strategy process, calling for the enactment of the strategy devised during the formulation stage. It is considered to be the most difficult stage of the strategy process, given natural challenges associated with putting often complex directives into practice.

Stressors A term referencing sources of stress (e.g., burdensome workloads, difficult co-workers).

Subculture An organizational culture, embraced by a particular subset of the greater workforce, which emerges based on some commonality shared by members (e.g., occupation, department, work location), unifying them in some manner which differs from that of the dominant culture of the institution.

Subordinate An individual who directly reports to a given manager.

Supervision A subset of management which generally focuses on a limited array of managerial activities centered primarily on personnel oversight.

Tactics Action steps which aid in the accomplishment of strategy.

Team A small group of individuals whose members work in an especially close and collaborative fashion in pursuit of a particular goal or objective for which they hold themselves collectively accountable.

Transparency The practice of being open and honest in all matters of institutional operation.

Unity of Command A principle of management suggesting that employees should receive orders from only one superior.

Values The mindsets and beliefs which drive an organization's operation, typically presented in a values statement.

Values Statement A document which succinctly presents the core standards, ideals, and principles that guide and direct an organization's pursuit of its designated mission and vision.

Verbal Communication A form of communication that makes use of written or spoken words to interact with others.

Vision (1) What an establishment desires to become; an aspiration typically presented in a vision statement. (2) A quality held by an individual who possesses the ability to accurately analyze and understand current scenarios and foresee with a high degree of accuracy how these scenarios will evolve over time, ultimately affording a strategic mindset.

Vision Statement A document which succinctly presents the aspirations of an organization. It essentially communicates that which an organization intends to become at some point in the future. It nicely complements the mission statement, which references present day pursuits, by presenting a vision for tomorrow.

Visionaries Individuals who possess an uncanny ability to examine their environments and identify avenues and opportunities which can be exploited for gains of some sort.

Want Something desired, as opposed to a requirement or necessity.

Whistleblower A reference for an individual reporting a claim of misconduct.

Workplace Stress The emotional tension or strain experienced by employees as a result of highly challenging circumstances and situations faced in their given work environments.

Index

The manufacturer's authorised representative in the EU is Springer
Nature Customer Service Centre GmbH, Europaplatz 3, 69115 Heidelberg,
Germany. If you have any concerns regarding our products, please
contact ProductSafety@springernature.com

Printed and bound by CPI Group (UK) Ltd, Croydon, CR0 4YY
27/04/2026
02097562-0006